♦

ESSENTIAL OILS are one of the great untapped resources of the world. The concentrated essences of various flowers, fruits, herbs, and plants have been used for centuries all over the world, but in modern times we have forgotten the power of these ancient medicines of the earth, preferring instead to use the products of perfume and chemical companies which imitate the natural fragrances and medicinal and cleansing properties of essential oils. Because the essential oils are so sweet-smelling, many people suppose their value is essentially one of charm and fragrance—but this is a mistake. Modern scientific research has proven that essential oils are potent, with remarkable medicinal properties. These substances are very complex in their molecular structure, and very powerful. The essential oil of oregano, for example, is twenty-six times more powerful as an anticeptic than phenol, which is the active ingredient in many commercial cleansing materials.

Unlike chemical drugs, essential oils do not remain in the body. They leave no toxins behind. And essential oils make much more sense as air fresheners than commercial products, as they cleanse the air by altering the structure of the molecules creating the smells, rather than masking the unwanted smells. When we are looking for alternatives to toxic products in our homes and in our lives, essential oils are a convenient, practical, and pleasant solution.

♦

THE COMPLETE BOOK OF ESSENTIAL OILS AND AROMATHERAPY

THE COMPLETE BOOK OF ESSENTIAL OILS AND AROMATHERAPY

◆

Valerie Ann Worwood

NEW WORLD LIBRARY
San Rafael, California

Published by New World Library
58 Paul Drive
San Rafael, CA 94903

Cover painting: Chantal Saperstein
Text design: Christi Payne Fryday
Typography: TBH/Typecast, Inc.
Word processing: Deborah Eaglebarger
Proofreading: Katherine Sullivan

First published in the United Kingdom 1990 by Macmillan London Limited

Library of Congress Cataloging-in-Publication Data

Worwood, Valerie Ann, 1955–
The complete book of essential oils & aromatherapy / by Valerie Ann Worwood.
p. cm.
Includes bibliographical references and index.
ISBN 0-931432-82-0 (acid free paper)
1. Aromatherapy. I. Title.
RM666.A68W67 1991
615'.321—dc20 91-20111
CIP

ISBN 0-931432-82-0
First New World Library printing, September, 1991
Printed in the U.S.A.
10 9

This book is dedicated to my daughter
Emma Daisy
and my mother
Vera

The material in this book is not meant to take the place of diagnosis and treatment by a qualified medical practitioner. All recommendations herein contained are believed to be effective, but since actual use of essential oils by others is beyond the author's control, no expressed or implied guarantee as to the effects of their use can be given nor liability taken.

A special thank you goes to Julia Stonehouse
for her work and confidence in this book

and to

The unseen Hand that guides me, in all I do.

♦ CONTENTS ♦

WARNING

Not all natural plants or plant products are beneficial to health. Deadly nightshade can be poisonous and stinging nettles sting. The following essential oils should NOT be used under any circumstances.

Bitter almond
Boldo leaf
Calamus
Yellow Camphor
Horseradish
Jaborandi leaf
Mugwort
Mustard
Pennyroyal
Rue
Sassafras
Savin
Southernwood
Tansy
Thuja
Wintergreen
Wormseed
Wormwood

♦ INTRODUCTION ♦

THE FRAGRANT PHARMACY

When you enter the fragrant pharmacy a whole world of possibility is waiting for you. There you will find nature in one of its most powerful forms—aromatic liquid substances known as "essential oils" which are extracted from certain species of flowers, grasses, fruits, leaves, roots, and trees. These concentrated liquids are indispensable to medicine, and to the food and cosmetic industries. There are at present about three hundred of the essential oils, which between them constitute an extremely effective medical system. Many of these are the active ingredient in drugs prescribed by the orthodox Western system of medicine, or the inspiration for chemical copies. In food and drink essential oils are used to give natural flavor and aroma, and as preservatives. Manufacturers of cosmetics appreciate their cell-rejuvenating and beautifying properties, while the fragrance industry is more concerned with their delightful aroma and their mood and emotion-enhancing capacities.

Each single oil is used for many diverse purposes. For example, peppermint oil is an antiinflammatory used to treat rheumatism and arthritis; and it is prescribed by doctors for the relief of discomfort in the digestive system, under the trade name "Colperin." It is well known that peppermint is used by confectioners; and less well known that it is also an ingredient in aftershave lotions. It is across this wide spectrum that this book extends, explaining fully and for the first time the many uses to which essential oils can be put in the home. We shall see peppermint oil used for all the purposes mentioned above and many more besides, from a headache cure to a method of clearing an ant's nest or deterring mice from spending the winter in your roof.

Impressive though the medicinal qualities of essential oils are, *The Complete Book of Essential Oils and Aromatherapy* is not just a book in which to look up an illness and find the appropriate treatment. This is the household manual of the future and it provides answers to a very wide range of problems. These natural plant oils can be used to treat your child's flu, or called upon when you want to create a delicious and exciting new dish when the boss is invited to dinner. They will get rid of the fleas from your dog's coat as easily as the aphids from your garden plants. They will help you at work or play—at the same time as helping your tomatoes to grow. With essential oils you can take control of your life and environment, secure in the knowledge that your well-being will be improved. You can use them for all the same purposes that the medical professions and the food and beauty industries do . . . and more!

All who know the pure product and use it with understanding come to respect the essential oils. One cannot but admire their ability to operate effectively not only on the cellular, physical level, but in the emotional, intellectual, spiritual, and aesthetic areas of our lives also. If anything in this world is holistic, it is essential oils. However, it is not only because the essential oils treat a human being as a whole that they could be the *materia medica* of the future. They provide a system of medicine which is not only in total biochemical harmony with the human body, but also non-invasive to it in terms of heat and electromagnetism. In addition, their delivery system is so efficient that chemical drugs are made to look crude by comparison. The usual way of taking chemical drugs —orally—is the least effective method of taking essential oils because it involves passing the substance through the digestive system where it comes into contact with food and bacteria with which it could chemically interact. Essential oils, on the other hand, can be applied through the skin—in massage oils or by osmosis in the bath—or by inhalation in a variety of methods.

The extraordinary versatility of nature's essential oils is made possible by the fact that they come in a most convenient form. A few drops of pure lavender oil wiped on a burn effects the most remarkable cure as the skin returns to normal within days, whereas without it there would be a blistering patch and, eventually, a scar. You can return to the same little bottle when you have a headache—just one drop rubbed on the temples will bring relief. Because lavender is a natural deterrent of mosquitoes and moths, among other insects, it can as easily be dabbed on a ribbon and hung at the window to deter the former, or put on a cotton-wool ball and placed in the wardrobe to deter the latter. The natural antibiotic and antiseptic qualities of lavender oil make it not only a highly effective wash for cuts and grazes—on you or your pet—but also for tables, tiles, and fridges. The fact that it smells divine means that it's a delight to use anywhere and any time, and makes it a useful oil when creating an air freshener.

Essential oils are one of the great untapped resources of the world. Here we have a system of natural help that is far more than a system of medicine that can prevent illness and alleviate symptoms. These extremely complex precious liquids are extracted from very specific species of plant life and are in harmony with people and planet alike. By taking essential oils into our lives we find a way to provide our family and home with the protection and pleasure they need without polluting ourselves or our environment with chemicals.

These days the medicines and household goods we use are mostly chemical-based, and the food we eat and the air we breathe contain more chemicals than we would like. The cumulative effect of these, and the unknown effects as they react together within us, cannot be good for us, any more than chemical overload is good for the planet. Sooner or later we are going to have to find some alternatives and, for some of our problems, the alternative is literally right under our noses, drawing us to them with their sweet-smelling aroma—precious miracles and delights of creation, nature's essential oils.

♦ CHAPTER 1 ♦

MEDICINES OUT OF THE EARTH

The Lord hath created medicines out of the earth; and he that is wise will not abhor them.
ECCLESIASTICUS 38:4

YOU DO NOT NEED to have worked with essential oils on a daily basis over many years to come to the realization that nature has provided mankind with a tremendously powerful and diverse *materia medica*. Some of the healing that has taken place under their influence would be called miraculous if we didn't have the scientific basis for explaining how the oils work. But giving a scientific explanation for a remarkable phenomenon does not make it any less miraculous.

The holy anointing oil that God directed Moses to make from "flowing" myrrh, sweet cinnamon, calamus, cassia, and olive oil, would have been a powerful antiviral and antibiotic substance, the use of which gave protection and treatment to all those to whom it was administered. Cinnamon is a powerful antiviral and antibacterial agent as well as being antifungal. Myrrh is an effective antiseptic and one of the best cicatrisants—that is, it stimulates cellular growth—and its healing effects on open wounds, ulcers, and boils was legendary even before Biblical times.

There are about three hundred essential oils in general use today by professional practitioners, but the average household could fulfill all its likely needs with about ten. Each oil has its own medicinal and other properties. Modern-day research has confirmed centuries of practical use of the oils, and we now know that the fragrant pharmacy contains, apart from its antiviral, antibacterial, and antifungal qualities, essential oils which are antiseptic, antiinflammatory, antineuralgic, antirheumatic, antispasmodic, antivenomous, antitoxic, antidepressant, sedative, nervine, analgesic, hypotensol, hypertensol, digestive, expectorating, deodorizing, granulation-stimulating, circulatory-stimulating, and diuretic, and much more besides.

One of the most satisfactory aspects of using essential oils medicinally and cosmetically is that they enter and leave the body with great efficiency, leaving no toxins behind. The most effective way to use essential oils is not orally, as one might think, but by external application or inhalation. The methods used include body oils, compresses, cosmetic lotions, baths—including sitz, hand, and foot baths—hair rinses, inhalation (by steam, direct from the bottle or from a tissue), perfumes, room sprays, and a whole range of room methods. Although under supervision the essential oils can be prescribed for oral ingestion, this is in fact their least effective mode of entry because it involves their passing through the digestive system, where they come into contact with digestive juices and other matter which affect their chemistry. This limitation also applies to any chemical medications. The flexibility of medicinal use makes the essential oils of special benefit to patients whose digestive systems have, for whatever reason, been impaired.

Unlike chemical drugs, essential oils do not, as far as we know, remain in the body. They are excreted through urine and feces, perspiration, and exhalation. Expulsion takes three to six hours in a normal, healthy body and up to fourteen hours in an obese or unhealthy body. The method of excretion differs from oil to oil. For example, sandalwood and juniper can be detected by their aroma quite clearly in urine. Garlic, on the other hand, even if applied to the skin, will be passed out of the body through exhalation, whereas geranium, which is a beneficial circulatory oil, will be detected in the perspiration.

Essential oils are extracted from certain varieties of trees, shrubs, herbs, grasses, and flowers. The oil is concentrated in different parts of the plant. Vetiver oil is made from the chopped roots of the grass species *Vetiveria zizanoides*; bay oil is extracted from bay leaves. Geranium oil comes from the leaves and stalks, while cumin oil comes from the seeds, and ginger oil comes from the root-like stems which grow under or along the ground. Myrrh, frankincense, and benzoin oils are extracted from the resin of their respective trees. Mandarin, lemon, lime, grapefruit, and bergamot oils are squeezed from the peel of the fruits, while tonka bean is extracted, as you would guess, from the bean. Cinnamon oil comes from the bark of the tree, and pine oil comes from the needles and twigs of *Pinus sylvestris*.

Depending on the plant, the essential oil is stored in specialized oil or resin cells, glandular hairs, cells, or scales which have single or multi-cell pockets or tiny reservoirs or, in the case of fennel, for example, intercellular spaces.

The oil is extracted from the plant by a variety of means, depending again on the particular species. The most common method is steam distillation, although other important methods are solvent extraction, expression, enfleurage, and maceration. New methods are also being devised.

It takes a great deal of work to produce a tiny amount of essential oil. Sixty thousand rose blossoms are required to produce one ounce of rose oil, whereas in the lavender plant the essential oil is more abundant and 220 pounds will provide 7 pounds of oil. In the case of jasmine, the flowers must be picked by hand before the sun becomes hot on the very first day they open, whereas the sandalwood tree must be thirty years old and thirty feet high before it is cut down for distillation. Between these two extremes, a whole range of growing and picking conditions apply to the plants that will ultimately provide the precious essential oils. The price of each oil reflects these conditions, and because it takes eight million hand-picked jasmine blossoms to produce 2.2 pounds of oil, you can understand why that is one of the most expensive oils on the market.

The trade in essential oils is worldwide, with consignments passing between France, China, Brazil, Bulgaria, Turkey, Saudi Arabia, Ethiopia, Indonesia, the United States, Réunion, Australia, USSR, Israel, Britain, Thailand, Java, Guatemala, Egypt, Somalia, and Spain, among other places. The same species of plant grown in different countries under different soil and altitude conditions will produce oils which differ in their chemical makeup and therapeutic properties.

On average, an essential oil contains one hundred components. The chief of these are terpenes, alcohols, esters, aldehydes, ketones, and phenols, and although technology is allowing us to identify more of the components, there remain many more to be discovered. There are those who would argue that there is no difference between essential oils and reconstituted oils, but these are people who are concerned with the aromatic quality of natural essences because they want to copy them for artificial flavors and fragrances. There is, however, more to an essential oil than its aroma. But if we do not yet know all the chemicals that go to make up an essential oil we do know that they are noninvasive to the human body because we and they are made of the same material. The aromatic chemicals found in essential oils are derived from phenylpropane, and these are the precursors of amino acids which link to make the proteins which provide the building blocks for just about everything in the human body from the smallest enzyme to the skeleton. Another large group of chemicals found in essential oils are the terpineols which are formed from acetyl-coenzyme A, which in the human organism plays a crucial role in the production of hormones, vitamins, and energy.

As well as being noninvasive and nontoxic to the human organism, essential oils are noninvasive in terms of heat and electromagnetism. Each body cell is electrically charged and the effect of electricity, in all its forms, plays a part in the healing process. The dextrorotatory and lavorotatory (clockwise and counterclockwise) characteristics of essential oils have been known for a long time but need to be reassessed in view of the growing awareness about the importance of the body's electromagnetic fields. It could be that these aspects of the essential oils contribute towards stimulating the body's own natural healing mechanisms.

The positive effect of essential oils on blood circulation is well known. Through this they play an important part in bringing oxygen and nutrients to the tissues while assisting in the efficient disposal of carbon dioxide and the other waste products that are produced by cell metabolism. The general increase in blood flow improves the efficiency of the immune system and decreases blood viscosity. Indeed, there is not a part of the human body and brain that is not helped by good circulation.

Plants in general are chemical factories. They inhabit the interface between light and dark, sun and earth, drawing energy from each and synthesizing this into molecules of carbohydrates, proteins, and fats. These are the "crude fuels" which we and other animals break down to produce ATP (adenosine triphosphate), our "high-grade fuel." But essential oils are the high-grade fuel of plants, and by taking them into our body we ingest the best of the goodness plants have to offer. As a preventative prophylactic there is nothing better, and the fact that they are so delightful to use and so flexible in their methods of use makes them extremely pleasurable and easy to incorporate into our busy, modern lifestyles.

Because the essential oils are so sweet-smelling it might be easy to suppose that their value is essentially one of charm. This would be a mistake. These substances are very complex in their molecular structure, and very powerful. The essential oil of oregano, for example, is twenty-six times more powerful as an antiseptic than phenol, which is the active ingredient in many commercial cleansing materials.

The Timeless Apothecary ♦♦♦♦♦♦♦♦♦♦

Hippocrates, the father of medicine, said that "the way to health is to have an aromatic bath and scented massage every day." As far back as the fourth century BC he recognized that burning certain aromatic substances offered protection against contagious diseases and this is a method we can adapt and adopt at social gatherings today for the same reason, but with the advantage of specific scientific information about the antibacterial and antiviral properties of particular aromatic oils. Indeed, the history of perfume needs to be reevaluated in the light of our modern knowledge and the protective and health-giving properties of aromatic substances.

Our earliest written evidence that perfume was a commodity commonly available to the man or woman in the street comes from an Indian epic of 2000 BC, the *Ramayana*, which includes an episode in which the hero-prince, Rama of Ayodhya, returns after a period of exile to a triumphant homecoming in his village. Everyone, we are told, pours into the street cheering, including the lamp-makers, jewelers, potters, bath-attendants, wine-sellers, weavers, sword-millers, perfumers, and incense-sellers.

Some people might suppose that perfumes were used in early times to cover up bad smells caused by lack of hygiene, but apart from the fact that nature provided unpolluted rivers and streams long before the Industrial Revolution produced internal plumbing, there is a great deal of evidence that early civilizations were as concerned with cleanliness as we are. In 5000 BC the people of the city of Mohenjo Daro, in modern Pakistan, were "obsessed with cleanliness," according to archaeologists who found a communal bath measuring 39 feet by 23 feet in addition to wells in every house. The Egyptians took personal hygiene seriously, as shown by the earliest recorded recipe for a body deodorant in the Papyrus Ebers of 1500 BC. The Egyptian priests used aromatic substances not only for embalming their pharaohs but also in their role as "psychiatrists" for treating manias, depression, and nervousness. Oils were used in ancient Egypt and many of these came from China and India, where there is evidence to suggest that they were already in use for a thousand or more years before the pharaohs.

The Babylonians went so far as to perfume the mortar with which they built their temples—an art they handed down to the Arabs who built their mosques in the same aromatic way. In India the early temples were built entirely of sandalwood, ensuring an aromatic atmosphere at all times. Clay tablets from Babylonia dating from around 1800 BC detail an import order which included the aromatics cedarwood, myrrh, and cypress, all used as oils therapeutically today.

The ancient Greeks had a very high opinion of aromatics, attributing sweet smells to divine origin. In ancient myths, gods descended to earth on scented clouds, wearing robes drenched in aromatic essences. The Greeks believed that after death they went to Elysium where the air was permanently filled with a sweet-smelling aroma which rose from perfumed rivers. And in Roman as well as Greek bath houses, aromatic oils were extensively used, as prescribed by Hippocrates, for health.

Another of history's famous physicians, the Arabian Avicenna, who lived in Constantinople in the tenth century, wrote over a hundred books, the first of which was on the beneficial effects of the rose. Rosewater was one of the perfumes and essences brought back from the East by the Crusaders. By the time of the fourth crusade in 1202 France had taken perfume-making to its heart and was the established center in Europe. Throughout Europe in the fourteenth, fifteenth, and sixteenth centuries, many herbals were published which included recipes for making essential oils. Glove-makers used aromatic oils, and it is reported that these and others who used aromatics of various sorts were the only people to survive the ravages of the plagues that struck Europe during these centuries.

The scientific study of the therapeutic properties of essential oils was started by the French cosmetic chemist, René-Maurice Gattefosse, in the 1920s. While making fragrances one day in his laboratory, Gattefosse burned his arm very badly and thrust it into the nearest cold liquid—which happened to be a tub of lavender oil. He was surprised to find that the pain lessened considerably and that, far from developing into a normal burn reaction of redness, heat, inflammation, and blisters, his wound healed very quickly and left no scar. From then on, Gattefosse dedicated the rest of his life to researching the remarkable healing properties of nature's essential oils. It was he who coined the term "aromatherapy."

Quality Control ◆◆◆◆◆◆

For effective therapeutic use it is crucial that only pure essential oils be used—that is, natural plant essences which have been extracted by steam distillation, solvent extraction, expression, maceration, or enfleurage. It is quite pointless buying any other product, no matter how charming its aroma may be, because reconstituted products or chemical copies of natural essences simply do not work for medicinal purposes. However, because the medicinal properties of essential oils have hitherto been of no importance to the biggest consumer of essential oils, the perfume industry, a large variety of so-called essential oil products have been devised to meet the demand of an increased market and give the uniformity that nature cannot provide. In law, all these products come under the general heading of "essential oils," which can be confusing to the inexperienced buyer: "reconstitutions"; "nature identicals"; "isolates"; "perfume compounds"; and "aromas," such as "lavender aroma." Apart from the range of products that have been devised to take the place of essential oils in perfumery, there are essential oils which, when mixed with others, mimic the aroma of the essential oil whose name they carry. For example, carnation oil is very expensive and so black pepper and ylang-ylang are combined to create the aroma of carnation. This is all very well if perfumery is your concern, but no good at all if the carnation oil is required for a therapeutic purpose.

Unscrupulous suppliers, as well as selling those oils mentioned above, will dilute a pure essential oil in a carrier base and pass that off as pure natural essence. These fakes are easier to spot than any others because the base oil is oily, while essential oils for the most part are not. For this reason the term "essential oil" is something of a misnomer. Pure essential oils when dropped on blotting paper will impregnate it, then evaporate and disperse, leaving no oily patch. Other vegetable oils, on the other hand, will leave an oily mark. There are some exceptions to this rule: vetiver, for example, is viscous and more difficult to identify when diluted in a base oil.

When going into a shop to buy essential oils, you may not wish to take blotting paper with you to check the stock. But certainly, a range of essential oils should reflect accurately the variation in the wholesale prices of these products which are grown in such varying circumstances and subject to wide differences in transportation and production costs. For example, jasmine is ninety-two times the price of grapefruit on my current wholesale list, and sandalwood is four times the price of lime. No reputable essential oil supplier sells essential oils all at the same price.

Look for pure essential oils in shops that are concerned with nature and health, such as health food shops, rather than those concerned with the body and perfume. At the back of this book you will find reputable suppliers who deal in mail order inquiries and, for the beginner, it may be best to purchase from these sources until you get to know what the real thing smells like and, as you become more sure of your nose's ability to discern the good from the bad, seek a more convenient retail outlet. But although the best judge of quality is undoubtedly the human nose—and perfumers must study for years before their olfactory senses are developed enough to do a professional job—it is often the case that a synthetic aroma will smell more pungently of the raw material than the real thing. Do not then be influenced by strength, but rather by price, supplier reputation and, in time, your own experience and instinct.

Storage is important. The oils should be kept in brown or dark-colored bottles away from light, heat, and dampness. Keep the tops tightly closed when not in use. The therapeutic life of essential oils is about two years, although some would argue that they last longer than this. Certainly their antibiotic and other properties can still be utilized in nonbody methods such as air fresheners, kitchen surface wipes, perfumes, or celebratory and gift purposes, when their aromas are a crucial aspect of their use. Unfortunately, essential oils are not yet dated when sold, so it is impossible to tell how old they are when you buy them—another reason for going to a reputable supplier.

How To Use This Book ◆◆◆◆◆◆◆◆◆◆◆◆

Before we look at the various methods of using essential oils there are a few points about them which need to be understood.

Synergy

When the combination is more than the sum of the parts, there is a synergistic effect. By mixing together two or more essential oils you are creating a chemical compound that is different to any of the component parts, and these synergistic blends are very particular and powerful. An increased potency can be achieved with synergistic blends without increasing the dosage. For example, the antiinflammatory action of chamomile essential oil is greatly increased by adding lavender in the correct proportion. The interaction of particular essential oils upon each other gives a vibrancy and dynamism to the whole which could not be achieved by using a single component on its own.

The important point about synergistic blends is that the proportions should be correct, and sometimes it is necessary to make up more in volume than you need to use so that the smallest component oils can be incorporated into the whole in the right proportion. Diluted in a body oil, you may have a component part which is only 0.001 percent of the whole and yet that minuscule amount is integral to the whole.

Adaptogens

There are several essential oils that act as natural balancers. These adaptogens, as they are called, will instigate a reaction in the body that is appropriate to achieve a state of homeostasis or balance. The reactions affect the autonomic nervous system, the endocrine system, and blood pressure, among others. For example, hyssop normalizes either high or low blood pressure so that an equilibrium is achieved. Lemon works on the autonomic nervous system, acting as a sedative when needed, or as a tonic. Peppermint is another oil that could be found listed on both "relaxant" and "stimulant" lists, and this apparent contradiction can cause confusion unless you understand that these are adaptogens. Interestingly, there are other natural products that fall into this group which have been researched by scientists in Vladivostok, USSR, among them the herb mint and the root ginseng.

Chemotypes

The same species of plant can produce essential oils with different chemical components when grown in various conditions. For example, the common herb *Thymus officinalis* produces several oils for medicinal use, depending upon the soil, climate, and altitude in which it is cultivated. Thyme linalol, which is usually grown at high altitudes, is the only chemotype of thyme that can be used in the treatment of children. Because one species of oil-producing plant can break down into several chemotypes, each with different medical potentials, the list of useful plants is more extensive than first appearances might imply.

Methods of Use ♦♦♦♦♦♦

What follows is a list of just some of the ways in which essential oils can be used, with their recommended quantities. There are many other methods not listed which are described through the book—in the chapters on cooking, gardening, pet domestic animals, and celebrations, for example.

The following chart has been broken down into three sections: body methods, water methods, and room methods. Although the quantities for the room methods can seem quite small, these are sufficient, and to gauge how strong the aroma really is, prepare your method then leave the room, shutting the door behind you, and return in a few minutes. In this way your olfactory nerves will get a truer picture. Entering a room filled with tobacco smoke for the first time as opposed to being in such a room for a while also has this different effect because we adjust so quickly to aromas.

BODY METHODS

Method	Dosage	
Perfume	Variable	There are two methods: you can use either simply dissolved in alcohol or oil and apply to the body as you would a perfume, or incorporate them into a perfume (see "The Still-Room," chapter 14).
Tissue or Handkerchief	1 drop	Sniff when required.
Inhaled as a Vapor	2-3 drops	Pour hot water into a bowl, add the oil, cover your head with a towel and lean over the bowl with your face about 10 inches away and your eyes closed. Breathe deeply through your nose for about one minute.
Massage oil	As directed *or* a maximum of 5 drops to each teaspoon of base vegetable oil	Ask your pharmacist for a brown glass bottle—these have their volume imprinted on the glass on the bottom. Measure out your base oil. Use almond, hazelnut, peach kernel, apricot kernel, grapeseed, soya, peanut, etc. Add the essential oil—you may see this streak through the vegetable oil. To dissolve them thoroughly, turn the bottle upside down a few times and then roll it briskly between your hands. To ascertain how much to use for each massage, cup your hand and pour the oil into it, but not so much that it pours into the finger creases or over the edge of your hand. As a person's hand is in proportion to his body size, the amount held there will vary. One teaspoon is adequate for most bodies.

WATER METHODS

Method	Dosage	
Baths	As directed *or* a maximum of 8 drops	Run the bath, then add the essential oil. Close the door of the bathroom so the vapors don't escape. Soak for at least ten minutes, relaxing and breathing deeply. In some instances, the essential oil is first diluted in a vegetable oil—see page 139 in "The Body Beautiful."

WATER METHODS (cont.)

Method	Dosage	
Bidet	As directed *or* 2–3 drops diluted in 1 teaspoon vegetable oil	Use warm water from the tap. Run the water then add the essential oil and swish it around as well as possible so that globules aren't left on the surface as these could irritate mucous membrane.
Douche	Only as directed	Use boiled and cooled water from the tap or warmed, bottled spring water. Add the essential oil and shake the douche until the contents are thoroughly mixed.
Jacuzzi	3 drops per person	See "Bacteria Busters," page 386, for shared jacuzzis.
Sauna	2 drops per 2½ cups water	Use eucalyptus, tea tree, or pine oils. Mix in the water beforehand and throw on to the heat source as usual. Only use these essential oils because they enter the body with inhalation and exit by perspiration. They are all excellent cleansers and detoxifiers.
Shower	As directed *or* a maximum of 8 drops	Wash as usual. Now add the essential oil to your facecloth or sponge and rub it over yourself briskly as you continue to stand under the running water. Breathe in the aromatic steam deeply.
Sitz Bath	As directed *or* 2–3 drops	Run a bath to hip level or use a bowl which is large enough for you to be able to lower your behind into it. Add the essential oil and swish it around thoroughly so that no globules are left on the surface, where they could come into contact with delicate mucous membrane.
Hand Bath	As directed *or* 2–4 drops	Soak the hands for a maximum of ten minutes in a bowl of warm water.
Foot Bath	As directed *or* 2–6 drops	Soak the feet for twenty minutes in a bowl of warm water.

ROOM METHODS

Method	Dosage	
Candles	1–2 drops	Light the candle and wait until the wax begins to melt and then add the oils to the warm wax. Essential oils are inflammable so do be careful not to get them on the wick.

ROOM METHODS (cont.)		
Method	**Dosage**	
Diffusers	1–6 drops	These are especially made for use with essential oils. There are all sorts of diffusers, some heated by candle flame and others by electricity, but it is important that the surface of the bowl section is nonporous so that it can be wiped clean and another essential oil used later. The idea of a diffuser, whether made of clay, glass, or metal, is that it can heat the oils, so allowing their molecules to be released into the atmosphere.
Light Bulbs	1–2 drops	The heat generated by a light bulb can be used to release the molecules of essential oil into the atmosphere. There are various attachments made of nonflammable material or metal which can be used in conjunction with light bulbs; or add the oil to a standing lamp bulb when it is not switched on, and cool. Do not put the oil onto a light bulb which is already heated, as essential oils are inflammable. Use only 1–2 drops—no more—or the oil may drip down the bulb into the attachment.
Humidifiers	1–9 drops	Add the essential oil to the water.
Radiators	1–9 drops	Put the essential oil onto a cotton-wool ball and lodge it by the pipe or somewhere where it is in contact with heat.
Room Sprays	4 or more drops per 1 cup water	Use a new plant sprayer. Put in warm but not boiling water, add the essential oil and shake before use. It can be sprayed in the air as you would any spray or on the carpets, curtains, and furniture, but do not let the water fall on good wood.
Water Bowls	1–9 drops	Put boiling water into a bowl and add the essential oil. Close doors and windows and allow five minutes for the aroma to permeate the room.
Wood Fires	1 drop per log	Use cypress, pine, sandalwood, or cedarwood oils. Put 1 drop on each log and leave for half an hour before using, although the oil will retain its effectiveness for a very long time and so the logs can all be prepared in advance. One log per fire will be sufficient.

Vegetable or Base Oils ◆◆◆◆◆◆◆◆◆◆◆◆◆

Essential oils in the pure state are too highly concentrated to be used directly on the skin, and you will therefore find references to base oils throughout the book. The essential oils are diluted in a base oil, so that they can be massaged or rubbed onto the skin in the correct dosage. One drop of an essential oil may be all you need to use. That obviously will not go very far, but when it is diluted in a base oil it will cover quite a large area.

Base oils are vegetable, nut, or seed oils, many of which themselves have therapeutic properties. Vegetable oils are obtained from the seeds of plants that grow all over the world. There are several hundred different plants known to have oil-bearing seeds, but only a few are produced commercially. Vegetable oils are in the main produced for food, and are a good source of nutrients and energy. They enable the body to produce heat and are a good source of protein, as well as providing lubricants and cooking materials for industry and home use. The vegetable oils used in aromatherapy should be cold pressed, as the oils on your supermarket shelves may have been processed with a chemical agent.

Use the following measurements as a guideline when diluting the essential oils in a vegetable base oil.

Minimum-maximum drops of essential oil	*Into measurement of base oil*
0–1 drop	1/5 teaspoon
2–5 drops	1 teaspoon
4–10 drops	2 teaspoons
6–15 drops	1 tablespoon
8–20 drops	4 teaspoons
10–25 drops	5 teaspoons
12–30 drops	2 tablespoons

1 teaspoon = 5 ml
2 teaspoons = 10 ml
1 tablespoon = 15 ml

When buying essential oils, it is useful to know that approximately:

20 drops = 1/5 tsp essential oil
40 drops = 2/5 tsp essential oil
60 drops = 3/5 tsp essential oil
etc.

Sweet Almond Oil

Color:	very pale yellow
Obtained:	from the kernel
Contains:	glucosides, minerals, vitamins. Rich in protein.
Uses:	good for all skin types. Helps relieve itching, soreness, dryness, and inflammation.
Base oil:	can be used as a base oil, 100 percent.

Apricot Kernel Oil

Color:	pale yellow
Obtained:	from the kernel
Contains:	minerals and vitamins
Uses:	all skins, especially prematurely aged, sensitive, inflamed, and dry
Base oil:	can be used as a base oil, 100 percent.

Avocado Pear Oil

Color:	dark green
Obtained:	from the fruit
Contains:	vitamins, protein, lecithin, fatty acids
Uses:	all skins, especially dry and dehydrated; eczema
Base oil:	use as an addition to a base oil, 10 percent dilution.

Borage Seed Oil

Color:	pale yellow
Obtained:	from the seeds
Contains:	gamma linolenic acid, vitamins, minerals
Uses:	PMT, multiple sclerosis, menopausal problems, heart disease, psoriasis and eczema, prematurely aged skin. Good for regenerating and stimulating the skin. All skin types.
Base oil:	use a 10 percent dilution.

Carrot Oil

(an essential oil in its own right, but often used in base oils)

Color:	orange
Contains:	vitamins, minerals, betacarotin
Uses:	premature aging, itching, dryness, psoriasis and eczema. Rejuvenating; reduces scarring.
Base oil:	use a 10 percent dilution. Do not use undiluted on skin.

Corn Oil

Color:	pale yellow
Contains:	protein, vitamins, minerals
Uses:	soothing on all skins (as a base oil)
Base oil:	can be used 100 percent.

Evening Primrose Oil

Color:	pale yellow
Contains:	gamma linolenic acid, vitamins, minerals
Uses:	PMT, multiple sclerosis, menopausal problems, heart disease. Excellent in the treatment of psoriasis and eczema. Helps to prevent premature aging of the skin.
Base oil:	use a 10 percent dilution.

Grapeseed Oil

Color:	almost colorless or pale green
Contains:	vitamins, minerals, protein
Uses:	all skins
Base oil:	can be used 100 percent.

Hazelnut Oil

Color:	yellow
Obtained:	from the kernel
Contains:	vitamins, minerals, protein
Uses:	has a slight astringent action; good for all skins
Base oil:	can be used 100 percent.

Jojoba Oil

Color:	yellow
Obtained:	from the bean
Contains:	protein, minerals, a waxy substance that mimics collagen
Uses:	inflamed skins, psoriasis, eczema, acne, hair care, all skin types; highly penetrative
Base oil:	use a 10 percent dilution.

Olive Oil

Color:	green
Contains:	protein, minerals, vitamins
Uses:	rheumatic conditions, hair care, cosmetics; soothing
Base oil:	use a 10 percent dilution.

Peanut Oil (Arachis Nut)

Color:	pale yellow
Contains:	protein, vitamins, minerals
Uses:	all skin types
Base oil:	can be used 100 percent.

Safflower Oil

Color:	pale yellow
Contains:	protein, minerals, vitamins
Uses:	all skin types
Base oil:	can be used 100 percent.

Sesame Oil

Color:	dark yellow
Contains:	vitamins, minerals, proteins, lecithin, amino acids
Uses:	psoriasis, eczema, rheumatism, arthritis; all skin types
Base oil:	use a 10 percent dilution.

Soya Bean Oil

Color:	pale yellow
Contains:	protein, minerals, vitamins
Uses:	all skin types
Base oil:	can be used 100 percent.

Sunflower Oil

Color:	pale yellow
Contains:	vitamins, minerals
Uses:	all skin types
Base oil:	can be used 100 percent.

Wheatgerm Oil

Color:	yellow/orange
Contains:	protein, minerals, vitamins
Uses:	eczema, psoriasis, prematurely aged skin; all skin types
Base oil:	use a 10 percent dilution.

♦ CHAPTER 2 ♦

YOUR BASIC CARE KIT

Lavender ♦ Tea Tree ♦ Peppermint ♦ Chamomile
Eucalyptus ♦ Geranium ♦ Rosemary
Thyme ♦ Lemon ♦ Clove

IF I HAD TO CHOOSE the ten most versatile and useful essential oils for the average home medicine cabinet, these would be they. Although these oils are chosen first for their medicinal properties and their ability to deal with a wide range of health complaints, you will find that they also feature strongly throughout the book and are useful for a diversity of purposes from skin care to gardening and from home care to celebrations.

The treatments outlined in this section are straightforward yet effective. Some of the conditions listed here are discussed in more detail in other chapters of this book, so please refer to the index. Other useful additions to your care kit would be aloe vera, witch hazel, and rosewater. Aloe vera comes from the leaf of the cactus of this name and is a fine healing agent in itself for cuts, inflammations, and burns, as well as being a good carrying agent for the essential oils. It can be bought in gel or liquid form. Witch hazel is extracted from a shrub and is known for its astringent and antiinflammatory properties. Rosewater is a by-product of the distillation of the essential oil of roses and is used for its mild antiseptic and soothing properties. But let us now have a brief look at the ten essential oils that comprise the Basic Care Kit.

Lavender ♦♦♦♦♦♦♦♦♦♦♦♦♦

Lavender is capable of many important jobs and is a delight to use. Every home should have a bottle of lavender, if no other oil, because it is so very effective in the treatment of burns and scalds. Lavender oil is a natural antibiotic, antiseptic, antidepressant, sedative, and detoxifier which promotes healing and prevents scarring, and also stimulates the immune system and contributes to the healing process by stimulating the cells of a wound to regenerate more quickly. Although not known specifically as a circulatory stimulant, lavender oil certainly seems to allay the effects of clinical shock and as a mood tonic and antidepressant it helps to deal with the psychological shock of injury. It also has a multitude of other qualities which make it a truly indispensable oil.

Tea Tree ◆◆◆◆◆◆◆◆◆◆◆◆◆◆

The antiseptic action of tea tree is thought to be one hundred times more powerful than carbolic acid—and yet it is nonpoisonous to humans! The Aborigines have been using this indigenous Australian tree in their medications for centuries and today tea tree is the subject of a great deal of international research. Its impressive antiviral, antibacterial, and antifungal properties make it useful in a wide range of conditions. It is used in the treatment of candida and all sorts of infections, for ringworm, sunburn, acne, athlete's foot, toothache, and pyorrhea, among other things.

Peppermint ◆◆◆◆◆◆◆◆◆◆◆

Peppermint has been used by many ancient cultures, including the Egyptians, Chinese, and American Indians, no doubt because of its extremely useful health-promoting properties. It is an excellent digestive, it helps the respiratory system and circulation, it is an antiinflammatory, and an antiseptic. These qualities make it a good oil in the treatment of indigestion, flatulence, bad breath, flue, catarrh, varicose veins, headaches and migraines, skin irritations, rheumatism, toothache, and fatigue. It even keeps mice, fleas, and ants away!

Chamomile ◆◆◆◆◆◆◆◆◆◆◆

There are several types of chamomile essential oil. Chamomile German is an excellent variety and its beautiful deep dark blue color, due to its high azulene content, comes as a bonus. Another excellent variety, chamomile Roman, is particularly good for the treatment of nervous conditions and insomnia. Beware though of chamomile Maroc (*Ormenis multicaulis*) which is not a true chamomile and cannot be used as such.

Although chamomile is antibacterial, antiseptic, and disinfectant, it is most valued for its antiinflammatory properties. These apply to internal conditions like rheumatism, as well as to external inflammations. Chamomile is indispensable if you have children because it can be used for teething troubles and in the bath to ease nerves and tetchiness. (See Chapter 9 for its many other uses in child care.) Chamomile is used in the treatment of burns, including sunburn, psoriasis, eczema, asthma, hay fever, diarrhea, sprains and strains, nausea, fever, and all nervous and depressive states. Its analgesic, diuretic, sedative, and calming properties make chamomile an extremely desirable oil. For kicking the tranquilizer habit it is invaluable, and in anorexia nervosa it is extremely helpful. As if this weren't enough, chamomile is used in rejuvenation treatments.

Eucalyptus ◆◆◆◆◆◆◆◆◆◆◆

Eucalyptus has been distilled from at least 1788 when two doctors, John White and

Dennis Cossiden, distilled *Eucalyptus piperata* for its use in treating chest problems and colic. This was in Australia where the Blue Mountains of New South Wales are so called because of the extraordinary blue haze that exudes from the resin of the eucalyptus gum and envelops the entire landscape. In such a powerfully aromatic environment, the medicinal qualities of this ancient tree would be hard to miss.

Eucalyptus is a marvelously versatile and useful oil. It cools the body in summer and protects it in winter. It is antiinflammatory, antiseptic, antibiotic, diuretic, analgesic, and deodorizing. Research has proved its antiviral properties as well. It is best known for its effectiveness against coughs and colds but is equally effective in the treatment of cystitis, candida, diabetes, and sunburn, while also being useful in veterinary care and as an insect repellent. There is a wide range of eucalyptus varieties, any one of which would be a useful addition to a Basic Care Kit.

Geranium ◆◆◆◆◆◆◆◆◆◆◆◆

Geranium is one of my favorite oils because it works profoundly on the emotions and is useful in many medical conditions—and smells wonderful while it works so hard. The oil is extracted not from the familiar brightly colored geranium but from the species Pelargonium—Geranium Robert or "lemon plant"—which is very often displayed in abundance in Greek restaurants.

Geranium will make chilblains disappear overnight and brings a radiant glow when used in skin care. More importantly, it is a vital component in the treatment of endometriosis, is very effective for menopausal problems, diabetes, blood disorders, throat infections, and as a nerve tonic, and works well as a sedative. It is reputed to help in cases of uterine and breast cancer and if nothing else, would certainly help the patient to relax and cope with the pain. Geranium has many applications, from frostbite to infertility, and its antiseptic and astringent properties contribute to its general usefulness. Its delightful floral fragrance makes it a pleasure to use, either on its own or as a contributory oil in blends.

Rosemary ◆◆◆◆◆◆◆◆◆◆◆◆

Rosemary is both a physical and mental stimulant, which makes it a good oil to have in the morning bath, while also being excellent in the treatment of all muscular conditions, making it the perfect oil for a bath after a long tiring day. This antiseptic oil is used in the treatment of muscular sprains, arthritis, rheumatism, depression, fatigue, memory loss, migraine, headaches, coughs, flu, and diabetes, among other conditions. It is also very useful in beauty treatments, being used in hair care and acne and cellulite remedies. For the sportsman, cook, and gardener, rosemary is invaluable.

Thyme ◆◆◆◆◆◆◆◆◆◆◆◆◆◆◆

There are many types of thyme, some of which can be used safely in all situations and some which cannot. Thyme has notable antiviral, antibiotic, antiseptic, and diuretic properties and should be *used with great care*. Overuse of it can stimulate the thyroid gland and lymphatic system. Like many good things, it must be used in moderation. It should never be applied to the skin undiluted and should not be used on children unless it is within the chemotype Thyme linalol (see page 11).

Thyme is a vital component of the Basic Care Kit because of its powerful antiviral properties. When flu is around it is a wonderful oil to have on the room diffuser. It assists in the elimination of toxic wastes from the body. It is used in the treatment of a wide range of conditions including whooping cough, warts, rheumatism, neuralgia, fatigue, and acne. It is also extremely useful in antiseptic powders, hair and skin care regimes, and cooking. Just to make it a perfect all-rounder, thyme will discourage all manner of parasites and insects from invading your home.

Lemon ◆◆◆◆◆◆◆◆◆◆◆◆◆◆◆◆

When our adventurous seafaring ancestors sailed the high seas, fresh lemons saved them from getting scurvy. For modern stay-at-homes, the essential oil of lemon is just as useful as a water purifier. This antiseptic and antibacterial oil will perform many tasks when used in blends, including treating verrucas, insect bites, and tension headaches. It has a tonic action on the lymphatic system and a stimulating action on the digestive system. It will assist you to slim, help disperse cellulite, and keep wrinkles at bay. Its contribution to synergy makes it particularly useful in blends, while it is indispensable as a fragrancing and flavoring agent.

Clove ◆◆◆◆◆◆◆◆◆◆◆◆◆◆◆◆

Clove oil is antibacterial, antiseptic, and analgesic and is a good oil for the prevention of disease and infection. Being a spice it can easily be incorporated into your cooking. It is best known as a quick cure for toothache although it is equally useful in digestive problems and muscular disorders. It can be used in the treatment of asthma, nausea, and sinusitis, and as a sedative. Clove is a powerful oil that has been used for the sterilization of surgical instruments. It should not be used undiluted on the skin.

Applications for the Basic Care Kit ◆◆◆◆◆◆◆◆◆◆◆◆◆◆

In the column to the right of the lists that follow you will find essential oils other than those mentioned in the text which may also be used to treat these conditions.

Through the Basic Care Kit certain methods of treatment are referred to, such as compresses, steam inhalations, and ice treatments. For details of these methods please refer to the chart on pages 12–14 and pages 95–97.

The oils in italics are not in the Basic Care Kit but have been included for your information.

Abdominal Pain

OTHER ESSENTIAL OILS THAT COULD BE USED TO TREAT THESE CONDITIONS

Abdominal pain should be checked by a doctor if it persists and increases in intensity because it could be appendicitis or another condition that needs to be properly diagnosed.

UPPER ABDOMINAL AREA Apply the following oil over the painful area in a clockwise direction:

Pepperment	3 drops	Diluted in 1 teaspoon vegetable oil
Clove	2 drops	

Eucalyptus
Chamomile
Marjoram
Coriander
Angelica
Fennel
Anise

LOWER ABDOMINAL AREA Apply the following oil over the painful area in a clockwise direction:

Thyme	2 drops	Diluted in 1 teaspoon vegetable oil
Eucalyptus	3 drops	

Geranium
Peppermint
Rosemary
Patchouli
Ginger

Abrasions

Clean the area well with 5 drops of lavender diluted in a bowl of warm water. Apply one neat drop of lavender and leave to heal.

Tea tree
Red thyme
Neroli
Frankincense
Myrrh

Abscesses

Make a compress using the following oils and apply it to the area of swelling twice a day:

Lavender	2 drops
Tea tree	2 drops
Chamomile	3 drops

Eucalyptus
Red thyme
Lemon
Juniper
Sandalwood
Palma rosa

DENTAL ABSCESS Put 1 drop of chamomile on a cotton ball and apply directly to the abscess. Also rub over the jaw and cheek area with the following oil:

Lavender	3 drops	Diluted in 1 teaspoon vegetable oil
Tea tree	2 drops	

Lemon
Geranium
Fennel
Bergamot
Myrrh

OTHER ESSENTIAL OILS THAT COULD BE USED TO TREAT THESE CONDITIONS

Anal Fissure

Bathe the area with warm water to which you have added 5 drops of lavender and 2 drops of lemon oil. Also massage around the anal area with the following oil:

Chamomile	2 drops	Diluted in 1 teaspoon vegetable oil
Geranium	1 drops	
Lavender	3 drops	

Eucalyptus
Tea tree
Thyme
Myrrh
Neroli
Pettigraine

Athlete's Foot

Make up a mixture of 2 drops of tea tree and 1 drop of lavender, dip a cotton-wool ball into it and smear it between the toes and around the nails. Also make up the following massage oil and rub it over the feet, paying special attention to the toes:

Tea tree	5 drops	Diluted in 1 teaspoon vegetable oil
Lemon	1 drop	

Thyme
Lavender
Tagetes
Hyssop

Bilious Attacks

Inhale from a tissue on which you have put 1 drop of peppermint and 1 drop of lemon oil. Also make an oil by adding 2 drops of peppermint to 1 teaspoon vegetable oil and use it to rub over the gall bladder area (around the right, lower rib cage) and stomach.

Rosemary
Clove
Ginger
Rose
Fennel
Cardamom

Black Eyes

Dilute 1 drop of geranium and 1 drop of chamomile in 2 teaspoons witch hazel and blend together well. Now add this to 1 tablespoon ice-cold water, mix well, and soak some cotton-wool pads in it. Close your eye and apply a pad to the eyelid and surrounding area.

Lavender
Rose

Bleeding

For bleeding from an open wound apply a compress to which you have added the following:

Geranium	1 drop
Lemon	1 drop
Chamomile	1 drop

Hyssop
Palma rosa
Cypress
Rose

OTHER ESSENTIAL OILS THAT COULD BE USED TO TREAT THESE CONDITIONS

NOSE BLEED Lie flat on your back, pinch the nostrils, then inhale the following oils from a tissue:

Lemon	3 drops
Lavender	1 drop

Rosemary
Chamomile
Cypress
Rose
Palma rosa

BLEEDING GUMS Make up the following mixture, add it to a tumbler of warm water, and use as a mouthwash. *Do not swallow.*

Lemon	2 drops	Diluted in 1 teaspoon brandy
Lavender	1 drop	
Eucalyptus	2 drops	

Tea tree
Myrrh
Rose
Cypress

Blepharitis

Inflammation of the eyelids—see Conjunctivitis.

Rose
Fennel

Blisters

Apply neat 1 drop of lavender and 1 drop of chamomile. Pat in thoroughly but carefully.

Tea tree
Lemon
Tagetes
Myrrh

BLISTERS FROM BURNS AND SCALDS DO NOT PIERCE. Put 1 neat drop of lavender oil onto the blister and then hold an ice cube on the blister for at least ten minutes. Cover with a piece of dry, clean gauze. Repeat up to three times a day. (See also Burns.)

Tea tree
Eucalyptus
Yarrow

Boils

Bathe the area with 2 drops of lavender and 2 drops of tea tree diluted in a small bowl of **hot** water. If the inflammation is severe, add 1 drop of chamomile. Bathe twice a day.

Chamomile
Thyme
Lemon
Parsley
Nutmeg
Oregano

OTHER ESSENTIAL OILS THAT COULD BE USED TO TREAT THESE CONDITIONS

HOT COMPRESSES These can be applied to draw out the pus. Put 1 drop of red thyme onto a hot compress and apply twice a day. After the pus has been dispelled apply a little of the following oil over the affected area twice a day:

Lavender	3 drops	Diluted in 1 teaspoon vegetable oil
Red thyme	2 drops	
Tea tree	2 drops	

Bruises

Make up two bowls of water, one hot and one cold, and add the following to both:

Lavender	2 drops
Rosemary	3 drops
Geranium	1 drop

Soak a washcloth in each bowl and apply them alternately to the bruised and surrounding area. Then apply a small amount of the following oil:

Geranium	2 drops	Diluted in 1 teaspoon vegetable oil
Rosemary	2 drops	
Lavender	1 drop	

Chamomile
Parsley
Cypress
Hyssop

Bumps

Treat as for Bruises.

Niaouli
Basil
Ginger

Burns

Apply ice-cold water for at least ten minutes. Then immediately put 2 drops of neat lavender oil directly onto the burn. Put 5 drops of lavender on a dry, cold compress and cover the area. (See also page 72.) Repeat as needed.

Chamomile
Eucalyptus
Yarrow
Niaouli

CIGARETTE BURNS Apply 1 drop of lavender to the burn.

Carbuncles

Treat as for Boils.

OTHER ESSENTIAL OILS THAT COULD BE USED TO TREAT THESE CONDITIONS

Oregano
Cinnamon
Ravensara

Catarrh

Use the bowl method of steam inhalation. Put the following oils on top of the water and inhale for at least ten minutes. Keep your eyes closed.

Rosemary	1 drop
Peppermint	2 drops
Tea tree	1 drop

Also rub your chest and back with the following oil:

Tea tree	2 drops	Diluted in 2 teaspoons vegetable oil
Rosemary	2 drops	
Eucalyptus	5 drops	
Thyme	1 drop	

Use the essential oils on tissues also, and inhale when needed. Use any of the following: rosemary, thyme, eucalyptus, tea tree.

Lavender
Clove
Pine
Frankincense
Nutmeg

Chapped Lips

Apply to the lips:

Chamomile	2 drops	Mixed well with 2 teaspoons aloe vera gel
Geranium	2 drops	

Alternatively, use the following oil.

Eucalyptus
Rose
Sandalwood
Neroli

Chapped Skin

Make up the following oil and massage over the chapped area, including the face if affected:

Geranium	10 drops	Diluted in 2 teaspoons vegetable oil
Chamomile	10 drops	
Lemon	5 drops	
Lavender	5 drops	

Rose
Sandalwood
Carrot
Neroli

Chilblains

Apply 1 drop of neat geranium oil to the affected area, usually the toes or fingers. Do this for two days then massage with the following oil:

Geranium	5 drops	Diluted in 1 teaspoon vegetable oil
Lavender	1 drop	
Rosemary	1 drop	

OTHER ESSENTIAL OILS THAT COULD BE USED TO TREAT THESE CONDITIONS

Tea tree
Chamomile
Lemon
Ginger
Black pepper

Cold Sores

Put 1 drop of geranium oil on a cotton ball and apply it directly to the sore, if possible as soon as it is suspected. Repeat every day. Also, massage the whole of the body including the face and neck with the following:

Geranium	10 drops	Diluted in 2 tablespoons vegetable oil
Lavender	10 drops	
Thyme	2 drops	
Lemon	8 drops	

Tea tree
Chamomile
Rose
Hyssop

Common Colds

Use the following oils in a hot bath. Lie back and inhale deeply:

Thyme	2 drops
Tea tree	2 drops
Eucalyptus	1 drop
Lemon	3 drops

For the steam inhalation method, use one drop each of the following: thyme, tea tree, lavender, and clove.

Carry with you a tissue on which you have placed one drop each of red thyme, peppermint, eucalyptus, and clove, and inhale deeply whenever possible.

Massage around the chest, neck, and sinus area (forehead, nose, and cheekbones) with the following:

Lemon	1 drop	Diluted in 1 teaspoon vegetable oil
Eucalyptus	2 drops	
Rosemary	3 drops	

All the oils in the Basic Care Kit
Oregano
Cinnamon
Clove
Basil

OTHER ESSENTIAL OILS THAT COULD BE USED TO TREAT THESE CONDITIONS

Conjunctivitis

Add 1 drop of chamomile to 1 teaspoon witch hazel and mix as well as possible. Then add to 2 tablespoons rosewater and leave it for at least seven hours. Strain through a paper coffee filter and use with a compress on the eyelids (keep eyes closed).

Constipation

Massage in a clockwise direction over the lower abdomen three times a day with the following:

Rosemary	15 drops	Diluted in 2 tablespoons vegetable oil
Lemon	10 drops	
Peppermint	5 drops	

Constipation can have underlying causes—check dietary habits.

Patchouli
Cedarwood
Angelica

Convalescence

If you have a convalescent at home it may well be worth investing in other essential oils that help nerves and strength but which are not within the scope of the Basic Care Kit. The following, which are in the kit, are all helpful and can be used in massage oils, in the bath, or in a room diffuser and other room methods:

Geranium
Lemon
Lavender
Rosemary
Chamomile

Mandarin
Palma rosa
Rose
Bois de rose
Ginger

Coughs

DRY COUGH Mix 2 drops of eucalyptus and 2 drops of lemon oil with 2 tablespoons honey. Take 1 teaspoon of this and dilute in a wine glass of warm water. Sip it slowly.

Massage over the back and chest with:

Eucalyptus	3 drops	Diluted in 1 teaspoon vegetable oil
Thyme	2 drops	

For the steam inhalation method use 3 drops of lavender.

Chamomile
Tea tree
Oregano
Sandalwood
Frankincense
Ginger

OTHER ESSENTIAL OILS THAT COULD BE USED TO TREAT THESE CONDITIONS

COUGH WITH MUCUS Follow the treatment outlined above except for the drink. For this mix the following essential oils into the tablespoon of honey:

Eucalyptus	2 drops	Blend together and use 1 drop only
Thyme	1 drop	
Tea tree	1 drop	

Cuts and Wounds

Bathe the area with warm water to which you have added the following:

Lavender	5 drops	To each 2 cups water
Tea tree	2 drops	

Put 3 drops of lavender on a piece of gauze and place it over the cut. Renew it twice a day and expose the cut or wound to air on the third day if possible.

Cypress
Myrrh
Rose
Palma rosa

Diarrhea

Diarrhea may be caused by a whole range of conditions which generally fall into the three categories of food-related, nerve-related, and viral-related. In all cases, drink large quantities of water. Follow the same treatment but use the oils which are appropriate to your particular condition:

FOOD	NERVES	VIRAL
Peppermint	**Lavender**	**Tea tree**
Eucalyptus	**Geranium**	**Red thyme**
Thyme	**Lemon**	**Lemon**
Chamomile	**Chamomile**	**Lavender**
Tea tree	**Peppermint**	**Eucalyptus**

Use these oils to make a massage oil or follow the formulas below. These quantities are to be diluted in 1 teaspoon vegetable oil. Massage over the whole of the abdomen area.

FOOD

Chamomile	2 drops
Peppermint	3 drops
Eucalyptus	1 drop

Cypress
Frankincense
Orange
Basil
Marjoram

OTHER ESSENTIAL OILS THAT COULD BE USED TO TREAT THESE CONDITIONS

NERVES

Chamomile	1 drop
Eucalyptus	2 drops
Lavender	3 drops

VIRAL

Thyme	3 drops
Lavender	2 drops
Tea tree	1 drop

Make a drink by adding 1 drop of the relevant essential oil to a teaspoon of honey and diluting it in a glass of warm water. Sip slowly.

Food-related:	Peppermint
Nerve-related:	Peppermint
Viral-related:	Eucalyptus

Diverticulosis

The inflammation, pain, flatulence, and discomfort of this condition are effectively eased by using the essential oils, but nutritional habits must be examined to ensure there is no recurrence of the problems. Rub the following oil over the abdomen twice a day:

Basil
Marjoram
Hyssop
Sage

Peppermint	2 drops	Diluted in 1 teaspoon vegetable oil
Chamomile	1 drop	
Rosemary	3 drops	
Clove	1 drop	

Also, mix 1 drop of peppermint with a teaspoon of honey and dilute in a cup of hot water. Sip slowly.

Earache

Persistent pain and earache could indicate a perforated ear drum or an infection and you should get a medical diagnosis.

For general earache, warm a teaspoon of olive oil and add to it 1 drop of lavender and 1 drop of chamomile; blend well. Soak a piece of cotton wool in this and use it to plug the ear.

OTHER ESSENTIAL OILS THAT COULD BE USED TO TREAT THESE CONDITIONS

Also use the following oil to massage around the ear area, up the neck, and across the cheekbone:

Chamomile	3 drops	Diluted in 1 teaspoon vegetable oil
Lavender	1 drop	
Tea tree	1 drop	

Applying a warm compress to the cheek and ear area after massaging also eases the pain.

Eucalyptus
Tea tree

Ear Infections

Treat as for Earache but using different essential oils. For the ear plug substitute 3 drops of tea tree and 2 drops of lavender. This is the substitute massage oil:

Tea tree	3 drops	Diluted in 1 teaspoon vegetable oil
Thyme	1 drop	
Lavender	2 drops	

Chamomile
Eucalyptus
Niaouli
Marjoram
Juniper

Fainting

Untie any tight clothing and raise the legs higher than the head. Hold the open bottle of essential oil under the patient's nose: use lavender, rosemary, or peppermint.

When consciousness is regained, give the patient a drink made by adding one drop of lemon essential oil to a teaspoon of honey and dissolving it in a cup of hot water. This should be sipped slowly. Also, put 2 drops of any of the essential oil listed above onto a tissue, which should be inhaled.

Angelica
Marjoram
Neroli
Rose

FAINTING FROM EXHAUSTION OR FATIGUE Treat as above, followed as soon as possible by a warm bath to which you have added the following:

Chamomile	2 drops
Lavender	1 drop
Geranium	1 drop

Bed rest should follow immediately.

As above

OTHER ESSENTIAL OILS THAT COULD BE USED TO TREAT THESE CONDITIONS

Fever

See "Your Basic Travel Kit," Chapter 3.

Fibrositis

Massage well into the affected area:

Rosemary	2 drops	Diluted in 1 teaspoon vegetable oil
Lavender	1 drop	
Peppermint	1 drop	
Clove	1 drop	

It is helpful to apply this massage oil after a cabbage compress has been applied. Iron a large outer leaf from a cabbage to release the vitamins and enzymes and apply while still hot to the area. Leave for fifteen minutes.

Also use the combination of essential oils above undiluted in hot baths—4 drops per bath.

Chamomile
Thyme
Clary-sage
Marjoram
Ginger
Black pepper
Frankincense

Frostbite

Massage up to 5 drops of neat geranium into the affected area. Alternatively, use lavender. When the person is warm, massage the area with:

Geranium	4 drops	Diluted in 1 teaspoon vegetable oil
Clove	2 drops	

Hyssop
Ginger

Frozen Shoulder

Frozen shoulder can often be eased by using the treatment for Fibrositis. The cabbage method (see page 96) should be used every day and followed by a massage using this formula:

Clove	3 drops	Diluted in 2 teaspoons vegetable oil
Chamomile	3 drops	
Thyme	3 drops	

Rosemary
Lavender
Black pepper
Ginger
Nutmeg

Gingivitis

OTHER ESSENTIAL OILS THAT COULD BE USED TO TREAT THESE CONDITIONS

Tea tree
Myrrh
Bergamot

Inflamed gums are thought to be the cause of more teeth being lost than through tooth decay. Prepare a mouthwash by adding 1 teaspoon of the mixture below to a glass of warm water. Swish well around the mouth; do not swallow.

Thyme	3 drops	Diluted in 1 teaspoon brandy
Eucalyptus	2 drops	
Chamomile	3 drops	
Peppermint	3 drops	

Also mix 3 drops of chamomile and 2 drops of lavender into 1 tablespoon of aloe vera gel and smooth a little over the gums.

Grazes

See Abrasions.

Halitosis

Anise
Coriander
Fennel
Myrrh

The problem of bad breath is often caused by factors other than breath itself. These are the oils that help:

DIGESTIVE PROBLEMS

Peppermint 2 drops
Lemon 2 drops

GUM DISEASE

Tea tree 2 drops
Thyme 2 drops

GENERAL

Lavender 4 drops

Dilute the 4 drops of essential oil in 1 teaspoon of brandy and then put in a tumbler of warm water and use as a mouthwash.

Hay Fever

Peppermint
Clove
Rosemary

Put 1 drop each of chamomile and lemon essential oils onto a tissue and inhale. Add the following combination to baths:

Chamomile 2 drops
Lemon 2 drops
Lavender 1 drop

OTHER ESSENTIAL OILS THAT COULD BE USED TO TREAT THESE CONDITIONS

Massage the neck, chest, and back with:

Chamomile	2 drops	Diluted in 1 teaspoon vegetable oil
Geranium	1 drop	
Lemon	1 drop	

Because hay fever affects people in different ways, treatment is often a case of trial and error. Experiment with the essential oils.

Headaches

Several essential oils in the Basic Care Kit can ease headaches but as these arise from a variety of causes, look under the appropriate heading.

GENERAL HEADACHES, FOR NO APPARENT REASON Massage around the temples and the base of the skull, along the hair line, with 1 neat drop of the following combination of oils then blend with 1 drop of vegetable oil:

Lavender	3 drops
Peppermint	1 drop

Or use lavender or peppermint on their own.

Rosemary
Chamomile
Rose
Marjoram
Coriander

GASTRIC HEADACHE This is often caused by eating the wrong foods. Mix 1 drop of peppermint oil with a teaspoon of honey dissolved in a glass of warm water, and sip.

Make up the following combination of oils:

Rosemary	1 drop
Peppermint	2 drops
Lavender	1 drop

Use 1 drop of the combined oils to massage the back of the neck. Either inhale 1 drop on a tissue or use 3 drops in a steam inhalation.

Chamomile

NERVOUS HEADACHE Follow the treatment as for General Headaches but use these essential oils:

Lavender	3 drops	Combine and use 1 drop
Chamomile	1 drop	

Rosemary
Clove

OTHER ESSENTIAL OILS THAT COULD BE USED TO TREAT THESE CONDITIONS

Also massage over the solar plexus (upper abdomen) in a clockwise direction using the following:

Geranium	1 drop	Diluted in 1 teaspoon vegetable oil
Lemon	2 drops	
Lavender	3 drops	

SINUS HEADACHE See Sinusitis.

TENSION HEADACHE As for Nervous headache.

Heartburn

Add 1 drop of peppermint to a teaspoon of honey and dissolve in a cup of warm water; sip slowly. Also rub the upper abdominal area with the following:

Eucalyptus	2 drops	Diluted in 1 teaspoon vegetable oil
Peppermint	3 drops	

Clove
Lavender

Hiccups

Put 1 drop of chamomile oil in a brown paper bag and hold it over your nose and mouth. Breathe in deeply and slowly through your nose.

Lavender
Lemon
Anise
Fennel

Influenza

There are many identified and unidentified viruses which are given the name "flu." Viral attacks that involve fever, tiredness, coughs, colds, muscular pain, and exhaustion are all likely to be given this label.

Treatment needs to be quick and is aimed at raising immunity levels as well as combating the virus. Depending on the severity of the attack it may also be wise to consult the "Bacteria Busters" list of oils on page 386. In the Basic Care Kit there are several oils which do have a profound effect on such viral infections.

If you are shivery and cold and feel that you have the onset of something more, take a warm bath to which the following oils have been added:

Tea tree	5 drops
Lavender	2 drops
Thyme	2 drops

Chamomile
Oregano
Cinnamon
Ravensara
Eucalyptus radiata

OTHER ESSENTIAL OILS THAT COULD BE USED TO TREAT THESE CONDITIONS

Then massage your whole body with the following oil:

Tea tree	2 drops	Diluted in 1 teaspoon vegetable oil
Eucalyptus	3 drops	

And go to bed.

Bedrooms should be sprayed with thyme and lavender, or use one of the other room methods to diffuse these oils throughout your living area. Drink plenty, and make a special drink by using 1 drop of the following blend of oils, adding it to a teaspoon of honey and diluting it in a cup of hot water.

Clove	1 drop	Combine and use 1 drop per drink
Lavender	2 drops	

Sip the drink slowly.

See other sections in this book for more specific advice on how to treat your symptoms.

Insect Bites

Remove the stinger if applicable and apply neat lavender to the site. See "Your Basic Travel Kit," page 56.

Chamomile

Laryngitis

Use steam inhalations with the following oils added:

Chamomile	2 drops
Lavender	3 drops
Thyme	1 drop

Massage all over the neck area and behind the ears with the following:

Chamomile	5 drops	Diluted in 1 teaspoon vegetable oil
Thyme	1 drop	
Lemon	2 drops	

To reduce the soreness, make a drink by adding 2 drops of lemon and 1 drop of lavender to 2 teaspoons of honey and mixing it into a wineglassful of rosewater which has been boiled.

Geranium
Ravensara
Ginger
Parsley
Sage
Pine

Lumbago

Put the following oils onto a hot compress and apply to the lower back:

Rosemary	3 drops
Clove	1 drop
Eucalyptus	1 drop

When the compress becomes cold replace it with another. Do this at least three times a day.

Massage the lower back and into the crevice of the buttocks, but not as far as the anus, with:

Peppermint	3 drops	Diluted in 2 teaspoons vegetable oil
Rosemary	5 drops	
Chamomile	2 drops	

Rest in bed.

OTHER ESSENTIAL OILS THAT COULD BE USED TO TREAT THESE CONDITIONS

Lavender
Ginger
Black pepper
Sage
Pimento
Nutmeg

Mouth Ulcers

Mouth ulcers are caused by a minor viral infection. If you have persistent ulcers refer to the "Bacteria Busters" list which includes oils you may use.

Make a mouthwash by adding 1 teaspoon of the mixture below to a glass of warm water. Swish well around the mouth but do not swallow:

Peppermint	2 drops	Diluted in 2 teaspoons brandy
Lemon	4 drops	
Geranium	2 drops	
Thyme	2 drops	

Blend the following together and use a little to smooth around the ulcerated area:

Chamomile	2 drops	Blend in 1 tablespoon aloe vera gel or liquid
Thyme	1 drop	

Lavender
Tea tree
Myrrh

Nettle Rash (Urticaria)

Apply up to 2 neat drops of lavender over the stung area as soon as possible. Make up the following mixture and smooth it over the rash:

Lavender	5 drops	Blend in 1 tablespoon aloe vera gel or liquid
Chamomile	5 drops	

Take warm baths to which one handful of Epsom salts and 4 drops of chamomile have been added.

OTHER ESSENTIAL OILS THAT COULD BE USED TO TREAT THESE CONDITIONS

Eucalyptus
Yarrow
Angelica

Neuralgia

Numbing the area with ice often relieves the pain initially so use a cold compress or ice treatment over the affected part. To relieve any inflammation follow by massaging with the following:

Lavender	5 drops	Diluted in 2 teaspoons vegetable oil
Chamomile	5 drops	
Clove	2 drops	

If the face is the area affected omit the clove and substitute 2 drops of rosemary.

Peppermint
Eucalyptus
Thyme
Nutmeg
Marjoram
Vetiver
Juniper

Palpitations

Put the following oils on a tissue and inhale:

Lavender	2 drops
Chamomile	1 drop
Geranium	2 drops

Massage over the whole of the torso regularly every night with the following:

Lavender	10 drops	Diluted in 2 tablespoons vegetable oil
Chamomile	10 drops	
Rosemary	3 drops	
Lemon	7 drops	

And before going to bed take a warm bath to which you have added 2 drops of both chamomile and lemon oil.

Valerian
Neroli
Rose
Angelica
Anise

Scalds

See Burns.

Shock

This can be treated as for Fainting, as well as by massaging the body before bed with the following:

Lemon	3 drops	
Geranium	2 drops	Diluted in 2 teaspoons vegetable oil
Lavender	1 drop	

Sinusitis

Use the following combination of oils in the steam inhalation method:

Rosemary	3 drops
Thyme	1 drop
Peppermint	1 drop

Make a blend using the following proportions and put 1 drop on a tissue and inhale.

Rosemary	2 drops
Geranium	1 drop
Eucalyptus	1 drop

Blend the oils below in these proportions. Use 5 drops only in each massage. Massage around the neck, behind and in front of the ears, over the cheekbone, the nose, and forehead.

Rosemary	5 drops	
Geranium	5 drops	Blend together and use 5
Eucalyptus	2 drops	drops per teaspoon
Peppermint	3 drops	vegetable oil

Sore Throats

See Laryngitis.

OTHER ESSENTIAL OILS THAT COULD BE USED TO TREAT THESE CONDITIONS

Chamomile
Valerian
Rose
Palma rosa
Basil

Tea tree
Basil
Juniper
Benzoin
Oregano
Niaouli
Pine

OTHER ESSENTIAL OILS THAT COULD BE USED TO TREAT THESE CONDITIONS

Splinters

Remove the splinter with a sterilized needle or pair of tweezers. Apply 1 neat drop of lavender.

Tea tree
Myrrh

Sties

First prepare the liquid needed for a hot compress. Boil 2 teaspoons rosewater and add to it 1 drop of chamomile essential oil. Strain this liquid through a paper coffee filter and leave to cool slightly.

Now put 1 neat drop of lavender on a cotton ball and smear it on the cheekbone, under the sty—keeping the eye well closed.

Soak a cotton-wool pad in the rosewater and chamomile liquid and put it on your closed eyelid. Leave until cool. Repeat the whole procedure twice a day for three days.

Also use the massage given for Sinusitis on page 40.

Synovitis

Massage the inflamed joint with the following oil:

Chamomile	10 drops	Diluted in 2 tablespoons vegetable oil
Eucalyptus	5 drops	
Rosemary	5 drops	
Lavender	3 drops	
Peppermint	7 drops	

Tea tree
Yarrow
Rose
Juniper
Ginger

Toothache

Put 1 drop of clove oil on a cotton ball and apply it to the gum around the tooth or into the crevices on either side. Massage the jawbone and cheek with:

Clove	1 drop	Diluted in 1 teaspoon vegetable oil
Chamomile	3 drops	
Lemon	1 drop	

In severe cases a hot compress can also help. Use 3 drops of chamomile in hot water and soak the material or cotton wool in this, then apply to the affected cheek area. If the nerves are not exposed, applying ice to the cheek can also bring relief.

Peppermint
Lavender
Clary-sage

Whitlows

Make up the following combination of oils:

Thyme	2 drops
Lemon	3 drops

Apply one drop neat around the affected area three times a day.

When the pus has been dispersed, follow the same procedure three times a day, but using 1 drop of this combination:

Lavender	2 drops
Chamomile	2 drops

OTHER ESSENTIAL OILS THAT COULD BE USED TO TREAT THESE CONDITIONS

Tea tree
Benzoin
Myrrh

◆ CHAPTER 3 ◆

YOUR BASIC TRAVEL KIT

**Lavender ◆ Peppermint ◆ Geranium
Chamomile ◆ Ginger ◆ Eucalyptus
Thyme ◆ Lemongrass or Citronella**

WHILE AWAY FROM HOME some of the circumstances we experience bring particular hazards to us and our families. We are not only going to eat food which may have been prepared in less than hygienic conditions and share toilet facilities with complete strangers, but expose ourselves to unusual weather conditions and come into contact with native insects. Most of us have experienced trips made gruesome because of travel sickness, or have spent hours in the local clinic waiting to be seen. But with your mobile fragrant pharmacy packed in your luggage you can be prepared for any eventuality and make sure that your vacation is not marred by any one of the many common upsets that beset families away from home. Even if you only take one or two bottles of essential oil away with you this may be all you need to deal with known, recurring problems—sensitivity to the sun, perhaps, or mosquitoes that are insensitive to you. Have a look at the chart on pages 58–60 to help you decide which are the most appropriate oils for your family and your destination.

The Journey ◆◆◆◆◆◆◆◆◆◆

Traveling is supposed to be one of life's great pleasures, but if you feel sick in a car or plane, you may wonder why. Peppermint oil has a marvelously calming effect on the stomach and is clearly an essential for an uneasy traveler. It is very strong, so use just one drop in a cup of hot water with sugar to taste, and sip it slowly before setting off on your journey. Alternatively, for children and grownups alike, put a mere smear of peppermint on a cube of sugar—this tiny amount will suffice for a long journey. The advantage of this method is that you can pop the sugar cubes into a plastic bag and into your pocket for when they are really needed.

Another excellent general travel oil is ginger, which is well known for alleviating seasickness but is equally effective for other types of travel sickness. Two drops of ginger oil placed on a handkerchief and inhaled works well, and a drop diluted in a little vegetable oil and rubbed over the upper abdomen also helps.

Midsummer traffic jams often make driving to the beach a hot and frustrating time, but passengers and driver alike are kept cool and calm by one drop of lavender, eucalyptus, or peppermint oil on one or two cotton-wool balls placed on the rear window shelf of the car. These oils are not only antibiotic and antiseptic but they soothe the nerves and keep them from fraying. They won't make the driver sleepy, but will keep him on an even keel, relaxed but aware. For more lengthy or tiring journeys the driver can put two drops of basil oil in his or her morning bath, or onto the facecloth after washing in the shower and rub it over the body. This will help to sharpen concentration and keep the driver alert.

Exhaust fumes can cause nausea, so roll up the windows if you are caught in a jam and put a drop of eucalyptus on a couple of tissues and place them around the car to counteract the smell.

Travel sickness is to a large extent caused by conflicting messages reaching the brain from the eyes, the balancing mechanism of the ears, and the stomach. It helps to look at an unmoving object on the horizon or, if you are in a plane or on a ship, to close your eyes. Children often become sick because they are focusing their eyes on things nearby them on the seat, so do get chairs which elevate them to the level of the window and encourage them to look at things in the distance by playing I-spy type of games.

Flying

Nowadays the majority of people fly to their destinations and this is a mode of transport that brings particular problems. The compressurized compartment causes dehydration and swollen feet and ankles, cramp, dry skin, headaches and, especially in tourist class, painful knees from having them pushed up against the seat in front! Avoid alcohol when traveling by air, and tea and coffee. Do drink plenty of water and fruit juices to keep your sugar level up. If you suffer from tummy problems your stomach may feel bloated and extended because gases in your stomach can expand during flights. To alleviate this, have a cup of peppermint tea before you leave the house—one drop of peppermint oil, mixed with a teaspoon of honey and dissolved in hot water.

If flying makes you anxious have ready a tissue with one drop of lavender and one drop of geranium in a little plastic bag in your pocket. When you are beginning to feel uneasy about the situation pull the tissue out and hold it to your nose for a moment. Take in big sniffs, lie back, close your eyes, and relax. This also works well for people who get irritable on plane journeys.

There are two methods of dealing with swollen feet and ankles, which can become particularly troublesome on long flights. Both work equally well, and need preparing in advance. For the first, you will need a piece of cotton — a small handkerchief is perfect—for making a compress. Wet it so that it's just damp and put 5 drops of lavender oil on it. Fold it up and put it in a small plastic bag and into your pocket. When your ankles swell during the journey, or at journey's end if they feel heavy and tired, apply the compress to your feet and ankles and gently massage them in an upward direction to the bottom of the calf, both back and front, for a few minutes. For the second method you'll have to retire to the toilet. Massage your feet and ankles in an upwards direction, as above, with an oil made from adding 5 drops of lavender or eucalyptus essential oil to a teaspoon of oil. If you are planning a world trip you'll need more than a teaspoon to see you through, so prepare a little bottle to take with you. I can assure you this works wonders and your traveling will not be marred by this silly inconvenience. I say "silly" because that's what you feel when you can't get your feet in your shoes!

If you are prone to getting cramps while traveling, make a compress as above but using geranium oil and hold the compress over the affected area—usually the calf of the leg or the foot. Also try the old Chinese trick of holding your big toes tightly between the thumb and forefinger.

Knees weren't designed to spend hours bent squashed up against the seat in front of you on a 747, and especially for tall men this can become a big problem on long, and even short, journeys. Again, use the compress method with 5 drops of lavender oil but rub it over your knees. Businessmen in suits might find this something of an embarrassment if done while actually sitting in their seat, but they can retire to the toilet where the trouser leg can be pulled up without anyone wondering what is going on!

Children on long flights can get fidgety and irritable—which can make your journey as uncomfortable as theirs. Have ready a small bottle containing 15 drops of chamomile in 2 tablespoons of a light nut or vegetable oil. When things start to get out of control, twist the child around on the seat so you can massage his legs and feet with the oil, tuck him in and he'll soon settle down. You will only have used a tiny portion of the oil but it will come in handy for other holiday problems.

As we take longer flights to hotter suns, jet lag becomes an increasing problem. Even two or three days of unhappy recovery time are too many in an already short holiday or important business trip—and then there is the journey home to look forward to as well! Jet lag occurs because your body time clock is out of synchronization with the new environment, but the essential oils seem to bring the two wheels of time together gently and slowly, avoiding fatigue and jarring of the nerves. There are several combinations of oils one can use, but a good one comprises peppermint and eucalyptus for the morning and lavender and geranium for the evening. Before you set out on your journey, have a bath using two drops each of peppermint or eucalyptus or, if you prefer to shower, put one drop of each on to a wet facecloth and wipe it over your body, once you have washed.

When you arrive at your destination, force yourself to stay awake and go to bed at local bedtime, although do have an early night. If you have a nap when you arrive to recover from the journey, you'll wake up in the middle of the night. Before you sleep, have a bath to which you have added one drop each of lavender and geranium oil. If it's not possible to take a bath, put a small amount of nut or vegetable oil in the palm of your hand, add one drop each of lavender and geranium and rub the oil around and up your neck, covering the shoulder blades, as much of the upper back as you can reach, the chest, and solar plexus region, inhaling deeply all the time. Also rub over your lower back and hips to relieve the travel pain and tension that comes from sitting for long periods confined to one chair, often without enough leg room.

This treatment will alleviate the symptoms of jet lag but for the best results it must be continued. So when you wake, put two drops each of peppermint and eucalyptus in your bath or one drop each on a wet facecloth, wiped over your body after the shower. Alternatively, use the oil method described above but with these morning oils. Try to stay awake during the day and again, go to bed early. Continue with this morning and evening routine for the second and third days after you arrive, or for as long as it takes for your body to adapt to local time.

If you are involved in serious intercontinental travel you would do well to add the fabulous oil of grapefruit to your travel kit. I recently took a twenty-six hour flight to Australia which arrived in the early hours, giving me a couple of hours' sleep before I had to appear on breakfast TV looking sparkling. Grapefruit saved the day—or, to be more precise, the morning! This was the first morning of a six-week tour packed with flights and interviews and I really needed all the help I could get from essential oils. When planning your essential travel kit it's important to know at what time of the day you are leaving and the local time of arrival. I planned to get straight to sleep on the plane and so before I left I had a relaxing chamomile and lavender bath. On the flight I slept as much as possible and drank plenty of water and fruit juice. At stopovers I got off and walked around. The whole time went by in a relaxed time-warp with sniffs of lavender and chamomile hankies. After my arrival at the hotel I got into a grapefruit and lavender bath and had a long soak, inhaling deeply the reviving aromas of the oils. I felt great by the time I arrived at the TV studio, and throughout the whirlwind tour I kept myself on my toes with a little help from my friends—grapefruit and lavender. Before setting off to the airport for that final long haul home, it was back to the chamomile and lavender combination to ensure a relaxing journey.

Another combination for travelers is peppermint and geranium. This works well for people returning home who, after having spent a week unwinding at their holiday destination, and a week getting totally relaxed, find that their two-week holiday has come to an abrupt end and they are back at their desks with that Monday morning feeling—only much worse! Getting back into the routine is very tough but a couple of drops each of peppermint and geranium will help you get over the shock of reality.

The Arrival ◆◆◆◆◆◆◆◆◆◆

When we travel to foreign lands we come into contact with bacteria and viruses against which we have no genetic immunological defense. Not only that, but we sleep and wash where strangers slept and washed the night before, and when some of the bacteria and viruses people carry with them are so dangerous, why take any chances of picking them up? With killer diseases on the rampage it is not being paranoid to take steps to ensure we don't come home with something longer-lasting than a tan.

Even if your toilet facilities look clean, that doesn't mean they have been disinfected. It doesn't take a minute to wipe the toilet seat—under as well as on top—with a tissue that has a neat drop of thyme essential oil on it. Even if your toilet is attached to your room, it may be wise to do this daily. Remember too the toilet flush knob and doorknob. If you are traveling in particularly suspect parts you might use a few tissues impregnated with thyme, lavender, and eucalyptus. These three together provide a very powerful bactericide and few dangerous microorganisms can escape their exterminating effect. Also, it never hurts to wipe around the basin and bath with an essential oil tissue.

Every bed in the world is teeming with minute life-forms which live off the dead skin cells we are constantly shedding, and mattresses soak up whatever fluids are put on them. This makes them a pretty hazardous area. As a precautionary measure, especially for your children, pull the bedclothes back and wipe the mattress with a tissue on which you have put a few drops of thyme, lavender, and lemongrass.

Last year I gave a traveling kit of oils to a young man who was planning to travel around the world on a shoestring and expected to stay in some pretty rough places. When he got back—after a safe and happy trip—he told me that when he arrived at the seedy dormitory-type hostels he was frequenting in places such as Calcutta, he would splatter a few drops of lavender on the mattress despite the amused looks of some of the hardened travelers around who thought he was just perfuming his sleeping quarters. In the mornings, while all the others were scratching themselves madly, he packed his gear up like Joe Cool and went on his way. Throughout his trip he didn't get one single bite from a bed mite—which must be a record many other young adventurers would envy.

Making a home away from home is easy with the essential oils because you will be taking with you several that you will already have been using at home and the aroma provides a comforting aura of familiarity and security when used in new surroundings. Of course this may not be as important to you as it is to your children, who often feel insecure while away from home. Things may be fine while they are going to the beach and running around the pool and enjoying all the new and wondrous things, but when Mom goes out—even just to the bar downstairs with baby listeners alerted—a small child can feel quite abandoned. At home alone in a familiar room a child hears the rest of the family talking, laughing, and moving about and can sleep perfectly well with all these noises. But left alone in a strange room with nothing except their furtive imagination and the banging of doors and the ominous whine of the elevator, fears of the bogeyman can become very real indeed.

Using familiar scents cannot stop the fears entirely but the essential oils do help in an as yet unexplained way to calm children at night, and perhaps their effectiveness is due to the theory of association. If you use something like the lovely aroma of geranium when you arrive to make the room yours by putting a few drops around the place, bathe in geranium yourself and, more importantly, give the children a geranium bath before bed, you'll be surprised how easily they settle down for the night in the pleasantly fresh room that smells just like home. When you are aware that the essential oils can be used in this way, to comfort the child through the sense of smell, use the oil you intend to take away with you around the home and in the child's bath for a few days before your departure.

The Sun ♦♦♦♦♦♦♦♦♦♦♦♦♦♦

Despite repeated warnings, in the press and elsewhere, that skin cancer is caused at least in part by exposure to the sun, we still flock in our millions to the beaches where we lie prostrate soaking in as much of it as we can. Malignant melanoma has a very high cure rate if caught early and the thing to look out for is changes in your moles. Specifically, go to your doctor right away if you develop a dark patch of skin or wart-like growth or if one of your moles becomes painful, itchy, grows in size, is large or has an irregular outline, has a mixture of shades of brown and black, has a red edge, is inflamed, or bleeds, or if it oozes any fluid or is crusty. This is quite a list and if you have a lot of moles it can by very worrying, especially as few of us really know the color and shape of those we do have, and therefore what changes they might have gone through. Lying on the beach more than half naked with nothing much to do provides the perfect opportunity to make a detailed note—and that means in writing—of the moles we do have. And as we seldom lie on the beach alone, our companion can examine the back of our body too. The commonest sites for melanomas, incidentally, are on the thighs, for women and on the backs, for men. This mole-map might just turn out to be the most useful souvenir you take home with you.

The nature of sunlight is changing as pollution destroys the ozone layer and lets in too much ultraviolet light. There's not a lot that we as individuals can do about that, but what we can do, and really should, is keep out of the sun between the hours of twelve and three and cover ourselves with a sunscreen of factor ten or more. But the fact remains that human beings need sun—we manufacture vitamin A within our bodies as a direct result of it. At the famous Bircher Benner Clinic in Switzerland sun is an important part of many treatments, and it is well known that lack of sunlight can cause depression in susceptible people, even making them suicidal. The skin disorders of psoriasis, eczema, and acne heal wonderfully in sunlight, and aches and pains just seem to vanish. We all know how sun makes us feel so much better all around—but in moderation, please.

Sunburn may be as severe as blistering and peeling or simply a feeling of tightness and soreness, but a burn is a burn and whether from prolonged exposure to the sun or from a hot iron, the most effective treatment for it is the miraculous oil of lavender. With all burns, it is crucial to get the heat out of the skin, so fill a sink or bath with cold water, add ice if possible, and immerse yourself as soon as you can. Stay under the water for at least ten minutes, then apply neat lavender oil all over the burned area, bearing in mind that one drop of lavender will cover quite a large area—you don't need to overdo it, simply make sure that the lavender has covered the surface. If you do this, by morning you won't notice a thing—but do be sensible and stay out of the sun for at least two days, even though the area looks perfectly healed. If you haven't got any lavender with you, use eucalyptus instead. And don't forget your sunscreen.

After a dose of sunbathing make sure you use an oil that contains essential oils—it will not only prolong your tan but will nourish your skin. Apply all over the body after showering or bathing:

AFTER-SUN OIL

Lavender	10 drops
Chamomile	5 drops
Bergamot	1 drop
Geranium	2 drops
Diluted in	
Almond oil	approx. 2 oz.
Sesame oil	2 tablespoons

Sesame seed oil is a natural sun filter and by using it in warm evening baths you will be protecting your skin from the early evening sun and cooling yourself down before going out to the hot, sweaty disco to dance the night away!

AFTER-SUN BATH

Chamomile	4 drops
Geranium	3 drops
Peppermint	1 drop

Diluted in 1 tablespoon jojoba oil

Dilute the oils in the jojoba oil and add it all to the bath. While there, gently massage the oil over the areas that have been exposed to the sun—thighs, bottom, chests, and breasts are usually the worst affected.

The following oil is very effective in the drying conditions of sunburn, such as experienced when skiing, sailing, or hiking. It is rather a thick oil but works really well in protecting faces exposed to the sun in the more invigorating types of weather and activities. Blend the ingredients together well and use the oil every night before sleeping and during the day use a sunscreen:

APRÈS SKI, SUN, SAIL, AND HIKE OIL

Chamomile	10 drops
Geranium	10 drops
Lavender	10 drops

Diluted in

Jojoba oil	1 teaspoon
Sesame seed oil	1 teaspoon
Evening primrose oil	1 teaspoon
Almond oil	1 tablespoon

Hair can also suffer from over-exposure to sun, sea, wind, and the chlorine in swimming pools. See "Essential Care for Hair," Chapter 8, for good conditioning treatments. Bald patches on the head should be well protected. Hair on the head provides natural protection from the sun, which is why African babies are born with it. But if you're not an African baby—wear a hat!

The Heat ♦♦♦♦♦♦♦♦♦♦♦♦♦

HEAT EXHAUSTION is not really likely to affect the majority of travelers, but not drinking enough water or replacing the body salt that is lost when temperatures soar into the 100's is dangerous. If you are feeling dizzy, faint, and nauseous—and you may not even feel thirsty—retire to the shade and drink as much water as you can. You should aim to drink at least three quarts during the day, with one teaspoon of salt added. Apply neat lavender or eucalyptus to the temples, back of the neck, and solar plexus (upper abdomen), and breathe deeply.

HEATSTROKE, SUNSTROKE, AND HYPERPYREXIA can start slowly. First there is a confused feeling, a headache, drowsiness, and a temperature. The skin becomes hot and dry and looks red and yet there is a feeling of coldness, and shivering. Basically the heat regulation system in the body has stopped working and caused the temperature to rise. This is a very serious matter and the temperature must be brought down immediately and treatment must be continued for at least forty-eight hours to ensure the crisis has passed.

Try to immerse the body in cold water to which you have added 4 drops each of eucalyptus and lavender essential oil. Alternatively, just pour water over the body and apply neat eucalyptus to the temples and the back of the neck. Applying ice to the underarms, the groin, wrists, and neck helps too—even if the only ice you can find is in your lemonade. Get the sufferer indoors as soon as possible and sponge him down repeatedly with ice-cold water and eucalyptus for at least forty-eight hours. A quick dowsing with water will only lower the body temperature by one-hundredth of a degree, which obviously will not do. The sponging must be frequent and prolonged. Plenty of liquids must be drunk, starting with three quarts of water to which is added half a teaspoon of salt per quart.

HEAT CRAMPS can occur after unaccustomed exercise, loss of water and salt. Drink a quart of water to which half a teaspoon of salt has been added and massage the legs with the following:

Geranium	2 drops
Eucalyptus	3 drops

Diluted in 1 teaspoon vegetable oil

PRICKLY HEAT is a rash of tiny blisters that look like little pink or red spots. It is caused by blocked sweat glands and is extremely itchy. It can affect any part of the body, and the best line of action is to keep as cool as possible, expose the area to air if possible, and only cover with light cotton clothing if not.

Apply a splash to the area, made by diluting 6 drops each of eucalyptus, lavender, and chamomile to a teaspoon of alcohol (vodka is fine) and shaking it all in a cup of spring water.

Warm baths are very soothing if you add to them 4 drops each of eucalyptus and lavender essential oil.

If you get hold of any baking soda while you are away, or if you are at home when someone gets prickly heat, including this in the bath is the best solution. If you can use this method you only need lavender oil but—and this is important—add the lavender to the baking soda and mix them together well before putting it in the bath, don't just put them in separately. Below are the amounts you will need for various age groups. If treating a baby, make sure that the folds of the skin are kept dry (when not being bathed). Use warm water in the following baths:

BABY UNDER TWO

Baking soda	¼ cup
Lavender	2 drops

TWO TO SEVEN YEARS

Baking soda	½ cup
Lavender	2 drops

EIGHT TO TEN YEARS

Baking soda	½ cup
Lavender	3 drops

TEN YEARS TO ADULT

Baking soda	1 cup
Lavender	4 drops

Fevers

A fever is a rise in normal body temperature and anything above 37° C (98.4° F) falls into this category. Fevers developed on vacation are usually the result of viral or bacterial infection. Typhoid, malaria, tic fever, and even lassa fever are quite common in tropical climates, and are usually passed by insect bites or parasites. But even on the Costa Brava you can get sandfly fever and fevers from the micro-bugs in contaminated water supplies. Hepatitis can be caught by contact with someone who has the disease. With a fever, it is very important to get a correct diagnosis.

A body that is feverish can go through many changes from shivering and coldness to heat, sweating, and delirium. General toxemia can arise in typhoid, for example. The feverish person must be kept in bed—rest is generally the best cure. You can help to bring the fever down by keeping the body cool with sponging. Add the essential oils of eucalyptus, peppermint, or lavender in the water you use to sponge the body down.

Give the patient plenty of liquids, including fruit juices, and make sure he has plenty of fresh air. Spray the room with thyme and use it yourself if you are nursing someone—4 drops in a bath.

Tummy Trouble ◆◆◆◆◆◆

I asked an intrepid traveler who never has tummy trouble—even up the Sepik in Papua, New Guinea, not known for its four star hotels—what the secret is. "Only drink bottled water, even if that means taking a crate of your own, never have ice in drinks, avoid all uncooked food, and take a Swiss army knife." That, apparently, is so you can cut the skin off fruits. It might seem a bit much to wash your teeth in Evian water but it's a lot less embarrassing than having diarrhea and spending your holiday sightseeing the toilet roll holder on the back of the bathroom door!

It is amazing the number of people who get tummy trouble when staying at deluxe hotels, and this may be due to the attractive but hazardous lunchtime buffet—a veritable breeding ground for bacteria and an interesting landing-stage for flies. The simple fact of having new foods can cause diarrhea, as can heat.

DIARRHEA, in its mild form, usually only lasts up to forty-eight hours. The main danger of it is dehydration and you should drink extra fluids, including fruit juices. (Women should also remember that diarrhea reduces the body's ability to absorb the birth control pill.) Lemon essential oil will help to purify the water in which you should wash all fruit and vegetables. After each bowel movement drink the dehydration blend. Don't think about cutting out the sugar; it is there to promote the absorption of the salt:

DEHYDRATION BLEND

Bottled water	1 quart
Sugar	8 teaspoons
Salt	½ teaspoon
Lemon essential oil	8 drops

Drink one glass at a time

A warm bath with four drops each of geranium and ginger essential oils often helps to alleviate diarrhea, and at the very least it will make you feel better.

FOOD POISONING usually shows up within forty-eight hours of having eaten the offending meal. It may be caused by bacteria, carried by humans or flies, or by rotten food. Nausea, vomiting, pain, and diarrhea are the most likely effects, and fever and illness can develop.

It is important to rest in bed and drink plenty of fluids—make up the dehydration blend above. Massage the whole body with the following:

Geranium	5 drops
Lavender	5 drops

Diluted in 1 tablespoon vegetable oil

To stop the circulatory shock that results from vomiting and purging, take baths with geranium and ginger—2 drops of each. Also, apply ginger to the whole of the abdomen—5 drops per teaspoon of vegetable oil. Castor oil is one of the best cures for food poisoning. It doesn't have the loveliest taste but this can be disguised by dissolving it in a glass of water and lemon juice. You need one to two tablespoons of it and you can also take it by mixing it with peppermint oil—one drop per tablespoon.

BACILLARY DYSENTERY is carried in contaminated water and food and spread by flies and other carriers, and also by human contacts. *It is infectious.* It must be treated by a doctor, as saline injections may need to be given. The sufferer must be isolated and the room sprayed with thyme and lavender. Add the following oils to the bath (the doses are high but these are necessary):

Thyme	5 drops
Lavender	5 drops
Ginger	4 drops

If muscle pains occur use the three oils above in a massage oil, in equal parts. Lavender may ease the headache and high temperature but if it doesn't, use peppermint oil instead—put one drop on your fingers and rub along the base of your skull and around your temples.

Little Things That Bite ◆◆◆◆◆◆◆◆◆◆◆◆◆

Most people traveling from the northern hemisphere to the southern are acutely aware of the discomfort and dangers that can be brought about by the smaller living creatures on this earth—and small creatures seem to make up for what they lack in size by being particularly aggressive. But traveling is a hazardous business whichever direction you go in, and those who have spent a holiday trying to avoid the blackfly in northern Canada know that going north can be as uncomfortable as going south.

As you will see from reading this section, dangers are as likely to come from walking in the mountains, or taking forest walks, or swimming in the sea, as from sunning yourself on a beach infested with sandfly or having a drink on the veranda when the mosquitoes are out. The danger may be less likely in terms of frequency, but more likely in terms of degree. So wherever you go take your travel kit with you, or at least the oil or couple of oils that are most applicable to your environment. They take up so little room that it's foolish not to take them, because by the time you get back to your hotel room it may be too late.

Even in the green and pleasant land of Britain you can get bitten by a snake. A number of harmless-looking plants cause nasty rashes and many more cause allergic reactions in some people. Fish, jellyfish, and sea urchins conspire to make a swim in the ocean, if not a horror moving on a par with *Jaws*, at least enough to ruin a precious holiday. The list of insects that bite is almost endless and includes bees, wasps, fleas, bedbugs, gnats, midges, sandflies, water-ticks, hornets, and that pernicious spreader of the world's number one killer disease, the mosquito. All the oils in the travel kit have antiseptic properties and can be applied directly to the skin if you get bitten by any insect, and the sooner the better, but try to acquaint yourself with the more specific action and remedies recommended in this section so that you are well prepared to deal with those little creatures that bite and sting.

Prevention

As far as insect bites are concerned, prevention is a fairly straightforward matter and a much better option than cure. As a general rule use lemongrass or citronella to keep insects at bay, using the airborne methods—the room methods of steam bowls, heat source, paper strings at the windows, on light bulbs, both inside and out, or on ribbons hung from trees or any other atmospheric method outlined in this book. To deter insects from landing on your skin, as a general rule, lavender is a better option.

If you have a plant-spray with you (new or used only for essential oils), use that to spray lemongrass or citronella diluted in water around the room. If you have your own en suite bathroom, let the water run steaming hot into the bath and put a couple of drops on that before going out for the evening and leaving the steam to waft through the open bathroom door and into your bedroom. Also put a couple of drops onto the hot tap so that its heat releases the aroma molecules into the atmosphere. Alternatively, fill any convenient containers such as cups or glasses with hot water from the bathroom or, preferably, boiling water from a kettle, put a couple of drops of essential oil on the surface of the water, and place them strategically by windows or other places where unwelcome visitors may enter your room.

You can also use lavender, thyme, or peppermint to do this, or make up the very effective synergistic blend below:

INSECT DETERRENT SYNERGISTIC BLEND

Thyme	4 drops
Lemongrass	8 drops
Lavender	4 drops
Peppermint	4 drops

It is worth making up quite a bit of this synergistic blend and taking it with you because it can be used in several different ways. Overnight, or during your afternoon siesta, put 2 drops of essential oil on a cotton-wool ball or tissue and leave it somewhere near your bed. Mosquitoes are the most aggravating little night raiders and can be dealt with by practically any essential oil, but lavender and red thyme are the best. To discourage insects from disturbing your meal on the balcony, cut up lengths of ribbon or paper—tissue paper will do—and put one drop of essential oil on each piece and hang them around the balcony. Hanging these aromatic strips above a window will make an insect think twice about entering your room.

Used in massage oils in the days before going on vacation, and during it, the essential oils will discourage most insects from dining on you. The synergistic blend above can be used to good effect for that purpose. Dilute 2 drops in 2 teaspoons of oil for a body rub or simply add the neat essential oil to any lotion or cream you may have.

You can make a water-based splash by adding 5 drops of the blend above to 1 tablespoon of witch hazel and then diluting it in 4 tablespoons of water. Shake the ingredients together well in their container before putting onto your body. Instead of the witch hazel, you can substitute an alcohol such as vodka, but use 2 teaspoons instead of the tablespoon. Splash the liquid onto your body and smooth it over the surface of the skin.

Before going out in the evening put on some oil-based body rub, and if you are prone to being bitten the simple solution is to prepare in advance an oil of 2 tablespoons base vegetable oil to which you have added 30 drops of lavender oil and rub a little of that on the parts of the skin that are exposed. You can do the same before going to bed to protect you during the night. This amount will last you the whole holiday and more. If you are in a rush before leaving home, just throw the lavender oil into your case along with a small plastic bottle and fill it with a local vegetable oil when you arrive, following the 5 drops per 1 teaspoon base oil rule.

The ankles are a prime target for mosquitoes and certain other little creatures. A walk along the beach, for example, can be less than romantic when the sandflies are out. Covering the ankles with cotton socks is a simple and effective measure and you can make sure that your legs are left bite-free by putting a neat drop of lavender oil or citronella on the top of your socks. Alternatively, put the drops of essential oil on the bottom of your trouser leg or on the cotton of your espadrilles.

Bites and Stings: General Action

Animal bites are not poisonous but they carry the risk of rabies, which is a very serious condition indeed. All animals have the potential to be infected, not only dogs and cats. Ticks feed on blood and spread infection, and the best course of action is to make yourself as unpalatable to them as possible. Only certain areas of the world are infested with ticks and for the majority of readers care must only be taken during the summer holidays in foreign, sunny climes. In Britain bites from snakes are usually nonfatal but the farther south you go the more risk there is of serious danger. The problem with snake bites is that they may or may not be dangerous and unless you are a snake expert, you just don't know. That's why expert help must be sought immediately.

Stings can be given by a whole range of living things, from insects to fish, sea creatures, and plants, such as the aptly named stinging nettle. Usually the effects are confined to a localized area of reaction with swelling, redness, soreness, and rash, but in an allergic reaction there can be effects throughout the whole body. In all cases of stings, whether from insects, fish, or plants, an antidote needs to be applied.

Infection is a risk with many bites and stings. Sandflies, for example, carry phlebotomus fever. Without a doubt, prevention is the best line of defense and a few moments spent in applying an oil, cream, or lotion might just save you a great deal of time and inconvenience, not to mention danger, later on. Essential oils are well known for their ability to keep you sting-free and are the active ingredient in many brand-name products. When you use the real thing—the natural product unhampered by chemical solvents and the like—you have tremendous flexibility in their use. The same little bottle can give protection in a room, on the balcony, in a car, on the body, and even on your clothes. And then, if you are unfortunate enough to encounter trouble, the essential oils can help you to deal with it. Before looking at particular situations, let's have a look at the general action to be taken.

In many cases you will need a disinfectant wash, especially if you have a brood of unruly and accident-prone children! The following blends are extremely effective and can either be made up before you go, or on the spot, if required.

DISINFECTANT WASH
SYNERGISTIC BLEND

Lavender	10 drops	(2)
Thyme	20 drops	(4)
Eucalyptus	10 drops	(2)

TROPICAL DISINFECTANT WASH
SYNERGISTIC BLEND

Lavender	10 drops	(2)
Thyme	20 drops	(4)
Eucalyptus	5 drops	(1)
Oregano	5 drops	(1)

Use 8 drops of either blend in a bowl of water for washing. If you do not have the synergistic blend prepared, use the number of drops in parentheses to a single bowl of water.

ANIMAL BITES If the skin is broken you should go to the hospital because you may need a tetanus injection. In any event, wash the area with a mild soap and warm water in which you have added either AV1 (see page 408), thyme, or lavender essential oils, or, if you have it ready, one of the synergistic blends above. Then cover the wound with a bandage, piece of gauze, or plaster to which you have added 4 drops of lavender and 3 drops of thyme.

INSECT STINGS If there is a visible sting, remove it but try not to squeeze and break the venom bag which may be attached. Apply 1 drop of neat lavender oil directly to the site of the sting. Continue to apply neat lavender, a drop at a time, every five minutes or as soon as the drop can be seen to be absorbed, until a total of 10 drops has been reached.

PLANT STINGS As soon as you are stung, apply 1 drop of neat lavender or eucalyptus over the area and wash with cold water as soon as you can. Afterwards, apply another drop of essential oil.

FISH BITES Dry the area and apply 1 drop of neat lavender oil. Continue to apply neat lavender, a drop at a time, every five minutes or as soon as the drop can be seen to be absorbed, until a total of ten drops has been reached.

SWELLING First apply neat lavender to the area, then neat chamomile. One drop can be rubbed to cover quite a large area—use as many drops as you need. If the swelling is excessive as a result of an allergic reaction it should be seen by a doctor as soon as possible. On your way there apply 1 drop of chamomile to the neck area, every fifteen minutes—to a maximum total of 4 drops.

And now to more specific advice on different types of bites and stings.

Rabid Bites and Scratches

Rabies is a viral infection that is transmitted by the saliva of an infected animal, usually stray dogs and cats. Little kittens popping their heads over the tops of cardboard boxes may look very sweet in the market but don't even think about touching them or going near. Licks on a small cut or open wound and licks to the mouth, nose, or lips can also transmit the virus, so make sure your children are well aware of the dangers. Wash thoroughly as outlined for animal bites, then apply thyme and the strongest alcohol you have. Get to the hospital as soon as possible.

Fish

Poisonous fish and marine animals carry their venom mainly in their tentacles and spines. These can be extremely painful to extract and the risk of infection is always a problem, especially in polluted waters.

Any visible spines should be removed and the area bathed in salt water; then apply neat thyme.

For stings, wash the area in cold water and apply neat chamomile immediately.

PORTUGUESE MAN-OF-WAR The stings are extremely painful and cause shock, cramps, and vomiting. Remove any of the remaining tentacles and wash the area with whatever water you have. Then apply neat lavender all over the area and as the tissues absorb it, apply some more. When you get home wash the area with soap and water and apply chamomile, and continue applying lavender and chamomile every three hours for twenty-four hours. Keep the person warm and in bed or rested. Give plenty of warm liquids and Rescue Remedy (a homeopathic preparation that is widely available). Massage the whole body with the following oil once a day:

Eucalyptus	10 drops
Peppermint	2 drops
Geranium	10 drops

Diluted in 2 tablespoons vegetable oil

JELLYFISH The small common jellyfish can give a slight sting with a reddening effect. Wash the area thoroughly as soon as you can with soap and water and apply 1 drop of chamomile or lavender oil and then ice.

SEA URCHINS If you happen to be unlucky enough to tread on a sea urchin the most important thing is to get all the spikes out. As these are extremely brittle and break easily, do be careful about it—and make sure that whatever you use to dig them out is sterilized first. After removing all the spikes and washing the area thoroughly apply 1 drop of neat thyme every three hours, for twelve hours.

If the spikes prove difficult to get out buy a papaya and use the inside of the skin as a poultice. The enzymes in the fruit help to dissolve the traces of spike left in the skin and also soothe the area. The pain can be treated by using equal parts of these three oils:

Chamomile	10 drops
Lavender	10 drops
Eucalyptus	10 drops

Diluted in 2 tablespoons vegetable oil

Alternatively, use 2 drops of each—a total of 6 drops—to a teaspoon of oil.

STINGRAYS Treat these stings as for sea urchins but apply lavender oil immediately, in addition to the thyme. The pain can be intense and last for up to forty-eight hours.

Bees

Bee stings are painful and may cause fever and headaches; an allergic reaction can further cause swelling, redness, and rash. Try to remove the sting and apply a cold compress of chamomile to the area. Leave it for several hours if possible but if the sting is in an awkward place just hold the compress to it for as long as possible. In both cases, apply 1 drop of neat chamomile three times a day for two days.

Wasps

Being alkaline, it helps if wasp stings are treated with cider or wine vinegar: into 1 teaspoon put 2 drops each of lavender and chamomile essential oil, mix well and dab onto the bitten area three times a day.

Spiders

Dilute 3 drops of lavender and 2 drops of chamomile essential oil in a teaspoon of alcohol. Blend together well and apply to the area three times—over one day should suffice.

THE BLACK WIDOW Lavender essential oil is reputed to neutralize the poison of this very nasty spider. Apply 10 neat drops to the area every two or three minutes until you get to the hospital.

Ticks

You will only notice the tick by its swollen body attached to your skin. *Do not* pull it out. A cigarette placed on its body will make the tick drop off, or 1 drop of thyme will also do the trick. Then apply 1 drop of neat lavender every five minutes, to a total of ten, to avoid infection and reduce pain and swelling.

Hornet Bites

Follow the treatment recommended for bee stings, or use lavender neat, three times a day.

Gnats and Midges

Dilute 3 drops of thyme in 1 teaspoon of cider vinegar or lemon juice and apply to the bites. This will stop the irritation. As an alternative, dab on neat lavender.

Bedbugs and Fleas

The important factor to avoid here is the risk of infection. Bathe the bitten areas and apply neat lavender. Alternatively, dilute 3 drops of thyme in cider vinegar and apply over the bitten area. Eucalyptus is another option—use as you would lavender.

Chiggers and Jiggers

These are burrowing insects which attack mainly through the feet. They lay their eggs in burrows under the skin and also spread infection. If red lines appear up the leg or there is swelling in the lymph glands see a doctor. Add 10 drops of thyme to a teaspoon of any alcohol and apply it to the area every three hours. The next day and thereafter apply neat lavender three times a day.

Sandflies

Sandflies can cause phlebotomus fever which usually lasts about three days after the bite. Apply neat lavender as soon as possible after the bite and to prevent fever massage the whole of the body twice a day for a week:

Lavender	10 drops
Eucalyptus	10 drops
Thyme	10 drops

Diluted in 2 tablespoons vegetable oil

If you cannot get a container for this quantity quickly, use 3 drops of each oil in 2 teaspoons of vegetable oil.

The parasite carried by sandflies is responsible for this and for oriental sore (or Leishmaniasis) which can cause long-term ulceration of the nose and mouth with chronic illness, fevers, and lesions that look like leprosy. Avoid all areas where sandflies are breeding and wear protective creams and oils wherever they are to be found.

Mosquitoes

The area you are visiting determines the severity of a mosquito bite. Malaria is carried by the Anopheles mosquito which now lives in over one hundred countries and is emigrating to more while at the same time becoming resistant to the usual medications. Dengue fever is a viral infection carried by another type of mosquito. It stands to reason that as several serious viral and bacterial diseases are transmitted by mosquitoes, other as yet unidentified transmissions may be taking place. As you can never know who that mosquito diving around your room bit before he started taking a swipe at you, it is only sensible to take all precautions possible to avoid getting bitten yourself. And when you put on your protective oil don't forget your face—it might be life-saving as well as face-saving!

If you have already been bitten use neat lavender oil on the bite. If you've been bitten over a large area take 1 cup of cider vinegar or the juice of 2 lemons and add to it 10 drops of lavender and 5 of thyme.

Put this mixture in a bath, swishing the water around before you get in. Afterwards, apply neat lavender oil to all the bites. Each night rub your body with the oil formula given for sandflies above, adding 5 drops of lemongrass to the mix.

Snakes

Lavender has long been used effectively against the venom produced by the adders in mountainous regions of Europe, and it is about the best essential oil to use from the travel kit until you can get help. You will want to identify the snake but do not be tempted to touch it or take any gambles in an attempt to kill it. Few people going on vacation will have read up on the local snakes, although if you have been bitten you will wish you had. If the skin has two distinct puncture marks the odds are that it is poisonous, but if you can see small rows of teeth marks and the skin is not punctured then you are probably lucky. In any case, get help quickly. Wash the bitten part with whatever liquid you can find, anything to try and remove the poison by washing. But *do not move* the bitten part as this might disperse the venom. Apply lavender essential oil—as much and as often as you want to—this is an *emergency.* Tie a bandage around the leg or arm to slow down the circulation.

Plants

Plants contain many irritants in species such as stinging nettles, poison ivy, and so forth. These can cause urticaria—white blotchy areas on the skin with raised wheals of flesh. Intense itching is also another problem. Apply soap and water as soon as possible to wash the area and then apply eucalyptus, lavender, or chamomile, either neat or on a compress. A cold compress with 2 drops of one of these essential oils often stops the irritation within a few hours.

Pollution ◆◆◆◆◆◆◆◆◆◆◆◆◆

When we travel away from home the attraction is invariably the sun and the sea. And yet the sea may cause all kinds of problems, because these days the world's seas are dumping grounds for all manner of toxic waste, human and animal sewage, metals, contaminated hospital waste, and the radiation that results from underground nuclear explosions.

In my local seaside town children have been paralyzed by a virus caught, it is thought by some, as a result of swimming in the sea, and in the Mediterranean conjunctivitis, rashes, and strange inflammations are commonplace. If you develop any unusual condition as a result of swimming, treat it as a viral infection—better safe than sorry!

The Basic Travel Kit Emergency Reference Chart ◆◆◆◆◆◆◆◆◆◆◆◆◆◆◆◆

ANIMAL BITES
Thyme, Lavender, Eucalyptus, Chamomile

BLISTERS
Geranium

BRUISES
Chamomile, Geranium, Lavender

BUMPS
Lavender, Chamomile

BURNS
Lavender

CHILLS
Ginger, Geranium

COLDS
Eucalyptus, Ginger, Thyme

CONSTIPATION
Peppermint, Thyme

CONTINENTAL TUMMY
Ginger, Lavender, Chamomile, Peppermint

CRAMP
Geranium, Ginger

DRY, FLAKY SKIN
Geranium, Lavender

EXHAUSTION, PHYSICAL
Lavender, Chamomile, Peppermint, Geranium

EXPOSURE, COLD
Ginger, Thyme, Geranium

EXPOSURE, HEAT
Eucalyptus, Peppermint, Lavender

FEVERS
Eucalyptus, Peppermint, Lavender

FRACTURES
Ginger, Thyme, Lavender, Geranium

GRAZES, CUTS
Lavender, Thyme, Eucalyptus

HAY FEVER
Chamomile, Eucalyptus

HEADACHES
Peppermint, Lavender

HEAT EXHAUSTION
Lavender, Eucalyptus

HEATSTROKE
Lavender, Eucalyptus, Peppermint, Chamomile

INDIGESTION
Peppermint, Ginger

INFECTIONS
Thyme, Lavender, Chamomile, Eucalyptus

INSECT BITES
Lavender, Chamomile, Eucalyptus, Thyme

INSECT REPELLENT
Lemongrass, Thyme, Lavender, Peppermint

ITCHING, SUMMER
Eucalyptus, Peppermint

JET LAG
Lavender, Eucalyptus, Geranium, Peppermint, Lemongrass, Grapefruit

MUSCLES, OVER-EXERCISED
Thyme, Lavender, Eucalyptus, Ginger

PRICKLY HEAT
Geranium, Chamomile, Eucalyptus, Lavender

RASHES
Lavender, Chamomile, Eucalyptus

SLEEPLESSNESS
Chamomile, Lavender

SPRAINS, STRAINS
Ginger, Thyme, Lavender, Chamomile

SUNBURN
Lavender, Peppermint, Eucalyptus, Chamomile

SUNSTROKE
Eucalyptus, Lavender

SWELLINGS
Eucalyptus, Lavender

TOOTHACHE
Peppermint, Chamomile

TRAVEL SICKNESS
Ginger, Peppermint

VOMITING
Peppermint, Lavender, Ginger

WINDBURN
Lavender, Chamomile, Eucalyptus

WOUNDS
Lavender, Chamomile

◆ CHAPTER 4 ◆

OCCUPATIONAL OILS FOR THE WORKING MAN AND WOMAN

Our working environment is usually the place over which we have least control. Fluorescent lights bear down on us as we work, already red-eyed from the inadequate air-conditioning system. The man two desks away has got a bad case of flu and can't stop sneezing. The woman between you is smoking. The air in the office is stale, and getting staler. You have a headache, feel tired, your ears are blocked, and there is pressure in your head. Look at the clock . . . . only five hours and twenty-two minutes more of trying to look efficient and bright.

But sitting in a modern office, even looking into a flickering VDU screen all day, is not the most hazardous way of spending one's working life. Traffic police and city taxi drivers breathe in more than their fair share of lead pollution; farm workers have high exposure to pesticides; various industrial dusts cause all manner of lung problems, from bronchitis to pneumoconiosis and asbestosis and the new "hard metal disease." The factory line produces more Repetitive Strain Syndrome than Wimbledon produces tennis elbow, and young commodity brokers are literally burned out by thirty.

Later on in this chapter we shall be looking at remedies for many of the common illnesses that derive directly from the working environment—including the emotional ones—and finding ways of dealing with pre-exam or preinterview nerves. But let us first cheer ourselves up by looking at some of the essential oils that can transform the working environment and make it fit for the working man and woman.

OILS TO CLEAR BACTERIA AND VIRUSES

Lavender	**Eucalyptus radiata**
Rosemary	**Cypress**
Tea tree	**Bergamot**
Niaouli	

OILS TO COMBAT STALE AIR

Lemon	**Grapefruit**
Lavender	**Eucalyptus lemon**
Rosemary	**Cypress**

OILS TO HELP CONCENTRATION

Basil	**Bergamot**
Cardamom	**Grapefruit**

The Office ♦♦♦♦♦♦♦♦♦♦♦♦♦

Working in an office can damage your health—and that's official. In "The Office Environment Survey" funded by the Health Promotion Research Trust, 80 percent of the 4000 workers questioned reported feeling unwell as a result of working in a particular office. The most commonly reported symptoms are listed below, along with the essential oils I recommend that you use to dispel them in a room method:

Lethargy	**Grapefruit, Eucalyptus lemon**
Stuffy nose	**Tea tree, Rosemary**
Dry throat	**Grapefruit, Lemon**
Dry and itchy eyes	**Tea tree (in humidifier)**
Headaches	**Lavender**

All the above are more likely to occur in air-conditioned offices, and according to Dr. Alan Hedge, lecturer in environmental psychology at Aston University in England, people who work in offices with apparently sophisticated air-delivery systems have twice as many colds, coughs, and sore throats as those who work in offices with natural ventilation. Humidifiers that are faulty are breeding grounds for bacteria, and we have all heard about the buildings that spread Legionnaire's disease to their poor unsuspecting occupants. Other contributors to "sick building syndrome" are dust extractors which give off a discharge, carpet cleaning fluids, the chemicals used in furniture and furniture veneers, and poorly maintained photocopiers which emit ozone and nitrogen dioxide. Things really get out of hand when all these elements interact with each other and you end up with a building that causes all the usual problems plus itchy skin, rashes, nose bleeds, tightness in the chest, and shortness of breath.

There are, however, things you can do to make your life safer. If the sun is hitting the veneer on wooden furniture it might be causing a gas to be emitted and that might be the cause of your allergy or sore throat. Simply moving the furniture around might help. Keep an eye on the maintenance schedule for all the office equipment and if necessary have a word with your union health and safety representative. Use natural ventilation wherever possible and ionizers where not. Large-leaved green plants improve the quality of the air, and provide a resting place for your eyes and mind when they are reeling from the buzzing electrics in the concrete jungle.

The essential oils could have been made for alleviating many of the "office induced" illnesses. They combat bacteria and viruses, which is so vital in the winter months when whole offices can go down one after the other, like skittles, with flu. Indeed on this score alone, if bosses were to invest in room diffusers and a few antiviral oils they would get their investment back within a week.

Essential oils can help in other ways besides lessening absenteeism through viral and bacterial illnesses, in ways that make productivity and efficiency greater while making everyone feel a lot better. Use any of the oils listed at the beginning of this section, or those in "Two Brains For the Price of One" (page 68), which enhance the right-hand side of the brain—the creative, inspirational side—either singly or in combination. The permutations are almost endless, so experiment and create different formulas for different days. Monday morning might need a different combination to Friday afternoon, for example! Most of the room methods can be used in an office. If you have air-conditioning, a humidifier is vital—but as humidifiers can cause more problems than they solve, it is essential to use the oils with them. You can use the essential oils in the small humidifiers that hang on radiators or sit on the floor, in room diffusers, water bowls, on cotton-wool balls on a radiator or other source of heat, or in the light bulb or plant-spray methods. Even in a large, open-plan office your own little area can be catered to. If you do share space, the aroma sensitivity of your office mates will have to be taken into consideration because aromas can conjure up strong emotional reactions. You might love the smell of cardamom, but it might remind them of an incident they would rather forget, so they will not like it. Do get feedback on the aroma effects of those around you, because with nature's essential oils there is so much choice that everyone can be happy.

The citrus essential oils smell very pleasant and few people object to them. An excellent combination would be equal parts of lavender and grapefruit—lavender is an antibiotic with slight antiviral properties which also creates a calm and tranquil atmosphere, while grapefruit stops you falling asleep on your paperwork and clears up stale air. Together they smell great, please almost everyone, help concentration, and allow inspiration to take place.

The Home ◆◆◆◆◆◆◆◆◆◆◆

Being a housewife is a major occupational hazard. Apart from the fact that most accidents happen in the home, housewives are particularly prone to falling into the tranquilizer syndrome which is a major hazard in itself. This is a complex subject involving assumptions made by the medical profession, as well as stress. It is interesting, for example, that women are twice as likely as men to be diagnosed as depressed. The sheer repetition and infinite nature of housework—immortalized in the expression "a woman's work is never done"—is indeed wearing, and all those who have experienced child care will agree that it is undoubtedly the hardest work they have ever done. Appropriate oils for use around the home can be found throughout this book. There are those for accidents in the home in "Your Basic Care Kit," oils that make the household tasks altogether more pleasant in "Fragrant Care for Your Home," ways of making mealtime a more interesting experience in "Cooking with Essential Oils" and the stress sections in this chapter.

The Factory ◆◆◆◆◆◆◆◆◆◆

The factory environment can be debilitating for a miscellany of reasons. Injury, dust, dirt, and grease are obvious hazards to health but there are also the hidden effects of radiation and electrical activity and the vibrational energies produced by the presence of crystals. Working with chemicals is dangerous because even if the short-term effects are known and deemed harmless, the long-term effects are rarely known. In addition, it is the combinations of chemicals that so often prove dangerous, and even if a chemical has been given safety clearance, its effect in conjunction with the 100,000 possible others has not. Monotony and boredom create their own problems, as does the pressure of being in the same area as many other people.

Adequate ventilation and dust-extraction systems are vital in the modern factory and everyone should be vigilant to ensure that they are being properly maintained to work efficiently. This is most especially the case when working with asbestos or one of the new hard metals—cobalt and titanium, for example. Every factory floor should be cleaned with industrial vacuum cleaners rather than brushes, and throughout the day rather than just once at the end of the shift. Make sure your health and safety union representative knows which chemicals are dangerous and which are not—people working with wood preservatives, for example, should avoid those that contain lindane (a nerve poison), TBT, or PCP (Pentachlorophenol). Get as much information as you can from the organizations listed in the appendix at the end of this book about the chemicals and metals you work with. It is known that better protected working conditions should be provided for many categories of workers, but those in the precision tool, airplane, and weapons industries should take special note if they don't want to become one of those who suffer from the latest industrial hazard, hard metal disease.

Most factory floors are too big to utilize the usual room methods when using essential oils but even if the size of your working space seems daunting, the essential oils can be applied to the corner of a tissue or handkerchief put in your top pocket so that the corner hangs out and allows the aroma at least to clear your own body space.

What you need on the factory floor is something to help you relax but at the same time enhance concentration. This isn't a contradiction. Think how impossible it is to concentrate when you are uptight—it is relaxation which facilitates concentration. (This relaxed and concentrated state is rather like driving a car along a familiar road, and it is at this time that we often get our flashes of inspiration.) Lavender and grapefruit are excellent oils on the factory floor for this reason. They can be used singly, with slightly different effects, or in an equal mix. Geranium makes a good addition. All these oils increase blood circulation and oxygen supply and calm the nerves.

If you work in an oily, greasy environment the best oil to use is cedarwood, which breaks these molecules down and clears the air. If noise pollution is the problem, cypress is the best remedy because it seems to work as a shock absorber, calming down the nervous system. The noise ceases to jar and you come to ignore it.

The Hospital ♦♦♦♦♦♦♦♦♦

Essential oils are a major component in the European system of medicine known as phytotherapy and are used extensively there in every aspect of patient care. In Britain and the United States many of the packaged air fresheners used in hospitals have essential oils as their active ingredent, but because we are so bombarded with long, scientific-sounding names, this fact is often disguised. Read the labels, and you'll see what I mean.

As antibiotic and antiviral air fresheners the essential oils obviously have a positive role to play in any hospital but they are also used to kill pain, help the patients sleep, and enhance the effect of sedative drugs, thus allowing lower doses to be used. At the Churchill Hospital in Oxford, England, many of the Alzheimer's patients treated with essential oils have become more alert and the general noisiness of patients with dementia has been lessened as they feel calmer. The geriatric ward at St. Stephens Hospital, London, has been using essential oils in diffusers. In a ward in another hospital in Oxford, patients were given a choice of conventional drugs or essential oils for pain relief and to help them sleep, and invariably they chose the essential oils. What is so interesting about this is that here we have a situation in which the patients are the best judge of the effectiveness of the treatments offered—only they know how much pain they are suffering and how well they sleep—and they are opting for essential oils. As a side benefit, the aroma of the oils makes the whole environment smell wonderful, surely a great improvement on the usual hospital smell!

Here are some antiviral essential oils which will not only help keep everyone "as well as can be expected," as the saying goes, but also uplift the spirit in their own special, subtle way. Simply spray in a clean or new plant-spray or put a few drops on a bowl of boiling water:

ANTIVIRAL OILS FOR THE HOSPITAL WARD

Oregeno	**Inula odorata**
Tea tree	**Cinnamon**
Niaouli	**Red thyme**
Cypress	

If you are not a patient but on night duty and need something to keep you alert but relaxed, put one of the following on boiling water in a bowl and allow the molecules to waft around. Not only will it help you in your office but it will soothe the patients in the ward too.

Geranium	helps emotionally
Lavender	clears the air, antibacterial, etc.

A mixture of geranium, lavender, and bergamot will alleviate anxiety and depression, while a mixture of lavender and grapefruit will keep the staff on their toes, even-tempered, and relaxed as well as benefiting everyone with its refreshing, uplifting, and stimulating aroma.

The Land ◆◆◆◆◆◆◆◆◆◆◆◆

Those who work the land have humanity's greatest asset in their hands and under their feet. It is their responsibility to think of the future—for the sake of their children and ours. Most people now agree that monoculture farming methods which rely on chemicals, rather than the inherent goodness of the land, are bad not only for the land itself and the workers who have to handle pesticides, herbicides, and fungicides on a regular basis, but for the consumers of produce so grown. If you are what you eat, most of us are by now to a certain degree pure chemical! Inter-growing so that the natural protective mechanisms of plant life can operate, feeding the land organically so that its nutrient qualities are retained, and utilizing the essential oils as growing enhancers (in both size and taste) and guardians against pests, would be the best action for anyone concerned enough about the environment to take personal steps to protect it. For more on the subject, refer to "Gardens for the Future."

Interviews and Exams ◆◆◆◆◆◆◆◆◆◆◆

What perfume or aftershave you are wearing when you go for a job interview is a crucial factor in "impression management," as it is known in research circles. The interesting thing is that it makes a great deal of difference whether you are being interviewed by a man or a woman. Men aren't impressed with men who wear aftershaves at all, perhaps because of male rivalry, and, surprisingly perhaps, they consider women who wear perfume at interviews to be frivolous and unbusinesslike. Female interviewers are much easier to please and consider perfume and aftershave an integral part of good grooming. But there are perfumes and perfumes, and nobody is going to be impressed if you wear a heavy, hypnotic type of perfume that you might also use on a seductive date. If you wear one of these fragrances you might get asked out, but you won't get the job.

Clearly, if you want to manage the impression you make, the aroma you wear at an interview is an important component of the overall picture. And because odor alters people's perception of each other on the subconscious level, it might even be more important than the qualifications you have in your hand. "I just didn't like him/her" is a pretty wishy-washy reason to turn an applicant down but it happens and, according to research, with predictable regularity. In view of all this it might be better not to wear a fragrance at all at interviews—especially if you are a man—but we wear fragrances to please ourselves as well as other people and, most importantly, to give us confidence. Somehow a balance has to be struck and using essential oils is the perfect way to do it.

Certain essential oils are confidence boosters, working through the limbic system of the brain, and their aromas are subtle so if they are detected on the subconscious level by the interviewers, they will have their confidence raised too. This is all to the good. In view of what we know about the negative impact of the heavy scents, it makes good sense to stick to the light, floral type of aroma so even if it is perceived on the conscious level it won't make a negative impression. Rather, you will come across as fresh, clean, and confident. Below is a guideline of which essential oils to use, and not to use. Just use them as you would a perfume—a dab behind the ears—or put a drop on your handkerchief in your top jacket pocket. And if, some time later, you ask why you got the job and you're told "We just liked you," don't be surprised!

THE RIGHT OILS FOR THE JOB

Lemon	**Neroli**
Bergamot	**Coriander**
Melissa	**Verbena**
Pettigraine (lemon or orange)	

THE WRONG OILS FOR THE JOB

Rose Maroc	**Jasmine**
Ylang-ylang	**Vetiver**
Narcissus	

Here is a synergistic blend of oils which will boost confidence, increase your powers of memory, and allow you to concentrate—even if you are a nervous wreck. This is perfect for an interview or exam alike. Mix the component parts together and use 6 drops in your bath before you go to the interview or exam, or put 3 drops on a wet washcloth and rub all over your body in the shower. Inhale the aroma deeply to get the full effect:

SAILING THROUGH INTERVIEW
AND EXAM FORMULA

Grapefruit	8 drops
Basil	5 drops
Bergamot	5 drops
Lavender	2 drops

The evening before an important interview or exam can be dreadful. The anticipation makes you more and more nervous so that you end up lying awake hour after ghastly hour. To nip this syndrome in the bud and give yourself the refreshing sleep you need use the following formula in a bath, followed by a massage:

THE NIGHT BEFORE
"SWEET DREAMS" SYNERGISTIC BLEND

Chamomile Roman	2 drops
Geranium	6 drops
Sandalwood	4 drops
Lemon	3 drops

Make up a concentrate in these proportions: Use 6 drops in a bath just before bedtime
and
5 drops in 2 teaspoons of vegetable oil for massage

There is no point spending the evening before the interview or exam going over your speech, again and again, or trying to cram more facts into your already nerve-jangled brain. You've done the basic work, so now try to get yourself into mental shape so that you can deliver the goods you already have in a nice orderly fashion (rather than spilling them in a disheveled mess all over the interview room or exam paper). Try to forget the whole thing and instead spend the time doing something you enjoy: watching TV, reading a book or, whatever. Then take your "Sweet Dreams" bath, preferably while listening to relaxing music which will help to drown out your anticipatory thoughts. Now massage yourself, or have someone massage you, with the same formula, as above. Close your eyes and float away to a place where people aren't subjected to the torture of interviews or exams. In the morning use the "Sailing Through" formula.

The essential oil of basil is tremendous for helping one concentrate and think straight, and using it in a room diffuser or by simply inhaling while cramming during the week before an exam will really keep you on the ball. I know you're not supposed to cheat in exams, but a drop of basil on a tissue sniffed before and during the exam will give you a head start—and nobody, except you, will be any the wiser!

If you are under sixteen years old use the following formula in a nightly bath for at least a week before the exams; it will keep your nerves under control. If you are reading this with your child in mind, don't tell them it's for "nerves"—that puts the idea that they are nervous into their head—but instead say it's to relax and make them feel good. Which it is. Use 2–4 drops in each bath:

PRE-EXAM SYNERGISTIC BLEND
FOR THE UNDER SIXTEENS

Lavender	5 drops
Chamomile	3 drops
Geranium	3 drops
Mandarin	5 drops

Make into a concentrate

On the morning of the exam put 2 drops of grapefruit and 1 drop of lavender in a bath and go for it!

Self-Hypnosis for Relaxation ♦♦♦♦♦♦♦♦

Some people get into such a state during exams or interviews that they couldn't remember the name of their own sister, if asked. Self-hypnosis is a technique they could find useful, but it is not only for them. Many jobs are extremely stressful and many of us need a mental oasis to recoup the mental faculties we lose during the course of the working day. Self-hypnosis for relaxation is as relevant for the commodity broker who would prefer not to be burned out by thirty as for the teacher of a rowdy bunch of teenagers and the mother with a toddler.

Self-hypnosis is a technique of suspending normal consciousness for a limited period of time in order to relax and allow the mind and body to recharge. This state of suspension allows complete relaxation and is, even if done only for a few minutes, extremely revitalizing. Some people find it easier than others to suspend the dominant left brain, but with practice everyone can achieve it. And once you have mastered the technique, self-hypnosis can be reached without all the preliminary procedure. Certain essential oils help the process.

ESSENTIAL OILS TO FACILITATE SELF-HYPNOSIS

Narcissus	**Osmanthus**
Neroli	**Geranium**
Palma rosa	**Patchouli**
Jonquil	**Clary-sage**

Or use one of the following synergistic blends:

HEAVY SYNERGISTIC BLEND

Narcissus	1 drop
Palma rosa	3 drops
Osmanthus	1 drop

LIGHT SYNERGISTIC BLEND

Clary-sage	5 drops
Geranium	2 drops

First, make sure you are comfortable and still. There should be no noise, at least while you are learning the technique. Place 1 or 2 drops of one of the above essential oils on a piece of tissue and inhale. It helps if you place a few drops on a source of heat as well to infuse the atmosphere of the room.

Now focus your attention on an object—something light and bright—and keep concentrating. Slowly count from one to fifty, while all the time maintaining your focus on that object. Close your eyes now and imagine the object in your mind, trying to see it as clearly as possible. Tell yourself that your eyes are heavy and that you couldn't possibly open them until five, ten, or fifteen minutes have passed. Feel relaxed and at ease with yourself.

When you open your eyes you will feel very relaxed indeed—able to tackle anything and anyone.

Two Brains for the Price of One ♦♦♦♦♦♦♦♦♦♦

The human brain has two distinct parts—left and right—which govern, respectively, the logical, analytical jobs and the creative, inspirational aspects of human endeavor. The majority of people rely on the left-hand side to get through life and can function quite adequately with the skills the left-hand side provides—speaking, reading, and writing, for example. Others use the right-hand side predominantly and are the artists of the community. Whichever side we rely most heavily on, we tend to under-use the other. So those who have developed the left-hand side of their brain tend to be accountants, lawyers, and teachers who cannot paint a portrait while those who have developed the right tend to be musicians and artists who cannot understand a balance sheet. This is of course a generalization, but you and I both know plenty of people who will say "I'm no good with technical things" while looking at the video machine and those who say "I can't draw a thing" when they haven't even tried to draw anything since they were a rebellious teenager in the art class at school. But are these mental blockages inherent or the result of teaching practices which tend to emphasize in a particular person those talents which first show themselves? Might we all not benefit from using both sides of the brain equally, not only so that we can perform logically and artistically but so that each side of the brain could feed off and charge the other side?

Leonardo da Vinci is the classic example of someone with a powerful two-sided brain—the most marvelous artist with tremendous logical talents that enabled him also to be a brilliant mathematician, architect, engineer, and inventor of flying machines, submarines, hydraulics, and weaponry. He has been called "the complete man," but we can all to some extent be complete in this same way—Renaissance men and women capable of doing diverse things and able to enjoy life and work to the fullest.

Most people know which side of the brain they favor and it is interesting that the logical person who uses the left side of the brain is usually right-handed while the right-brain, artistic person is usually left-handed. (As you probably know, the right side of the brain controls the left-hand side of the body and vice versa.) The majority of people in our society are right-handed, leaving the inspirational, creative part of the brain largely under-used and undeveloped. It is this right-hand side of the brain that most of us need to develop.

The duality of human nature has for millennia been recognized by Eastern systems of thought, and balance between the two sought so that the interaction can stimulate a more effective performance in all sorts of activities. In Western society the group who have taken these lessons most to heart have probably been sportspeople, who add to their very disciplined and logical training methods those specifically designed to bring out the inspirational—and of such methods tennis and golf stars have been made. Men and women all over the world have read books such as *Drawing on the Right Side of the Brain* by Betty Edwards (Jeremy P. Tarcher), and have learned to draw, paint, or play music when these talents had previously totally evaded them. Clearly, much can be achieved by training the brain.

First, sit or lie down quietly and imagine that you have a small glowing, colored light in your head. The light can be of any color. Place the light inside your head just over the left eyebrow and slowly allow it to explore all over the left side of your brain. Then imagine it crossing over and exploring the right-hand side of the brain. Then get the light to travel along the line that separates left and right, back and forth. Again, let the light explore left and right, and down the center. Do this every day for a few minutes. Also, if you are right-handed try to use your left hand instead.

When you feel harassed at work picture in your mind a scene of great tranquility and transfer that scene from one side of the brain to the other, back and forth. This can also be done for success—imagine yourself achieving the particular job you are trying to get done, whether it is getting through a pile of paperwork, finishing a Ph.D., or decorating the house. See yourself with the job finished, complete with satisfied grin, and transfer that image back and forth from one side of your brain to the other. You will find that this simple device can motivate you into getting the job done.

You might be wondering what part essential oils play in all this and may be surprised to learn that certain oils stimulate the right-hand side of the brain (as others stimulate the left-hand side). Here then are the oils which you can use at work or when developing the right-hand side of the brain. Use 1-4 drops in a room diffuser or in one of the other room methods:

THE RIGHT SIDE, "BRAIN TRAIN" OILS

Bergamot	**Geranium**
Neroli	**Birch**
Pettigraine	**Palma rosa**
Grapefruit	**Coriander**
Chamomile Roman	**Melissa**

Go for the brain train with these synergistic formulas:

THE RIGHT SIDE, "BRAIN TRAIN"
SYNERGISTIC FORMULAS

FORMULA 1

Palma rosa	8 drops
Pettigraine	4 drops

FORMULA 2

Geranium	4 drops
Grapefruit	6 drops

FORMULA 3

Neroli	4 drops
Coriander	4 drops

FORMULA 4

Melissa	6 drops
Chamomile Roman	2 drops

Indirect Perfuming ◆◆◆

Over the past few years indirect perfuming has become a serious concern of businesses who are trying to find ways of increasing the efficiency of their staff and the satisfaction of their clients. All over the world scientific laboratories are experimenting on the effects of aroma and coming up with results that will one day affect you and me as we go about our work and play. For example, Dr. Robert Barron at Purdue University, Lafayette, Indiana, has confirmed that aromas in the workplace affect the efficiency with which people perform tasks—not only do the workers feel in a better mood and project a more positive frame of mind, they actually think more clearly and intuitively. Airlines are looking at the possibility of indirectly perfuming their airplanes with aromas that will make the passengers more relaxed. Shimizu, the third largest construction company in Japan, now incorporates an "Aroma Generation System" into the air-conditioning of new offices and hospitals. They tailor-make the aromas to the clients' needs and already have a standard twenty aromas in their catalogue. Shimizu's faith and investment in the power of aroma is based on research carried out by Japan's largest fragrance manufacturer Takasago, among others. They found that people operating computers and word processors made 54 percent fewer keying errors when the air was diffused with lemon, 33 percent fewer with jasmine, and 20 percent with lavender. "Perfume dynamics," as it is called in Japan, means that workers in Japanese banks now work with a lemon atmosphere and their customers are being soothed with lavender.

America is not far behind. Henry Walters, chairman of International Flavors and Fragrances in New York, has been quoted as saying they "envision a zillion different possibilities." In his view the new field of indirect perfuming is as full of potential as the "beginning of antibiotics." As IFF is the world's largest producer and supplier of fragrances (which appear in the dishwashing liquids, detergents, and perfumes you and I buy every day) you can be pretty sure that sooner or later we are going to be feeling the effect of all that enthusiasm as we go about our work and business. And the younger generation had better watch out—it could already be planned to pump stimulating aromas into the classroom to wake them all up!

You may not be too happy about the idea of your boss putting aromas into your space to increase your efficiency or even reduce your stress. And what will happen to the lunchtime pub trade if appetite suppressors come into use and the lunch break becomes a thing of the past? Where will it all lead? Of course we cannot know, but if the ethical considerations seem mind-boggling to us now, in times to come we may consider mental and emotional management through aroma no more of an infringement on our personal rights than the introduction of new technologies or working conditions such as fluorescent lighting and air-conditioning, which are known to have a bad effect on those who are obliged to work in them. It may simply be that job application forms will have an extra question—"Do you have any objection to perfume dynamics being operated in your workplace?" We may even see trade union "aroma representatives."

But if lack of choice may become an issue in indirect perfuming in the future, we have a choice in the matter right now. Certainly there is no doubt that aromas affect one's performance at work, so why not take advantage of the reality in ways that will make your job more enjoyable and productive? You can choose the essential oils to use from the various sections of this chapter and use them in a plant-spray, room diffuser, or atomizing ring, or just on cotton-wool balls with a few drops added on a heat source. Desk lamps are useful for this as they are nearby so we get the full effect ourselves.

Indirect perfuming has particular advantages for both male and female workers. As it has been shown in psychological testing that men wearing a personal scent brings out rivalry in other men, it may be better to diffuse the atmosphere instead. They might get jealous of your working space—but that's harmless enough and takes the heat off you. Women's perfumes are usually advertised with sexual connotations, and wearing a scent in the office can give the wrong impression to the males around. But a scented office gives the whole place a charming aura—and there's nothing wrong with charm. Women working in a man's world could utilize the oils of basil or sandalwood which do not smell at all like feminine perfumes and which, respectively, give an intellectual boost and enhance the "active principle." But for everyone, whatever their working situation, the essential oils have much to offer in terms of indirect perfuming. So just experiment and find the perfect ones for you. Most of us have to spend about forty hours a week in the workplace so we might as well make the very best of it.

Burns ◆◆◆◆◆◆◆◆◆◆◆◆◆◆◆◆◆◆

A hospital burns unit is as likely to see a burn from contact with corrosive materials, electricity, radiation, or boiling liquids as from contact with fire. Many of these cases are the result of accidents at work. The depth and severity of a burn is something that should be assessed by a hospital. The classifications of first, second, and third degree burns depend upon the depth of the burn rather than the area concerned, and sometimes a burn can be more serious than it appears. Electrical burns can be particularly misleading because the damage can extend for some distance beneath the skin. A dangerous element of all burns is shock, which can develop some hours after the accident. The degree of shock depends upon the area of the burn. If 10 percent or more of the skin area has been affected the shock will probably be serious enough to need hospitalization, so don't play the hero and just go home to rest because things could get worse. Infection is another danger with burns.

Four essential oils provide excellent treatment for first degree burns and shock:

ESSENTIAL OILS FOR TREATING BURNS

Lavender
Yarrow
Chamomile Roman
Chamomile German

Any of the above used singly has a remarkable healing capacity on burns, clearing them up in no time, removing the pain, and in many cases preventing blistering and scarring. Using them in a synergistic blend can be even more effective.

ELECTRICAL BURNS These are usually worse than they look so make sure you get a medical opinion on them. Before you do anything, however, it is vital to immerse the affected area in cold water as soon as possible. Burns of any description involve a process known as denaturation which is the killing of protein, the material of which living matter is composed. If you can imagine the tissue beneath your skin as egg white subjected to heat and see it turning from the liquid form to the hard white form of a cooked egg you will understand why it is so crucial to stop this process as soon as possible. Keep the burned area in the cold water for a good ten minutes, even if the pain is subsiding. The point being—you want to get all the heat out of the area as soon as possible to prevent further damage to the living tissue beneath your skin.

On no account put butter or vegetable oil on the skin as this will only keep the heat in and make the burn worse. Having cooled the burn in cold water you should cover the area with a compress. This can be made from gauze, if you have it, or a piece of sterile material—if someone has a clean ironed hankie use that if that is the best you can do. But if you can't find something really clean it is better not to use anything. Soak the material in ice-cold water, add the essential oils and apply it to the burned area. Use 1 drop of essential oil for each square inch of skin affected. Use any of the above on their own or the synergistic blend given below. If burns are a hazard in your workplace, this formula should be ready and waiting in the first-aid box:

BURNS SYNERGISTIC BLEND

Lavender	10 drops
Chamomile German	10 drops
Chamomile Roman	5 drops

Mix together in these proportions

As the lavender is antibiotic this also reduces the risk of infection.

Corrosive Burns ♦♦♦♦♦♦

Follow the advice given on page 72. Although most chemicals will have a neutralizing agent, interaction between the two usually generates more heat and could just make things worse. Wash the area thoroughly in cold, running water from the tap. Then apply the essential oils neat and cover with a cold, wet, clean cloth.

Burns can also be treated with a blend of aloe vera and essential oils. Use 2 drops of the synergistic blend to 1 tablespoon aloe vera and apply to the burned area three times a day. Take 1000 mg. of vitamin C daily to assist the healing and alleviate the effects of shock. You'll need to replace the fluids that have been lost through shock, so have plenty of drinks and include honey, glucose, or sugar in them.

Back Problems ♦♦♦♦♦♦♦♦

It has been estimated that in Britain alone thirty million working days are lost each year through backache. The worldwide figures for lost production must be staggering and yet nobody has come up with a solution to the problem of chronic back pain. Instead we are told that it is an inevitable result of our forefathers having got up from the all-fours position very many millennia ago. In other words, it's just something you have to put up with.

One of the most exasperating aspects of back pain is that unless you are actually in spasm nobody can actually see you have a problem, and telling the boss you are in agony so can't come into work can be met with disbelief. On the other hand, when you tell someone you have back pain they invariably say "Oh, I have that too" and proceed to launch into a monologue about how ghastly theirs is!

Sometimes back pain is due to specific physical reasons such as a slipped disc, and for this remedies can be found. But more often than not it is just the pain of strain. Slouching over a keyboard for fifty-two weeks of the year leads to trouble, or lifting boxes the wrong way. Bad posture, digging the garden, and staggering home with the shopping after a long day's work can all cause problems. Falls and whiplash can reappear as back pain years later, and a number of degenerative diseases cause back pain too.

But the spine is one of the most important parts of the body and needs special care. It does, after all, house the spinal cord which is actually a part of the brain. Serious back damage can cause paralysis and a whole range of other problems. One of the best preventative measures involves strengthening the stomach muscles so that compensatory action doesn't need to be taken by the muscles that support the back. This exercise is especially important for those who have bad posture or bad muscle tone: lie on the floor with your arms crossed and slowly lift the upper half of your body, using only the upper and lower stomach muscles. Breathe out as you lift up and in as you roll down. Start slowly and increase to twenty of these roll-ups per day. Not only will they improve your posture and strengthen your back, they will also help you to lose weight.

There are many types of back pain: lumbago, which affects the lower back; sciatica, which causes pain in the buttocks radiating out to the thighs and legs; fibrositis, tender bundles of fibrous tissues within the muscle; arthritis; spondylosis; curvature of the spine; slipped discs; and pains caused by weak back muscles, weak abdominal muscles, and tension.

Essential oils can provide wonderful relief from chronic back pain. They penetrate deeply into the muscle tissues, encouraging contracted muscles to expand, they increase blood flow to the area, and allow torn fibrous tissues to be repaired by the body. Use these essential oils to best advantage in blends, 5 drops per 1 teaspoon base oil:

ESSENTIAL OILS TO TREAT BACK PAIN

Thyme (all types)	**Rosemary**
Balsam de Peru	**Ginger**
Camphor	**Lavender**
Chamomile (both)	**Juniper**
Vetiver	**Sage**
Benzoin	**Angelica**
Cypress	**Oregano**
Peppermint	**Basil**
Eucalyptus	***R1 Formula**

* R1 Formula is a prepared blend–see appendix for suppliers.

And here are three synergistic blend formulas that are very good for alleviating back pain:

BACK PAIN SYNERGISTIC FORMULAS

FORMULA 1

Rosemary	10 drops
Marjoram	10 drops
Sage	10 drops

FORMULA 2

Lavender	10 drops
Eucalyptus	10 drops
Ginger	10 drops

FORMULA 3

Peppermint	10 drops
Rosemary	10 drops
Basil	10 drops

All diluted in 2 tablespoons vegetable oil

Massage eases any type of backache. Get a friend to do it for you. If this is impossible, massaging the lower back yourself is relatively easy although you will find the upper back more difficult. But the oils can still be applied to the skin, where they will penetrate through to the tissues, by putting them on a sponge or cloth and attaching it to a back brush, or something similar.

Ice-massage is a very effective method of treating lumbago, sciatica, and fibrositis. Typists and clerical workers are prone to develop these conditions, which are often caused by sitting in one position for too long. They usually affect the upper back muscles and cause a chronic ache, often with the muscles going into spasm. Ice-massage is also very helpful on any area that feels inflamed. To prepare the ice you need several Styrofoam cups. Fill them with water and freeze, then cut the cup down so that the ice is protruding. Massage over the sore areas in circular movements.

Repetitive Strain Syndrome ◆◆◆◆◆◆

It seems that the human body was not designed to repeat the same movement over and over again, because when it does so it develops all sorts of problems, from writer's cramp to tennis elbow and even, now, space invader's wrist! "Repetitive Strain Syndrome" is a term used to describe a whole range of conditions which come from continuously using the same joints and muscles, whether typing, packing cases, operating machinery, or picking grapes in the fields. Over-using particular muscles can result in muscle fatigue, inflammation, and various sorts of damage to the bones, joints, cartilage, tendons, and tissue. Apart from pain and discomfort, one may experience stiffness and fatigue.

It is essential that the first symptoms of RSS are treated, as neglect can lead in later life to the development of conditions such as arthritis. Lessening your chances of developing RSS is important too and can often be achieved very simply by using ergonomic furniture, varying the working posture, and breaking up repetitive actions—although all this is easier said than done. And it's no use getting a new chair if you are still going to slump over the keyboard!

In countries where RSS is recognized as a compensatory injury at work it is keeping a lot of lawyers in brisk business. In Britain you may have trouble persuading your boss that you have a work-related condition and need time off work. This is one reason for getting a medical opinion. You also need an accurate diagnosis. In this section I cover seven conditions which could be classified as Repetitive Strain Syndrome, starting with tenosynovitis—a term often wrongly applied to other conditions in this group.

Tenosynovitis

Inflammation of the fibrous sheaths which enclose the tendons of the ankles and wrists is known as tenosynovitis. When these parts of the body become inflamed there is immediate pain and a dull ache which can travel up the forearms or legs. Other symptoms are cracking and grinding noises, numbness, tingling sensations, stiffness, and increasing weakness. Sometimes the joints swell. Tenosynovitis mainly affects people who use their hands and wrists for long periods of time—from pianists and computer whiz kids to carpenters, painters, and decorators.

Treat this condition as soon as you can. Use ice-massage on the affected area (see page 74) and massage frequently. Use the following formula or make your own from the list that follows:

TENOSYNOVITIS MASSAGE FORMULA

Peppermint	10 drops
Lavender	10 drops
Eucalyptus	10 drops

Diluted in 2 tablespoons vegetable oil

TENOSYNOVITIS ESSENTIAL OILS

Chamomile Roman	**Lavender**
Chamomile German	**Eucalyptus lemon**
Peppermint	**Eucalyptus peppermint**

Tendinitis

Inflammation of the tendons of the wrists can become a work hazard if the fingers and joints start to lock. Again, this is a condition that affects people who use their hands a great deal in their work. Symptoms usually start with a tingling numbness in the fingers and hand. Ice-massage the affected area and massage with the following essential oils:

TENDINITIS MASSAGE FORMULA

Rosemary	10 drops
Lavender	10 drops
Peppermint	10 drops

Diluted in 2 tablespoons vegetable oil

TENDINITIS ESSENTIAL OILS

Rosemary	**Eucalyptus lemon**
Lavender	**Eucalyptus peppermint**
Peppermint	
Ginger	

Ganglion

Typists and clerical workers are particularly prone to develop these harmless but unsightly swellings that appear on the back of the hand or wrist. Ganglions are cysts.

They look like a round nodule of jelly under the surface of the skin and will move around if pressed. They can be dispersed gradually by gentle massage and essential oils. When massaging, concentrate on the area of the swelling only. Make your own formula from the list of oils below, or use the synergistic blend—5 drops per 1 teaspoon of base vegetable oil. Massage three times a day.

GANGLION SYNERGISTIC BLEND

Ginger	8 drops
Basil	5 drops
Patchouli	10 drops
Juniper	7 drops

GANGLION ESSENTIAL OILS

Ginger	**Basil**
Juniper	**Patchouli**
Thyme linalol	

Writer's Cramp

You don't have to be a writer to get writer's cramp. Students cramming for exams, dressmakers, composers, engravers, and many others who hold their hand and forearm in one position for a long time are all at risk. The main symptom is cramp in the hand which can be bad enough to bring all work to a halt and it needs to be treated because, if left, it will get progressively worse. Massage is one of the best solutions but increasing your vitamin D and calcium intake also helps. Make your own massage formula from the oils listed below, or use the formula—5 drops essential oil per 1 teaspoon of base vegetable oil:

WRITER'S CRAMP FORMULA

Geranium	10 drops
Hyssop	5 drops
Cypress	15 drops

Diluted in 2 tablespoons vegetable oil

WRITER'S CRAMP ESSENTIAL OILS

Rosemary	**Geranium**
Hyssop	**Cypress**

Tennis Elbow

Repetitive use of a screwdriver can cause so-called "tennis elbow" as easily as can a few games on the courts. The trouble is caused by straining the muscles, specifically those on the outer side of the elbow joint and below the joint. Pain, stiffness, and swelling are the result. Again, ice helps greatly, but this time place crushed ice loosely in a plastic bag and put it around the elbow, using bandages or plaster to keep it in place. Also massage essential oils into the area, then work the oil down the arm and into the hand. Make your own formula from the list below or use the formula—5 drops per 1 teaspoon of base vegetable oil:

TENNIS ELBOW FORMULA

Eucalyptus peppermint	10 drops
Ginger	10 drops
Rosemary	10 drops

Diluted in 2 tablespoons vegetable oil

TENNIS ELBOW ESSENTIAL OILS

Rosemary	**Ginger**
Cypress	**Hyssop**
Eucalyptus peppermint	

Bursitis

Housemaid's knee, dustman's shoulder, and weaver's bottom are just some of the names used to describe bursitis. This is inflammation of the bursa, a clump of fibrous tissue which is encased in membrane whose job it is to reduce friction between the body's moving parts—between bone and ligaments or tendons, for example. Typists and others who use their fingers constantly are particularly at risk, although anyone who over-uses a specific bursa can expect to get complaints. Like us, bursae insist on fair working conditions!

The ice-cup massage technique is very helpful for bursitis. You should also exercise the area in any way you can, using movements you do not employ at work. For example, typists should splay their fingers and then relax them. Also massage the area using the following formula, or make your own from the list below using 5 drops per 1 teaspoon of base vegetable oil:

BURSITIS FORMULA

Juniper	5 drops
Chamomile Roman	10 drops
Cypress	15 drops

Diluted in 2 tablespoons vegetable oil

BURSITIS ESSENTIAL OILS

Juniper	**Cypress**
Ginger	**Hyssop**
Chamomile Roman	

Torticollis

"Wry-neck," as torticollis is sometimes called, comes from holding the neck in one position for hours on end. Watching the assembly line go by to check for errors is one job that may bring it on, especially if the head is turned to one side. If you sit in a draft you could end up with your head painfully stuck in one position.

The muscles affected are the two sternomastoids, the large muscles at the side of the neck which extend on either side behind the ear down to the sternum and clavicle. Apply ice packs, followed by warm towels. The cabbage-leaf treatment also helps a great deal (see page 96). Massage with the following formula, or make your own using the list below on the 5 drops per 1 teaspoon vegetable oil basis:

TORTICOLLIS FORMULA

Marjoram	10 drops
Basil	5 drops
Rosemary	15 drops

Diluted in 2 tablespoons vegetable oil

TORTICOLLIS ESSENTIAL OILS

Rosemary	**Basil**
Thyme	**Marjoram**
Chamomile Roman	

Visual Stress ◆◆◆◆◆◆◆◆◆◆

Your eyes are one of your most valuable assets and if you are a secretary, clerk, accountant, or lawyer, you are liable to strain them without noticing until one day the words don't quite focus and the figures seem to move. Visual stress symptoms may also surface as blurring, seeing colored lights or black specks, haze around objects, double vision, burning, soreness, dryness, aching, headaches, tiredness, a feeling of sleepiness, watering, red eyes, bags under the eyes, and the feeling of having something in the eye that never goes away. But the most commonly reported symptom is the inability to focus. When you are reading a book look up quickly at the TV screen and if it's blurred, you could have visual stress.

There are several things you can do to protect your eyes. Make sure your lighting arrangements at work and at home are as good as possible—when reading, for example, the light should be behind you, over your shoulder. Move your desk so that you get all the natural light there is. If you are experiencing visual difficulties you should have an eye test. There are some very good exercises for strengthening the eyes, and I recommend a book called *Better Eyesight Without Glasses* by W. H. Bates (ABC-CLIO). To strengthen your eyes—whether you are experiencing visual stress or not—splash them with cold water several times after you wash your face, morning and night. This is also marvelously refreshing. Bathing the eyes in ice-cold water often helps to relieve burning.

Essential oils can be of use but it is vital to understand that they should only be used to bathe the eyelids. To put essential oils into the eye itself is extremely dangerous, whether they are diluted in water or not. If you do have visual stress the following treatment can help, but be very careful indeed to keep your eyes closed throughout.

Make the eyelid bath by adding 10 drops of chamomile German (blue) to 1 tablespoon of disperser (which enables essential oils to become water soluble) or 2 teaspoons of alcohol (use brandy or vodka). Add this mixture to 5 ounces good mineral water. Shake well. Keep the mixture in the fridge and bathe the eyelids morning and night. If your eyes are really aching and you have a heavy head, soak a piece of natural material in the solution and place it over the eyes and head. Store your pieces of soaked material in the freezer compartment for when they are needed.

Marigolds make an excellent addition to the solution above and although they take a little time to prepare, it is well worth the effort if you are suffering from visual stress. With this method, the order of preparation is somewhat different. Mix the essential oils and disperser (or alcohol), then add 3 marigold heads, if you have them growing in the garden, or 2 teaspoons of dried petals. Leave to stand overnight. In the morning add the mixture to the mineral water and leave the bottle to stand in the fridge for at least five hours, then pour through a paper coffee filter. You will now have a clear liquid which makes an excellent eyelid bath.

Mental or emotional stress also causes eye strain and if you can alleviate this you may find that the eye problem goes too. Use the oils from the stress section in your workplace to scent the air and relieve tension.

The VDU ♦♦♦♦♦♦♦♦♦♦♦♦

On opposite sides of the VDU-hazards controversy are those who are concerned about your health and those concerned with their own wealth. I don't have to tell you who is for them, and who is against.

Anybody who works on a visual display unit should read the *VDU Hazards Handbook* produced by the London Hazards Centre Trust, even though it is depressing reading and may make you consider a new career. Even to summarize the comprehensive research contained in the handbook would take more space than I have here. The list of complaints from people who use VDUs is so long that there is bound to be something in there you suffer from, whether it's as important as the inability to conceive a child or as unimportant as pimples. Apart from the problems you would expect—to the eyes, hands, wrists, arms, shoulders, neck, back, skin, and ears—and the stress that results from the monotonous and isolated nature of much

VDU work, there is the whole can of worms relating to the subtle effects of radiation and electricity as they bombard you from a VDU. Keyboard operators working away on the nation's "invisible earnings" at the bank may themselves be incurring invisible losses they know nothing about, but which one day in the future may hit them like a bombshell.

The effects of radiation and electricity on the human organism is a subject still little understood. We are learning new things every day about electrobiology, and it is becoming clear that the human being is an electrical phenomenon and that the invisible waves passing through the atmosphere play a crucial role in human health—or ill health. We simply do not know what effects are suffered as a result of moving from the normal atmospheric electrostatic charge of 3 volts to that 18 inches away from a VDU screen—150 volts per square inch. And we know nothing about the long-term effects because VDUs haven't been around long enough.

One victim may be sperm. They are exceedingly vulnerable little cells and the impact of invisible rays on them may account for the unusually high numbers of deformed babies and miscarriages that occur in women who work with VDUs. According to the *VDU Hazards Handbook,* women who move away from the VDU when they find out they are pregnant may be too late, not only because their partner's VDU may already have caused damaged sperm and therefore a damaged fetus, but because a baby can be severely brain-damaged during the first 4-6 weeks of pregnancy, before the woman realizes that she is pregnant. It may therefore be wise to give up the VDU some time before starting a family. I have to say that there is no conclusive case for linking VDUs to these dangers, merely bits of evidence which seem to be pointing in that direction. But it is a serious subject and one that, if you work on VDUs, you may wish to explore further. You must inform yourself and draw your own conclusions from what you learn. That may be the only choice you have in the matter of VDUs at work.

The VDU is only one contributing factor towards the high positive charge found in many offices. The metal frames of modern office blocks, air-conditioning and air-carried central heating, and fixtures and fittings made of unnatural fibers are other factors. This atmosphere is very unnatural and, according to a great deal of research, is not good for health, including mental health. It is in this area that essential oils can help by redressing the balance. They increase the effectiveness of the negative ion effect, making things as good as they can possibly be in the circumstances. The following essential oils are those I recommend for use in the high-tech environment:

ESSENTIAL OILS THAT INCREASE THE EFFECTIVENESS OF NEGATIVE IONS

Cypress	**Cedarwood**
Lemon	**Grapefruit**
Orange	**Pettigraine**
Bergamot	**Patchouli**
Pine	**Sandalwood**
Bois de rose	

As you can see, the majority of oils on this list are from trees and what you are doing, in effect, is bringing the well-known beneficial effects of the forest into your own interior space. Use them in any of the room methods, preferably in a diffuser to save you trouble when replenishing your supply. When you get home, compensate for the negative effect all this technology and stress is having on your immune system by using the following:

ESSENTIAL OILS TO STIMULATE IMMUNE SYSTEMS

Geranium	**Rosemary**
Lavender	**Tea tree**

Myalgic Encephalomyelitis (ME) ♦♦♦♦♦♦♦♦♦♦♦♦♦♦♦♦

All over the world ME sufferers are coming forward and announcing that they feel utterly exhausted. Until the late 1980s the symptoms of ME were variously ascribed to hysteria, malingering, and depression because nobody could find a cause for the profound muscular fatigue and various other symptoms of which sufferers complained. Controversy still abounds, but the consensus of medical opinion now ascribes the symptoms to the presence in the body of one of the 74 enteroviruses. It seems that any one of these viruses can switch off the body's cells so that they cannot perform their usual function.

ME, or post-viral syndrome, has been called "yuppie flu" because it seems to affect so many high-powered young people in stressful jobs. But this is a misnomer because all sorts of people have it, from housewives and family doctors to dentists and cab drivers. The only thing sufferers have in common is that the condition develops after a viral infection of some sort—flu or food poisoning, for example. Instead of getting better, the sufferer becomes profoundly tired after the slightest activity and may develop any number of other symptoms, relating to practically every part of the body. It was the very varied nature of these symptoms which made it hard for the medical profession to see the common, basic problem; plus the fact that extreme exhaustion is difficult to test for and identify clinically. Many an ME sufferer has been told to "go home and take it easy," perhaps with a prescription for tranquilizers in their pocket too. Before ME became better understood, sufferers were made to feel as if they were edging towards a nervous breakdown, or just imagining things or malingering, when they were in fact suffering all sorts of debilitating physical problems. Besides the muscle fatigue, common problems are loss of concentration and memory, mental confusion, lethargy, insomnia, irritability, depression, impaired balance, sight and hearing, and headaches. The frightening thing about ME is that it can last for years. At present people are being told that if the symptoms continue for a year, there's a fifty-fifty chance that they will continue for another seven. No wonder depression is a symptom.

Essential oil treatment consists of fighting the battle on all fronts. You don't have to worry that your treatment for muscle fatigue will clash with the oils you are using to treat other symptoms because essential oils, unlike chemical drugs, do not have dangerous side effects if you take the wrong cocktail. Rather, they are like a team of good friends, all helping out in the best way they can when their particular attributes are needed. Take each day's symptoms as they come and invite your new friends to help you—whether singly or in a group, according to your needs at the time. Several of the main symptoms of ME are discussed separately here; for those that are not you will find other treatments throughout the book. But the one symptom you need to treat on a regular basis is the muscular fatigue, even though it may come and go.

Muscular Fatigue

If you've ever seen a cartoon of someone so exhausted that she fell asleep in her soup, it was probably an ME sufferer. Few of us, unless we have run a marathon or spent many nights awake with a sick and crying baby, can truly understand the profound nature of ME muscle fatigue. It can come and go quite suddenly and people experience it in different ways, and in different ways on different days. It may be like having lead weights for limbs, or an ache in the muscles like a bad flu attack, or aching bones, or just a general weakness. One patient was so weak all over that the comforter on her bed felt as if it were stuffed with lead shot.

If you have had ME for a long time you may have noticed a pattern to your fatigue; if so, use this information to your advantage and treat yourself with the oils before an attack is due. If you are unfortunate enough to be one of those who has continual muscle fatigue, choose a time when you have nothing to do except apply the oils. Keep the oils handy so that you can use them when the best opportunity presents itself. The aim is to avoid apathy taking over because then you won't be able to help yourself. Apply at least twice a day:

MUSCLE FATIGUE FORMULA

Thyme	5 drops
Rosemary	10 drops
Cypress	5 drops
Eucalyptus peppermint	10 drops

Diluted in 2 tablespoons vegetable oil

MUSCLE FATIGUE ESSENTIAL OILS

Red thyme	**Grapefruit**
Rosemary	**Eucalyptus peppermint**
Cypress	
Marjoram	

See also the list in "Sports," page 97.

Insomnia

It is very important that ME sufferers have enough sleep but, paradoxical as it may seem, insomnia is one of the problems they encounter. To be terribly tired yet unable to sleep is one of the worst aspects of ME and has been described as a kind of living death. These are the oils to use:

INSOMNIA ESSENTIAL OILS

Valerian	**Clary-sage**
Marjoram	**Sandalwood**
Chamomile Roman	**Lemon**

Massage the oils into the body before having an essential oil bath. Make a blend using a total of 30 drops from the list above to 2 tablespoons vegetable oil. For individual massages use 5 drops of essential oil to a teaspoon of vegetable oil or 10 drops to two teaspoons. Massage over the whole of the body, including the shoulders and neck. You can do this while the bath is running. Put 4 drops of your chosen essential oil or oils in the bath, which should be neither too hot nor too cold. Get in and just lie there and drift or, if you have the energy, read a book. Then go to bed. Repeat nightly, as often as needed.

Depression

The depression that so often accompanies ME comes from a chemical imbalance as well as from the fact that it's impossible to complete the tasks that were sailed through before the onset of ME. You seem to be weighted down by an invisible force while your friends clamber up the ladder of success and accomplish all the things you too had set out to do. Life seems to be passing you by. Meanwhile it can be difficult to explain the nature of your fatigue, and not everyone is convinced that you have a real physical problem rather than a mental collapse. You feel guilty about being so dependent on others and would love to be able to "pull yourself together," as the ignorant and unfeeling advise. You might be sitting on the sofa all day but you are definitely not taking it easy! If only people could understand.

No wonder you sometimes get depressed. Treat this with the same essential oils as in the stress list on page 85, although the following seem to help the ME sufferer more specifically:

ME DEPRESSION ESSENTIAL OILS

Grapefruit	**Rose**
Tangerine	**Geranium**

Loss of Memory

This is an extremely irritating factor in ME. Here you are, the one who used to get all the work done at double speed, unable to complete your pile of work and forgetting things too. But it's not old age, and you're not cracking up after all these years; it is that horrible enterovirus getting your brain chemicals in a twist again.

Learning to live with loss of memory is not easy and calls for adjustments in your life. Write down all the important and indeed nonimportant things you need to remember. Forget the "key word" lists you used to make, for when you have forgotten what they were about, they are useless. Be precise. Of course it is frustrating and irritating to watch the simple things of the past become a series of little uphill struggles (and big ones), but you can learn to adjust and some people will never know the difference. Try to become aware of your daily rhythms in terms of mental and muscular fatigue. If you can't hold a pen at four o'clock, write this down, along with the other lows and highs, and see if a pattern emerges. Work this pattern to your advantage by getting as much done when you have the energy. Here are the oils to help you get through that work:

ME CONCENTRATION AND MEMORY ESSENTIAL OILS

Rosemary	**Grapefruit**
Bergamot	**Lavender**
Basil	**Neroli**

Try always to have a small bottle of diluted oils in your desk drawer or wherever you work, and inhale as needed and apply to the temples and nape of the neck. You could also keep a small sprayer handy to spray around the office. You decide how to use the oils, in any way to best effect—perhaps in a shower in the morning, or apply them on the way to work. Here is a very effective synergistic blend you might like to try:

ME CONCENTRATION AND MEMORY SYNERGISTIC BLEND

Basil	8 drops
Grapefruit	10 drops
Lavender	7 drops
Rosemary	5 drops

Other Symptoms

There are possibly many other symptoms you are suffering from. Look them up elsewhere in this book and follow the treatment recommended. Feel free to use the formulas mentioned in this section in any way that is most convenient. The muscle fatigue formula can just as effectively be used in the bath, and the depression and concentration formula in a body rub. Do what works best for you.

ME is such an individual disease that you will have to work out your own essential oil treatment. For some, stress is a factor that must be managed. Do try the various relaxation techniques, including meditation. Sitting in a heap when your fatigue is at its height for the day doesn't count. Breathe correctly, get plenty of fresh air and fresh food. Don't overtire your body by making it work on chemicals and pollutants in food. If what you eat swims, flies, walks, or grows, fine; if it comes out of a packet, box, or tin, forget it. Increase your vitamin and mineral intake: vitamins B, D, and C are all useful, as are zinc, selenium, and geranium.

The Workaholic Heart

If you answer "yes" to the following questions, you are a workaholic. Do you think you are the only one who can do the job properly? Do you churn your work over in your sleep? Are you neglecting your family, friends, and hobbies? Is your sex life taking second place?

Workaholics have to learn to say "no." Enough is enough. The world will not come to a grinding halt if I don't work late tonight. The customer will not drop down a big black hole before tomorrow morning. Everything will be right where I leave it tonight. "I'm going home now." Practice saying it!

There's no denying that to get ahead today one must strive to become better and faster than everyone else. Competition is fierce and the accent is on the younger man or woman who has time, energy, and ambition to give the job one hundred and fifty percent. It's difficult to be laid back when these determined and talented people have an eye on your job. So the pressure is on—and it's on your heart.

Essential oils can help you cope and calm you down, but you have to be prepared to help yourself too. You really must carve out some time during the week to give your heart a complete rest and recharge. Having a regular aromatherapy treatment is the best way. At least learn to relax. Ask your partner to massage you or, if that's too passive for you, massage your partner instead—but in gentle, rhythmic movements, not speedy, insensitive slaps!

The following essential oils are good for workaholics because they are stimulating without being overstimulating while many of them also have relaxant properties. This is a difficult thing to explain. Perhaps you can think of it in terms of people—some are intellectually stimulating while at the same time you feel completely relaxed in their company. A vicar or guru might be the kind of person who falls into this group, or a very dear and bright friend. So, these are the workaholic's friends; use them at any time, anywhere, and anyhow:

THE WORKAHOLIC'S OILS

Geranium	**Basil**
Lavender	**Neroli**
Marjoram	

And here is a formula for the bath:

THE WORKAHOLIC'S BATH

Neroli	1 drop
Lavender	2 drops
Geranium	1 drop

You can use this in the morning bath, of course, but it's better to do the whole treatment after work when there is a slight chance you may be thinking of relaxing. Lie back in the bath and read a book, even a textbook if you must, or catch up on your professional trade magazines. Then spend a few minutes doing stretching exercises, like a cat. This helps to release the toxins from your muscles. Breathe deeply. Now massage your body with a combination of essential oils diluted in either base, vegetable oil, or a pure and simple type of body lotion. Whichever base you choose, use a combination of the oils listed above on the 5 drops per 1 teaspoon basis, or follow the formula below:

WORKAHOLIC'S MASSAGE FORMULA

Neroli	5 drops
Lavender	10 drops
Geranium	5 drops
Lemon	10 drops

Diluted in 2 tablespoons vegetable oil *or* lotion

Although workaholics generally have a neat and tidy appearance, their insides aren't usually in such terrific shape. Skin care in women is often neglected, and because of the stress workaholics often develop dry skin and greasy hair. (See Beauty section.) Just try to remember that you'll need your body longer than you need that job!

Stress ◆◆◆◆◆◆◆◆◆◆◆◆◆◆◆◆◆

Arguably, everyone in the whole world is under stress of some description. It might be positive stress, of the sort joggers voluntarily put themselves under, or the negative stress that comes, for example, from sitting in an open-plan office with a dozen telephones ringing at any given point in time. The kinds of stress and degrees of it are manifold, and so the oils we use and the combinations must reflect this diversity.

First of all, let us distinguish between positive stress, normal stress, and distress. Positive stress could be described as a "high," the excited tension you get when performing your job fast and efficiently. It is, indeed, this kind of high that makes people enjoy working in the first place: the sheer joy of being a human being accomplishing something, whether that's whizzing through the in-tray or writing a book. Positive stress makes us aim that little bit higher, leap over the pitfalls life presents to each and every one of us, and gives us the force to take on challenges. This is the kind of energy that increases stimulation, helps our energy level, and makes creativity flow. And as it contributes to our feeling good, we obviously don't treat it with essential oils. We don't need to.

Normal stress is a state during which the body performs its functions for survival in response to circumstances. For example, when you have a car accident the body is flooded with adrenalin which causes all kinds of physical phenomenon—everything goes into slow motion, for example, or pain cannot be felt. The out of the ordinary stress caused by accidents is all to the good because it increases your capacities and efficiency. Your heart may be pounding, you are shaking all over but somehow you manage to walk to the phone booth and call for help. "I don't know how I did it," you say later, looking at the gash in your leg, but you do know really—your mechanisms for dealing with survival situations took over and enabled you to do what had to be done at the time. You can collapse later, when the emergency has passed. These normal stress mechanisms are good—very good—and we don't need to treat them either.

Distress, however, is another thing. This is when the healthy stress becomes chronic, with the result that we have no energy, no will, only frustration at the ever-increasing pressure load. This is when essential oils are needed.

Here we look at the various types and degrees of stress and the oils which are best suited to deal with them. Of course different types can exacerbate each other, so that the environmental stress you suffer at work can cause mental stress which, when taken home, can lead to emotional stress.

ENVIRONMENTAL STRESS caused by, for example, bright lights over your desk; noise of machinery; the constant ringing of telephones; or too cramped office space.

Cedarwood	**Chamomile Roman**
Coriander	**Basil**
Geranium	**Bergamot**
Cypress	

CHEMICAL STRESS caused by, for example, too many cups of coffee; too many lunchtime drinks; too much junk food; too many aspirins or antibiotics; inhaling substances at the factory or office; pollution on the way to work; smokers in the office.

Lavender	**Clary-sage**
Patchouli	**Grapefruit**
Pettigraine	**Lemon**
Geranium	**Rosemary**

PHYSICAL STRESS caused by, for example, pushing your body to the limits; running in the office "fun run"; working out at the gym; driving long distances continually.

Rosemary	**Bergamot**
Chamomile Roman	**Thyme**
Marjoram	**Geranium**
Lavender	**Fennel**

MENTAL STRESS caused by, for example, trying to achieve; taking exams; anguish over uncompleted jobs; unemployment; financial worries.

Geranium	**Bergamot**
Lavender	**Grapefruit**
Sandalwood	**Cardamom**
Basil	**Patchouli**

EMOTIONAL STRESS caused by, for example, relationship problems; parental guilt; the inability to give or receive love; grief.

Geranium	**Vetiver**
Sandalwood	**Rose**
Palma rosa	**Cardamom**
Bergamot	

These different types of stress occur in varying degrees and the oils and formulas recommended take these levels of stress into consideration. Identify the degree of your stress from the categories below and then you can choose from the formulas and oils that follow the most effective treatment for your individual needs. Treat the first level before it develops into the second, and so forth. Mental health is as precious as physical health; indeed, the sharp distinction so often drawn between the two is misleading. They are at different ends of the same phenomenon but they are actually the same thing. The human being works as an integrated unit of body and mind, and to take care of one is to take care of the other.

LEVEL 1: starts as tiredness and develops into irritability, headaches, and insomnia.

LEVEL 2: depression, anxiety, muscular pain, chronic aches, persistent infections, guilt, apathy, helplessness.

LEVEL 3: persecution complex, agoraphobia, claustrophobia, despair, increasing guilt and depression, susceptibility to viral infections and bacterial invasion.

LEVEL 4: now the body is really crying "Help." Unexplained pain, heart problems, strokes, and high blood pressure may be experienced, along with all the other diseases that are thought to have their roots in stress, like ulcers and even, according to some opinions, arthritis. The immune system is further depressed, leading to all manner of physical problems.

First, here are some synergistic blends. Levels 1 and 3 are grouped together because these need sedatives and relaxants. At Level 2, however, you need something that will add an element of stimulation to prevent you slipping into Level 3. This is to get you out of the quagmire and motivated, and to stimulate your immune system to prevent infection. If you have reached Level 4, it's time for the heavier sedatives which are known as "hypnotics."

Only those synergistic blends at Level 2 and essential oils listed later under Level 2, the stimulant oils for stress-related disorders, can be used in an open workspace. All the blends and oils can be used in the atmosphere at work if you have a fairly closed office, and in any other method that you choose. At all levels of stress a bath after work every night is a must—use 6–8 drops of your chosen formula or oil. You may also make up a massage oil which can double as a body rub to put on before going to work. Also use it in a shower, if you have one, in the morning. Any of the room methods can be used at home, and at work perhaps the best solution is to have a bottle of oils ready with a plant-spray so you can spray your workspace when it's convenient—perhaps when everyone else has gone to the pub for lunch. You can, of course, also use the tissue or handkerchief method—you can pretend you've got another cold—or just sniff the bottle or put a dab of oil on the space between your nose and upper lip.

As Level 1 of stress is grouped with Level 3, let's start with the Level 2 synergistic blends that will, as well as helping you, benefit your fellow workers and boss too. The three general formulas are ideal for reducing stress levels throughout the workplace, enabling everyone to cope *before* they get stressed-out.

STRESS LEVEL 2 SYNERGISTIC BLENDS

FOR GENERAL USE

BLEND 1		BLEND 2		BLEND 3	
Bergamot	9 drops	**Grapefruit**	15 drops	**Neroli**	7 drops
Geranium	11 drops	**Rosemary**	11 drops	**Lavender**	3 drops
Ginger	10 drops	**Palma rosa**	5 drops	**Lemon**	20 drops

FOR SPECIFIC USES

APATHY/HELPLESSNESS		DEPRESSION/GUILT		ANXIETY	
Grapefruit	15 drops	**Geranium**	15 drops	**Lavender**	10 drops
Rosemary	10 drops	**Lavender**	5 drops	**Geranium**	10 drops
Lavender	5 drops	**Bergamot**	10 drops	**Palma rosa**	10 drops

MUSCULAR PAIN		INFECTIONS UNEXPLAINED ACHES AND CHILLS		DIGESTIVE PROBLEMS	
Lavender	10 drops	**Lavender**	10 drops	**Coriander**	15 drops
Rosemary	5 drops	**Ginger**	15 drops	**Grapefruit**	10 drops
Cypress	15 drops	**Cardamom**	5 drops	**Cypress**	5 drops

STRESS LEVELS 1 AND 3 SYNERGISTIC BLENDS

FOR GENERAL USE

BLEND 1		BLEND 2		BLEND 3	
Clary-sage	15 drops	**Marjoram**	15 drops	**Pettigraine**	17 drops
Lemon	10 drops	**Chamomile Roman**	5 drops	**Neroli**	5 drops
Lavender	5 drops	**Lemon**	10 drops	**Nutmeg**	8 drops

FOR SPECIFIC USES

TIREDNESS		IRRITABILITY		HEADACHES	
Lemon	10 drops	**Nutmeg**	10 drops	**Lavender**	10 drops
Clary-sage	5 drops	**Sandalwood**	8 drops	**Chamomile (both)**	10 drops
Lavender	15 drops	**Pettigraine**	12 drops	**Geranium**	10 drops

INSOMNIA		DEPRESSION		FEARS	
Marjoram	9 drops	**Geranium**	15 drops	**Rose**	15 drops
Vetiver	8 drops	**Neroli**	8 drops	**Chamomile Roman**	10 drops
Lemon	14 drops	**Nutmeg**	12 drops	**Pettigraine**	5 drops

DESPAIR		GUILT		LOW IMMUNITY (VIRAL INFECTION)	
Rose Maroc	15 drops	**Sandalwood**	20 drops	**Vetiver**	10 drops
Pettigraine	10 drops	**Chamomile Roman**	5 drops	**Lavender**	10 drops
Neroli	5 drops	**Clary-sage**	5 drops	**Geranium**	10 drops

Some of the essential oils used to treat Level 4 are the heavier "absolutes" and are very expensive. All the following formulas can be lightened a little by using lemon, bergamot, and pettigraine as substitutes. It does not decrease the effectiveness of the formulas if you add 1–2 drops of one of these three oils.

STRESS LEVEL 4 SYNERGISTIC BLENDS

FOR GENERAL USE

BLEND 1		BLEND 2		BLEND 3	
Narcissus	2 drops	**Michela alba**	7 drops	**Osmanthus**	3 drops
Rose	5 drops	**Tonka bean**	2 drops	**Hyacinth**	4 drops

FOR SPECIFIC USES

CHRONIC DEPRESSION		INCREASING ANXIETY		HEART MURMURS	
Osmanthus	3 drops	**Michela alba**	5 drops	**Rose**	8 drops
Jasmine	3 drops	**Jonquil**	6 drops	**Valerian**	9 drops

CHRONIC INSOMNIA		HYPERACTIVITY		IRRATIONAL BEHAVIOR	
Valerian	15 drops	**Narcissus**	4 drops	**Rose**	7 drops
Hops	10 drops	**Tonka bean**	3 drops	**Osmanthus**	1 drop
Rose	5 drops				

Making Your Own Formulas to Treat Stress

You can make your own synergistic blends using the levels of stress lists below, cross-referring to the oils relating to the various types of stress mentioned earlier. The oils can be used singly or in a blend of a maximum of three. You will see that four of the same oils appear in the first two lists—for stimulants and sedatives—and this is because used in moderation they are relaxants, while used in greater quantity they become stimulants. These adaptogens are marked with an asterisk.

STIMULANTS Although these are particularly useful in the Level 2 type of stress, to motivate and stimulate, they can be used in the other levels too.

Bergamot	**Grapefruit**
Lavender*	**Rosemary**
Lemon*	**Geranium***
Cypress	**Neroli***
Coriander	**Palma rosa**
Ginger	**Cardamom**

SEDATIVES/RELAXANTS Although these are particularly useful in treating Levels 1 and 3, they can be incorporated into a formula using the oils for Level 2, stimulants, above. Use an increased dosage if treating Level 3, so that whereas for example you would use a total of 30 drops to make a massage oil for Level 1 degree of stress, use a total of 40 drops if treating Level 3. Also, use the oils more often if you are suffering at Level 3, and reduce the dosage when the condition improves.

Nutmeg	**Geranium***
Marjoram	**Lemon***
Lavender*	**Chamomile (both)**
Sandalwood	**Neroli***
Clary-sage	**Rose**
Pettigraine	**Vetiver**

HYPNOTICS These oils are used to treat Level 4. They could be incorporated into formulas using the previous two categories of oils, but use only one hypnotic essential oil in those formulas. The term "hypnotic" means heavy sedative.

These oils and those in the section about developing the creative, right-hand side of the brain, page 68, are extremely useful in self-hypnosis techniques, page 68.

Although some of the oils in this group are difficult to find, they are extremely effective.

Narcissus	**Carnation**
Jonquil	**Jasmine**
Rose Maroc	**Valerian**
Hyacinth	**Tonka bean**
Osmanthus	**Hop**
Michela alba	**Vanilla**

Suffering stress as a result of work is in no way an indication of incompetence. Far from it. Indeed, it is very often those who volunteer for the front line in the "battle of the bucks" who incur the greatest injury through stress because that is where the pressure is greatest. As all our mothers told us, it takes hard work to succeed, and that takes its toll. Whether successful or not, men in particular are subjected to the "winners" and "losers" syndrome which exerts its subtle pressure on the psyche. Who can say whether it is more stressful to be clambering up the ladder of success and becoming a "winner" or sitting at the bottom and being described as a "loser"?

The work situation is characterized by a great deal of lack of choice, not least having to arrive at a particular location by a particular time. Every morning millions of us subject ourselves to tremendous stress waiting for buses that never come or come full up, standing like sardines in packed underground trains, looking for seats on commuter trains, or sitting in traffic jams on the roads into town. Before the clock strikes nine, half the people in the country are already a bundle of nerves!

But using the essential oils can help to alleviate the inevitable stress we suffer. There are many effective relaxation techniques to try, and counseling services to help you sort out your problems. A monthly massage or aromatherapy treatment helps many people to keep on an even keel, while many more benefit from yoga and other Eastern techniques of physical training. Sport and exercise help tremendously if you are not suffering from physical stress, and those people working out at the gym are effectively working off the tension they took on at work.

Make yourself a priority. Plan things around your personal requirements. Learn to say no. Don't try to be superhuman—delegate if you cannot allow things to be left until tomorrow. If the workload has built up and you are behind, take a clear day to get ahead of yourself. If possible, go into the office on a Saturday and try to clear your desk. Housework is an endless chore but if things are behind there, spend a whole day with the duster and clear the cobwebs away. Then you can relax and spend some time on number one. Call it therapy, if you like. Set a period of time during which you cannot be interrupted, take the phone off the hook and spend some time doing what *you* want. Not cleaning, washing, or paperwork, but finishing that book, practicing self-hypnosis, exercising, having a massage or bath or pampering your body. And however you choose to spend this time for yourself, make it a routine ritual, sacrosanct for your sanity. Find some time too for your real friends—even if that means driving to the other side of the state to see them for the weekend. Maintain the vital links of friendship and you overhaul life's safety net.

Take care of your body. Check your diet and cut down on tea and coffee which often lead to nervousness and headaches. Vitamin B complex is wonderful for combating stress, as is a dose of between 250 and 500 milligrams of vitamin C per day. Get some fresh air and exercise, because the effect of stress can deplete you of oxygen and make you feel sluggish. And getting out and about can be a great tonic. Enjoy the world. It's not all about struggle and work. Laugh as much as possible—laughing boosts the endorphin level and makes you feel good. Several hospitals in America take the physiological effects of laughter so seriously they have designed "laughter rooms" where patients can have their prescribed fun. It is true—laughter is the best medicine.

Performance Stress ♦♦♦♦

Performance stress can be caused by one-shot events or by the nature of the job. The idea of giving a speech at the wedding, presenting the company's annual report to the shareholders, giving a presentation to the prospective client, speaking at the women's guild, reciting the gospels in church, or giving the end of term speech at school induces tremendous stress in some individuals and a certain amount of stress in most of us. People who perform in front of others as part of their job may suffer performance stress every day. As they walk on the stage, performers know that there are hundreds if not thousands of people watching their every move and aware of their every mistake. For most performers, exactness is expected of them, whether it's in the notes they play, the dance steps they take, or the words they say. Almost all performers have the added stress of not knowing whether they will still be working in six months' time and able to pay the bills. No wonder performers of all types turn to beta-blockers, tranquilizers, alcohol, or cocaine to get them through the night.

Yet giving a performance requires a certain amount of stress. Many maintain that having the "butterflies" before a performance is necessary to provide the sort of energy that enables them to do a good job. The essential oils given here get rid of the sort of stress that undermines the confidence needed to perform while allowing the positive stress to fuel a good performance:

PERFORMANCE STRESS
ESSENTIAL OILS

Bergamot	**Rosemary**
Coriander	**Ginger**
Neroli	**Grapefruit**
Palma rosa	**Rose**
Benzoin	**Clary-sage**
Lemon	

SYNERGISTIC BLENDS FOR
THE PERFORMANCE

BLEND 1

Bergamot	10 drops
Palma rosa	15 drops
Clary-sage	5 drops

BLEND 2

Basil	15 drops
Ginger	5 drops
Coriander	5 drops

BLEND 3

Rose	5 drops
Grapefruit	15 drops
Neroli	5 drops

Use the essential oils in a bath or shower before the performance, inhaling deeply while you do so. Add a drop to a tissue to take with you and inhale when needed—again, deeply and slowly. Use 4–6 drops in the bath or 3 drops on a washcloth in the shower. The oils may also be used in a plant-spray around the environment you will be performing in—a recording studio, for example. If making a massage oil, use 5 drops of essential oil to 1 teaspoon base vegetable oil.

Burnout ♦♦♦♦♦♦♦♦♦♦♦♦♦

Well, you've done it. You've worn yourself to a frazzle and the cells that haven't seized up have gone on strike. The plant has been shut down. Congratulations! Instead of charging around achieving four things at once, rising at five a.m. and working until ten at night, you're now incapacitated by an overwhelming tiredness. Relaxation is impossible as your mind goes around in circles, getting nowhere fast. You seem to be a different person and you are beginning to wonder if you're cracking up. Your energy is completely and utterly depleted and you wonder if you will be able to get the milk in off the doorstep, yet alone get through the day.

Burnout is exactly what it sounds like, only instead of referring to an energy source which burns fast and furiously until nothing is left, it's referring to that energy source—you. It happens when the body and mind have been under stress for a long period. Commodity brokers and other whiz kids in the city suffer burnout with alarming regularity, and with millions of dollars hanging on their split-second decision making, it is not surprising. But mothers trying to juggle the requirements of a family may suffer burnout too, as can any one of us if we do not take care of our natural resources.

It is vital to build up your energy stores to avoid exhaustion. Exercise not only helps to keep you healthy enough to fight off fatigue, it also strengthens the heart and enables endorphins to be sent from the brain into the whole physical system, providing you with a sense of well-being. Rub the following synergistic blend oil over your body before exercise:

BURNOUT EXERCISE OIL
SYNERGISTIC BLEND

Grapefruit	5 drops
Cypress	4 drops
Geranium	2 drops

Mix together in these proportions and use 5 drops per 1 teaspoon vegetable oil

Relaxation is equally important but if you find that you can't relax, at least breathe in a way that will slow down your pulse rate. Open a window, inhale and take in large volumes of air, slowly filling the lungs, then exhale slowly. Do this several times, once a day at least. Self-hypnosis is a good way of reaching into what is out of your conscious control and is a method that can be used at any time of the day.

Lessen your workload wherever possible, and start and finish work at preordained times. Don't let anything interfere with this resolution—it can wait. You only have one body and that is your priority. The human energy system has been likened to a gas tank in a car—if you run out you can draw on the "reserve tank." People with burnout are relying on their reserve tank and need to cruise nice and gently until they can fill up again. If you continue to drive yourself at full throttle, you may run out of energy again before you reach further supplies. Bring yourself into lower gear with the relaxation oils:

BURNOUT RELAXATION
SYNERGISTIC BLEND

Sandalwood	8 drops
Palma rosa	5 drops
Lemon	9 drops

Mix together in these proportions

You can use this blend in any of the room methods, or in the bath while relaxing with a book. Make up a massage oil on the 5 drops per 1 teaspoon vegetable oil basis and ask a friend to massage you, or simply apply it to your body yourself.

To revive yourself at any time, use the following formula in any of the room methods, in the bath (4–6 drops), or shower. A foot bath is extremely effective—use 2–3 drops, or make a body rub using 5 drops per 1 teaspoon of vegetable oil.

BURNOUT REVIVER
SYNERGISTIC BLEND

Lavender	5 drops
Eucalyptus peppermint	8 drops
Grapefruit	7 drops
Rosemary	4 drops

Mix together in these proportions

After a warm bath, splash yourself all over with an ice-cold reviver. Make up a bottle specially for this—an empty plastic mineral water bottle is ideal—and add 3 drops of rosemary to 5 ounces water. Keep the bottle in the fridge so it's always cool when you require it. Shake the bottle well and splash all over your body. To disperse the essential oils more effectively you could mix them with a dispersant (see page 140) or 1 teaspoon of vodka before putting them in the water bottle.

Tired eyes respond well to a rest under cotton wool which has been soaked in an equal mix of cold water and witch hazel. See also the section "Visual Stress" on page 77.

♦ CHAPTER 5 ♦

ASSERTIVE OILS FOR SPORTS, DANCE, AND WORKOUTS

WHETHER YOU ARE a dancer who wants to keep supple or a runner who wants to win the race, the essential oils have something for you. They not only treat sports injuries but relieve pain and help to keep the muscles toned. They improve circulation and also protect you from other people's germs while in the close confines of the communal locker room. But they also help in the all important mental area too, improving concentration and giving a positivity that can mean the difference between winning and losing.

It is extraordinary that something as gentle as essential oils can be assertive as well, but they can. Indeed, their varied positive effects on the psyche as well as on the physical body make them an excellent therapy for all who push their body to the outer limits in the challenge of sport or the art of dance. This is not to say that the oils aren't strong (the verruca you caught in the changing room had better look out), but we are here talking about a wide range of qualities from a variety of precious oils.

Although sport is thought of as a healthy activity, sports centers should display a large sign on their door: "Sport can be injurious to your health." Tennis elbow is probably the most obvious sports injury but that is only one manifestation of repetitive strain syndrome which collectively describes a range of injuries. The problem begins with the nature of the sport, which may involve making the same movement repeatedly. The scope for this is enormous—serving at tennis, lifting a leg over hurdles, throwing a ball in baseball, hitting with the bat in cricket, swinging the club on the golf course, or doing the butterfly stroke. Using the same muscle or area of the body to make the same movement over and over again is also the result of personal style and that can be difficult to change—and if you are winning you won't want to change it. Dancers have no choice; they must move their leg or arm in a very exact way, whether there is pain or not, for the audience is watching. The various manifestations of repetitive strain syndrome may be treated as described for tennis elbow on page 76. Before reading that section, however, do refer to pages 74–77 where the methods employed in that section, and elsewhere in this chapter, are described in detail.

Injuries are often the result of over-extending oneself, and this in turn can be caused by the need to achieve the "high" created by endorphin release. The very real sense of well-being given by these natural opiates is fine when it gives you the incentive to get up on a frosty winter morning and go for your two-mile daily jog, but it becomes destructive when it acts like a drug and more and more exercise is needed to create the same level of "high." This is when people over-extend and a part of the body becomes strained. So do remember that moderation is best in all things—exercise included.

Professional sportsmen and women are not interested in moderation—winning is the name of the game—but for them essential oils have proved extremely helpful over the years. Indeed, I doubt that there has been an Olympic games at which essential oils weren't used either in preparatory or recovery treatments.

We can't all hope to win gold medals on the running track but jogging is an activity many people enjoy, and it's an easy sport for families to do together. It is important when starting out not to over-exert yourself because pounding those pavements puts great strain on muscles, ankle bones, and the skeletal frame, especially the lower back. Here then is a formula for people who are just learning about the strains of jogging and which is especially helpful for the lungs and respiratory system in general, and the muscular and skeletal frames. Before you go running rub the oil over your feet, ankles, calves, thighs, buttocks, lower back, and arms. The thyme will help to prevent sprains:

RUNNING FORMULA FOR BEGINNERS

Eucalyptus	10 drops
Rosemary	10 drops
Thyme	10 drops

Diluted in 2 tablespoons vegetable oil

If you want to build yourself up, make up another bottle using 15 drops of eucalyptus and 15 drops of rosemary to 2 tablespoons base vegetable oil and use it in addition, every day for two weeks, as an all-over body rub after the shower, after your run.

When you use the following competition oil bear in mind that the essential oils have an effect on the psyche too, so inhale the aroma deeply. The formula should be reserved for the occasion of the big race because aroma sensitivity can become jaded and you want the rarity value to give you that extra boost. The oil strengthens the muscular system and keeps the rhythm of the body flowing so that peak performance becomes easier. Rub the mixture all over your body before the event.

RUNNERS' COMPETITION OIL

Bergamot	5 drops
Basil	5 drops

Diluted in 2 teaspoons vegetable oil

Geranium oil provides an excellent remedy for "jogger's nipple" which is caused by the action of material rubbing on the nipple for long periods of time. The discomfort suffered by long distance male runners, as well as by women in all sports, can be quite considerable. Clearly, all sportswomen should wear a good-fitting bra, but for all who have developed this problem the answer is to add 5 drops of geranium oil to a teaspoon of vegetable oil and rub this around the area each day, especially before and after the sporting activity.

The thrust of competition has always fueled the determination of sportspeople to find preparations that will help their performance and keep their body in peak condition. In days past athletes bathed in mint and balm to strengthen muscles and sinews, while today it is more likely to be baths to which the essential oils of ginger and black pepper have been added. Nasturtium seed oil was used widely to ease tired, post-race muscles, whereas today physiotherapists and sports therapists choose eucalyptus oil, birch oil, wintergreen, tea tree, or rosemary oils. But nasturtium seed oil is still an excellent muscle decongestant, and although it is no longer generally available you can make your own. Crush a handful of nasturtium seeds in a pestle and mortar and add them to 1 cup soya bean oil. Leave this to stand for seven days, filter, and use as required.

Natural remedies go hand-in-hand with the standard methods of treating sports injuries and maintaining the well-being of the body which sport pushes to the limits of endurance, stamina, and skill. These methods are outlined in the next pages, and thereafter you will find various essential oil remedies and suggestions that will help you to be a winner in your particular field.

Methods of Treating Injury ◆◆◆◆◆◆◆◆◆◆◆◆◆◆◆◆

Heat

When heat is applied to an area of the body it dilates the capillaries and increases blood flow. Blood nourishes the tissues and can hasten healing, reduce muscular spasm, and reduce pain, but applying heat does carry the risk of seepage of blood and plasma to the injured area. If this were to happen healing would be prolonged and swelling and fluid retention would be increased. It is important therefore that heat is not applied to an injured area until at least twelve hours has passed.

Cold

Cold causes contraction of the small capillaries and this decreases the amount of blood collecting around a wound—which could prolong the healing time. The application of cold to an area of injury reduces bruising, swelling, inflammation, and pain.

RICE

"Rest, ice, compress, and elevation" are words so often repeated by physiotherapists and sports therapists that they have been shortened to form the word "RICE" which is drummed into anyone with an injury that needs care.

REST Resting an injury is extremely important to assure that no further damage takes place. And when you are advised to rest, that doesn't mean don't go dancing next Friday night, but rest now—immediately!

ICE The ice methods are so helpful in treating all sorts of injury that they are referred to throughout this book, not only for the treatment of sports injuries. Ice can stop internal bleeding, bruises, and inflammation and in so doing decrease healing time, if applied correctly. There are many methods. The Styrofoam cup method enables you to hold the ice to a specific part of the body without freezing your hands. Fill a Styrofoam cup with water and freeze it. When it is required, cut the sides a few inches to reveal a solid block of ice, which can be applied to the injured area.

Ice may also be placed in bowls or buckets into which you put the toes, feet, fingers, hands, or elbow, and other areas of the body affected. Top up as required. In physiotherapy departments ice is often put into a plastic bag, crushed, and then placed between two towels and wrapped around the injured area. Although this method has to be used in some circumstances, the dripping wet towels can be most uncomfortable.

Whichever method you use, apply the ice to the injured area for at least twenty minutes, then allow twenty minutes' rest before repeating the application. Continue in this way for three to four hours.

COMPRESS A compress can be made with a bandage or piece of material, folded to form a pad. This should be wrapped firmly over the area to prevent swelling.

Compresses can be hot or cold. Compression is often needed to reduce the level of blood flowing to the area but should never be so tight that it decreases circulation and causes the injured person to experience pain, numbness, or the skin turning blue.

ELEVATION By raising the injured limb higher than the heart, swelling and pain can often be prevented or lessened. Elevation is especially important for dancers. Use whatever you have handy to support the limb—pillows, cushions, or whatever.

Ointments

An ointment can be made which provides a carrier for the essential oils. In some cases the essential oils are more effective when used *during* a sporting activity in this way, than when used in a vegetable oil base.

Make the basic ointment in the following way. Using the bain-marie method, blend 4 tablespoons of anhydrous lanolin and 2 tablespoons almond oil. (This will give a total of 3 ounces.) When well blended together, mix in your chosen essential oils. Essential oil formulas are given for individual injuries and conditions which can be combined in this basic ointment.

Massage Oils

As a general rule, use 5 drops of essential oil to each 1 teaspoon of base vegetable oil. In the acute stage of injury, however, a higher dose may be needed than prescribed here. This may be up to double the usual amount. When the acute state has passed, revert to the 5-to-1 rule.

Compresses

During the acute stage of injury, unless specific directions have been given, use a total of 8 drops of essential oil on the compress—whether this is hot, cold, wet, or steamed.

Cabbage Leaf

Iron a cabbage leaf (see page 77) and leave it on the affected area while still warm. Apply for ten minutes and repeat if necessary.

Clay Poultice

Add 2 tablespoons of green clay to hot or cold water and blend until a thick and sticky paste is achieved. Then add the essential oils and mix well. Apply to the area and wrap with a bandage or piece of muslin.

Massage or Movement Cure

Massage is extremely effective in the treatment of muscular spasm and contraction, and used in sports injuries it can reduce fluid retention and swelling while stimulating blood circulation and lymphatic flow. Massage should always be gentle. Long, gentle, smooth strokes are the most useful for sports injuries. Use the flat of the hand, moving away from the injured part, but always in the direction of the heart—from hand to shoulder, foot to thigh, and so on.

Muscles ◆◆◆◆◆◆◆◆◆◆◆◆◆◆

Muscles can be toned with essential oils, used in conjunction with exercise. Add the oils to a bath or to a massage oil applied either before or after the bath. To keep muscles supple, put the essential oil onto a facecloth and rub onto the muscles in the shower before exercise. Use the following essential oils:

ESSENTIAL OILS FOR SUPPLE, TONED MUSCLES

Black pepper	**Juniper**
Ginger	**Thyme**
Rosemary	**Peppermint**
Lavender	**Grapefruit**
Cypress	**Orange**
Basil	**Lime**
Pettigraine	**Birch**

Aerobic exercise is helped and improved when using essential oils, which not only tone muscles but facilitate easier breathing and increased circulation:

ESSENTIAL OILS FOR AEROBICS

RESPIRATORY OILS	CIRCULATORY OILS
Eucalyptus	**Geranium**
Peppermint	**Palma rosa**
Rosemary	**Rose**

Over-Exercised Muscles

Over-exercised muscles cause pain and in some cases the inability to move without trembling as the muscles struggle to contract. Rest is the best remedy, followed by hot baths and massage. If pain continues to be a problem you may have an injury. Ice can reduce swelling, if there is any, and the pain caused by inflammation. Follow this with a hot bath into which you have put 3 drops of marjoram and 2 drops of lemon and soak for as long as possible. Afterwards massage with the following oil:

MASSAGE OIL FOR OVER-EXERCISED MUSCLES

Eucalyptus	5 drops
Peppermint	5 drops
Ginger	5 drops

Diluted in 1 tablespoon vegetable oil

Topical Analgesic Ointment

The following ointment can be applied to painful muscles. Combine the lanolin and rosewater in a bain-marie and when this mixture is cold add the essential oils and mix well:

Anhydrous lanolin	2 ounces
Rosewater	6 teaspoons
Clove	20 drops
Eucalyptus	20 drops
Thyme	10 drops

If you prefer a stiffer base, add ½ ounce of beeswax at the bain-marie stage.

Foot Care ◆◆◆◆◆◆◆◆◆◆◆◆

For all dancers, and most sportspeople, it is the feet that take the pounding, and caring for them is of paramount importance. Feet that are well cared for can withstand the pressure placed on the twenty-six bones in each foot as well as avoiding the very real pain of blisters, corns, and bunions.

Blisters can become infected, especially those on the toes, and they need to be seen to immediately. Lavender may sting, but 1 drop on an open blister will stop it from becoming infected. Corns develop over a period of time and become painful. Tagetes is the oil to use on these—massage 1 drop on the affected toe when the corn hurts. Dancers who use tagetes as a preventative are less likely to develop corns.

Massage the feet as often as you can to keep them supple and flexible and prevent injury. Dancers have different needs from those of athletes and their feet take more punishment: classical ballet dancers have to cram fragile toes into blocked ballet shoes, and modern dancers are expected to be agile on heels so high that most of us could only just walk on them. Here then are two formulas designed for specific foot needs: they are synergistic blends so make up a bottle of essential oil using these proportions:

FOOT OIL SYNERGISTIC BLEND FOR DANCERS

Tagetes	5 drops
Rosemary	3 drops
Benzoin	4 drops
Geranium	3 drops

5 drops to 1 teaspoon vegetable oil (for each foot)

FOOT OIL SYNERGISTIC BLEND FOR ATHLETES

Lavender	5 drops
Thyme	3 drops
Rosemary	4 drops

5 drops to 1 teaspoon vegetable oil (for each foot)

Walking, jogging, or running causes different pressures within the foot and a different oil is required. It has been found that female walkers use more force when their heel hits the ground so they might be wise to use padded heels.

FOOT OIL SYNERGISTIC BLEND FOR WALKERS, JOGGERS, AND RUNNERS

Rosemary	5 drops
Peppermint	3 drops
Lavender	4 drops

Blend together in these proportions and use 5 drops to 1 teaspoon of vegetable oil per massage

The constant heavy landing on the ground can not only make the feet sore and cause strain on the hip bones, it may also put pressure on the head as we try to keep it up high. This can result in migraines.

If you are feeling worn out, here is a tremendously relaxing remedy. Lavender is an excellent antibiotic and will help to heal any blisters and cuts. Take a large bowl and cover the bottom with a dozen or more small, round stones. Pour in enough hot water to cover your ankles and add 2 drops of lavender oil. Sit back, inhale the vapors, and then roll your feet gently over the pebbles.

The African marigold produces the essential oil of tagetes, which has been much researched and proven to be an excellent cure for bunions—so much so that there is now a Marigold Clinic in London. It can also be used for corns, calluses, or hard skin, and to strengthen the joints and feet. Make an oil using 30 drops of tagetes oil to 2 tablespoons vegetable oil and rub all around the bunion and the other toes, paying particular attention to inflamed areas or those that you want to heal. Use every night for as long as you continue to have inflammation or pain.

If your feet have been especially battered and bruised, or if you have a problem with corns, bunions, or inflamed joints, here is a formula which will both heal and strengthen:

FEET TREAT FORMULA

Red thyme	5 drops
Bicarbonate of soda	1 cup

Place in a large bowl of warm water and soak the feet in it

The following formula gives a wonderfully restorative treatment for feet. Use 3 drops of this synergistic blend in each bath and add 1 tablespoon of Epsom salts and 1 teaspoon of rock salt:

SPA FOOT BATH SYNERGISTIC BLEND

Peppermint	3 drops
Rosemary	1 drop
Tagetes	2 drops
Geranium	3 drops

Use 3 drops per foot bath

Alternatively, blend the whole formula with 3 tablespoons of Epsom salts and 3 teaspoons salt. Mix in the blender and use as needed in hot water, soaking the feet for ten minutes. Follow by using the appropriate foot massage oil.

Foot Problems

BLACK TOENAIL Toenails that turn black are caused by bruising under the nail which can be caused by a blow, ill-fitting shoes, or by stubbing your toe. Nails that have become loose should be taken off by a chiropodist if they are causing a problem. Use 1 drop of oil of hyssop under the toe, as far as you can get it, for the first three days. Then make up a toe massage oil by diluting 5 drops of hyssop in 1 teaspoon of vegetable oil.

BLISTERS See page 25. Alternatively, dilute 2 drops of tagetes oil in 2 drops of iodine and apply to the area. If your feet are susceptible to blisters, soak them in cold tea (this is an old dancers' trick). Make up a pot of strong tea and add it to a bowl of water.

BUNIONS See page 299.

CALLUSES See page 300.

CORNS See page 300.

INGROWING TOENAIL To stop an ingrowing toenail becoming infected massage daily with the following:

Lavender	10 drops
Tea tree	10 drops

Diluted in 1 tablespoon vegetable oil

FALLEN ARCHES If the arch causes pain and aching, massage the instep towards the heel of the foot with the following:

Rosemary	10 drops
Black pepper	5 drops
Ginger	10 drops
Clary-sage	5 drops

Diluted in 2 teaspoons vegetable oil

SWEATY FEET See page 270.

VERRUCAS See page 191.

Tips for Feet

Soaking the feet in a mixture of 3 drops of rosemary oil and 1 tablespoon of baking soda in a bowl of warm water will soothe away tiredness.

The ice treatment applies to feet as well as to other parts of the body: 3 drops of lavender oil in a bowl of iced water is excellent for swollen feet.

Stress and Sport ◆◆◆◆◆◆

By its very nature competitive sport is stressful, and a certain amount of positive stress can give the impetus for a better performance. But stress that is not burned off can lead to problems. Use relaxing baths to combat stress, both leading up to the event and after it, but before taking either of the recommended baths rub the body all over with the following:

PRE-BATH STRESS RUB

Patchouli	1 drop
Lemon	3 drops
Red thyme	1 drop

Diluted in 1 teaspoon vegetable oil

PRE-SPORT STRESS BATH
SYNERGISTIC BLEND

Rosemary	3 drops
Lemon	4 drops
Lavender	3 drops
Chamomile	2 drops

Blend together and use 4 drops in the bath

AFTER-SPORT STRESS BATH
SYNERGISTIC BLEND

Lemon	4 drops
Nutmeg	2 drops
Orange	2 drops
Clary-sage	4 drops

Use 4 drops in the bath

These baths and the pre-bath rub aid in the elimination of any traces of adrenal chemicals that can remain in the body if not burned off and lead to negative stress symptoms.

ESSENTIAL OILS FOR
INCREASED PHYSICAL PERFORMANCE

Grapefruit	**Black pepper**
Thyme	**Ginger**
Basil	**Pimento**
Lavender	**Rosemary**
Peppermint	

Use the above oils on their own or in combination, to a total of 2 drops only in baths and 10 drops to 2 tablespoons base oil for a massage oil. The smaller quantities have their beneficial effect over a period of time and as these measures are likely to be used over a longer period the small doses are better.

If you experience deep fatigue it is better to use an oil that relaxes as opposed to stimulates, as a sudden rush of stimulation can tire the body further. Use for example, marjoram instead of rosemary, and stick to low doses—only 10 drops of essential oil to 2 tablespoons vegetable oil.

Showers ◆◆◆◆◆◆◆◆◆◆◆◆◆◆

Taking a warm shower after a workout is one of the best things you can do, not only to make you feel good (all those negative ions you are inhaling are so beneficial) but to help eliminate the lactic acid that causes muscle ache. A shower with just soap and water cannot provide the deep cleaning your body requires, but using essential oils will help to eliminate waste products from the body, preventing sore and aching muscles.

Before taking a shower, rub the body with a clean washcloth on which you have put

3 neat drops of essential oil, rub it all over yourself and then shower in the normal way. A combination of equal parts of rosemary, lemon, and eucalyptus peppermint would be ideal for this purpose.

After showering, massage the muscles with a muscle relaxant oil or toning oil, depending on what you want to achieve.

ESSENTIAL OILS TO USE
BEFORE AND IN THE SHOWER

Lavender	**Eucalyptus lemon**
Rosemary	**Birch**
Lemon	**Niaouli**
Eucalyptus	**Juniper**
Eucalyptus peppermint	**Bergamot**

Saunas ◆◆◆◆◆◆◆◆◆◆◆◆◆◆◆

Saunas are extremely useful but they can leave you a little depleted unless you are able to roll in the snow afterwards! Oils to use in the sauna are those that promote the elimination of waste products and debris through the skin. Use them in the water that you throw on the coals or other heat source.

ESSENTIAL OILS FOR THE SAUNA

Eucalyptus	**Birch**
Pine	**Rosemary**
Lemon	**Lime**
Lavender	**Grapefruit**
Niaouli	**Bergamot**
Cypress	

Although not generally thought of as a sauna scent, the following synergistic blend is effective, gentle, and relaxing, and it has a very nice fragrance:

RELAXING SAUNA SYNERGISTIC BLEND

Sandalwood	10 drops
Lemon	5 drops
Geranium	2 drops

Make up in these proportions and use 4 drops at a time

And here is a formula that is more stimulating:

STIMULATING SAUNA
SYNERGISTIC BLEND

Pine	3 drops
Rosemary	3 drops
Niaouli	2 drops
Grapefruit	10 drops

Make up in these proportions and use 4 drops at a time

Eucalyptus lemon and eucalyptus peppermint are very good oils to use singly in the sauna—they clear the head and respiratory tract as well as helping to eliminate waste products.

Jacuzzis ◆◆◆◆◆◆◆◆◆◆◆◆◆◆

Relaxing in your own jacuzzi, with warm water bubbling on your back and essential oils relaxing you, is a very different matter from sitting in the chemical stew which is what most communal jacuzzis, with their constantly recycled water, resemble. Any of the oils listed in this book would be fine, and although the essential oils if used over a long period of time may cause a residue to build up in the pipes, this can be cleaned away with the usual cleansing program you should be using. If you are completely hooked on the idea of communal jacuzzis and want to ask the neighbors in to share yours, I suggest you acquaint yourself fully with the Bacteria Buster list of essential oils on page 386—and use them!

Hot Tubs ◆◆◆◆◆◆◆◆◆◆◆◆

Hot tubs are the tradition in Japan, where whole families will happily soak with their neighbors. The difference between Japanese and Western cultures, however, is that the Japanese wouldn't dream of getting into a tub without having washed thoroughly beforehand, and certainly not if they had any bacterial, viral, or fungal infections. In fact, if the manager of any such establishment is reading this, he or she might like to bear in mind that there are excellent oils for rheumatism and arthritis and a special tub could be put aside for sufferers of these conditions.

Locker Room Scents ◆◆

Locker rooms, changing rooms, and communal showers could have been designed for the continuation of many species of bacteria, viruses, and fungi. I dare say none of us would ever enter one if we had a microscope available to show just what a community of little microbes harbor and indeed flourish there.

The floors and benches in these places could routinely be washed down with antibacterial, antiviral, and antifungal essential oils—it would also give the whole place a lovely aroma—and with the choice available, something in keeping with the masculine or feminine would be no problem to find. To be realistic, however, such measures are unlikely to have been taken, and so it is wise to use essential oils on the areas one uses to keep oneself free of everybody else's "hangers on." Certain rules should be common sense. Never use anybody else's towel, for example—always use a fresh towel of your own. Put a small towel on the bench before you sit on it, and keep a towel for just this purpose, putting a few drops of protective essential oil on it before you set off to the gym or wherever. Wear shoes that you have already dusted with a bacteria buster powder to avoid the spread of fungal infections. Don't eat food in locker rooms and try to avoid putting your fingers in your mouth. Wash your hands thoroughly before leaving. Try to get the windows opened to ensure a fresh circulation of air. If you have your own locker, spray it with antibacterial oils, and if you share it with others put a tissue with essential oil in a corner and leave it there. As so many sprays and body preparations are used in locker rooms, nobody will care or even notice if you spray around a bit. There are many essential oils you can use but the ones that follow are quite acceptable aromatically in public changing rooms. All have antiseptic and antibacterial properties, while those marked with an asterisk also have antiviral properties.

LOCKER ROOM BACTERIA BUSTERS

Niaouli	**Lavender**
Pine	**Lemon**
Ravensara*	**Oregano***
Thyme	**Cinnamon***
Eucalyptus	**AV1 (Dermatect)***
Bergamot	

BACTERIA BUSTER DUSTING POWDER

Pure talcum powder	3½ ounces
Ravensara	20 drops
Pine	20 drops
Eucalyptus	20 drops
Cinnamon	10 drops
Bergamot	20 drops

Mix in these proportions

Put the talcum powder in a blender and drip the essential oils, already mixed together, into the talc through the hole in the lid of the blender. Blend until all the particles are evenly distributed, package and use as required.

LOCKER ROOM SPRAY AND WIPE

Cinnamon	20 drops
Lemon	20 drops
Pine	20 drops
Thyme	20 drops
Oregano	10 drops

Blend the essential oils and add to 1 tablespoon vodka or pure alcohol. Use 10 drops in 3 ounces water.

Shake well before use in the sprayer. If using as a wipe, use the same dilution as for the spray but pour it on the cloth you use to wipe down surfaces.

A–Z of Sports and Dance Injuries ♦♦♦♦♦♦♦

ABDOMINAL WALL STRAIN Injury to the muscles or tendons of the abdominal wall and lower abdominal area.

Use the ice method for the first day. From the second day add 4 drops of rosemary on a hot compress and place over the affected area. Repeat three times a day. Also massage the area gently using equal proportions of ginger and thyme—5 drops per 1 teaspoon of vegetable oil.

Likely Causes: High jump, Long jump, Contact sports, Stretching, Javelin, Discus, Throwing, Weight lifting, Dance

ACHILLES TENDINITIS Inflammation of the achilles tendon. This limits movement and the area may be hot and painful. For the first three days use a cold clay poultice to which you have added 3 drops each of chamomile and lavender. Thereafter use a hot clay poultice to which you have added 3 drops of ginger and 2 drops of chamomile. Also massage the area with a teaspoon of vegetable oil to which 3 drops of chamomile and 2 drops of lavender have been added.

The cabbage method also helps.

Likely Causes: Running, Jogging, Jumping, Dance, Aerobics, Kicking

ANKLE AND HEEL CONTUSION Bruising of the tissues and skin as a result of a direct blow to the area. There is pain and swelling. Use the ice method at least three times a day for three days, and in between massage all over the foot and ankle, three times a day, with the following:

Hyssop	10 drops
Cypress	10 drops
Geranium	8 drops
Lavender	2 drops

Diluted in 2 tablespoons vegetable oil

Likely Causes: Hockey, Football, Rugby

ANKLE SPRAIN A slight tearing or stretching of the ligaments in the ankle. Use the ice method, then massage the whole of the foot and ankle and the leg to the calf muscle, using the following oil:

Ginger	20 drops
Nutmeg	17 drops
Cloves	3 drops

Diluted in 2 tablespoons vegetable oil

Keep the ankle bandaged to prevent further damage.

Use ice packs for three days (followed by the massage), three times a day, and if the pain continues begin to apply alternate hot and cold washcloths, to both of which you have added 4 drops of peppermint. Use steaming hot washcloths and ice-cold ones, and apply them alternately several times. Do this three times a day. The best thing of course is to rest the ankle, but dancers may not be able to do this and they should follow the alternative hot and cold washcloth treatment every five minutes.

Likely Causes: Almost any sport or dance

ARM STRAIN A strain or injury to the muscles or tendons of the upper or lower arm. Use the ice method followed by massage of the area with the following formula, three times a day for two days:

Ginger	20 drops
Black pepper	5 drops
Nutmeg	5 drops

Diluted in 2 tablespoons vegetable oil

Likely Causes: Contact sports, Throwing, Weight lifting, Dance (male)

BACK: SLIPPED OR RUPTURED DISC A break in the ligaments surrounding a vertebral disc. This should be treated by a doctor, but intermittent additional care can be as follows. During the first three days use ice packs over the painful area to reduce inflammation. Afterwards apply the following oil gently to the area:

Rosemary	10 drops
Peppermint	10 drops
Eucalyptus	5 drops
Ginger	5 drops

Diluted in 2 tablespoons vegetable oil

Depending on the type of injury, after the initial three-day period it may prove a more effective method of pain control to move on to alternate hot and cold compress (or washcloth) treatment. Put 2 drops each of basil and peppermint essential oil on the compresses, followed by gentle massage oil treatment three times a day for as long as required.

Likely Causes: Tennis, Bowling, Gymnastics, Weight lifting, Dance

BACK: STRAIN, GENERAL Follow the treatment as for slipped disc, but during the acute stage hold against the painful area an ice bag wrapped in a towel for at least ten minutes, have a break, and start again.

Likely Causes: Contact sports, Lifting sports, Dance, Gymnastics

BREAST CONTUSION Bruising of the breast; pain in the breast. Massage the area using the ice method four times a day and afterwards gently smooth the following oil over the damaged area:

Chamomile	5 drops
Geranium	10 drops
Cypress	10 drops
Hyssop	5 drops

Diluted in 2 tablespoons vegetable oil

After two days, hot compresses or washcloths with 2 drops of chamomile added can be used. Afterwards apply the massage oil. If you are a woman, wear a protective and supportive bra.

Likely Causes: Contact sports, Dance

BUTTOCK CONTUSION Bruising of the buttock skin and tissue caused by a fall or direct blow. Use the ice method four to six times a day and after three days transfer to hot compresses. After each application, use the following oil, gently massaged into the affected area:

Cypress	10 drops
Geranium	5 drops
Hyssop	5 drops
Rosemary	10 drops

Diluted in 2 tablespoons vegetable oil

Protect the damaged area.

Likely Causes: Contact sports, Dance, Falls, Horse riding, Ice skating, High jump

CARPAL TUNNEL SYNDROME A nerve disorder in the hands and arms. Massage *both* hands, arms, and shoulders twice a day with:

Marjoram	10 drops
Lavender	10 drops
Eucalyptus	10 drops

Diluted in 2 tablespoons vegetable oil

CHEST MUSCLE STRAIN Strain and injury to the muscles in the chest area. Use the ice method four to six times a day and after forty-eight hours use the heat method. Twice a day throughout, massage with the following oil:

Ginger	10 drops
Eucalyptus	10 drops
Peppermint	5 drops
Nutmeg	5 drops

Diluted in 2 tablespoons vegetable oil

Soaking in a hot bath often relieves the symptoms; add 2 drops each of lavender and rosemary.

Likely Causes: Contact sports, Weight lifting, Dance (male)

EAR INJURY Use the ice method to relieve discomfort and use the analgesic ointment on page 97.

ELBOW CONTUSIONS Bruising of the skin and underlying tissue of the elbow. Apply the ice method for three days, four to six times a day, and after each session massage gently using the following oil:

Hyssop	5 drops
Ginger	6 drops
Cypress	10 drops
Eucalyptus	9 drops

Diluted in 2 tablespoons vegetable oil

The compress or washcloth heat method with 2 drops of eucalyptus can be used after three days.

Likely Causes: Contact sports, Falls, Blows

ELBOW SPRAIN Caused by overstretching the ligaments in the elbow joint. Rest the elbow in an ice pack, keeping it there for fifteen minutes, three times a day. Between times, massage with the following oil:

Ginger	15 drops
Nutmeg	8 drops
Clove	6 drops

Diluted in 2 tablespoons vegetable oil

Hot water elbow baths also help, as do alternate hot and cold baths. In these place 2 drops each of rosemary and lavender.

Likely Cause: Contact sports

ELBOW TENDINITIS (TENNIS ELBOW) Inflammation of the muscles, tendons, bursa, or tissues of the elbow area which often causes pain in the arm as well. In cases such as this heat is usually the best answer. Apply a hot washcloth or compress which has been soaked in 1 quart of hot water with 5 drops of peppermint. Apply this to the area three times a day and afterwards massage the whole of the arm from the wrist to the shoulder gently with the following oil:

Peppermint	10 drops
Eucalyptus	10 drops
Chamomile Roman	10 drops

Diluted in 2 tablespoons vegetable oil

Likely Causes: Tennis, Ball games, Throwing

FACE CONTUSION Bruising of the skin and underlying tissue on the face. Apply an ice pack over the injured area immediately and at least three times a day for fifteen minutes. Afterwards, massage the whole facial area with the following oil:

Lavender	5 drops
Geranium	10 drops
Cypress	5 drops
Hyssop	5 drops
Rosemary	5 drops

Diluted in 2 tablespoons vegetable oil

Twice a day, morning and night, apply direct to the area a cold cotton-wool compress on which 3 drops of chamomile have been placed.

Likely Causes: Contact sports, Fencing, Baseball

FINGER SPRAIN Overstretching of the ligaments between the finger joints. Place the fingers in a bed of ice for at least ten minutes then massage over the whole hand with the following:

Ginger	20 drops
Black pepper	5 drops
Nutmeg	5 drops

Diluted in 2 tablespoons vegetable oil

After twenty-four hours use alternating hot and cold compress treatment, four times a day. After the compresses, apply the massage oil.

Likely Causes: Contact sports, Catching, Throwing, Gymnastics

FOOT BURSITIS The soft sacs on the pad of the foot filled with fluid are known as bursa and can become inflamed. This condition develops over a period of time and treatment should be started as soon as it is suspected. Soak the foot in a cold foot bath three times a day. Afterwards, massage the whole of the foot with the following oil:

Peppermint	30 drops

Diluted in 2 tablespoons vegetable oil

Rest as much as possible.

Likely Causes: Dance, Aerobics, Competitive sports

FOOT CONTUSION Bruising of the skin and underlying tissue. Treat as for Foot Bursitis above, but massage with this oil:

Hyssop	5 drops
Cypress	15 drops
Geranium	10 drops

Diluted in 2 tablespoons vegetable oil

Likely Causes: Dance, Aerobics, Blows to foot

FOOT GANGLION (SYNOVIAL CYST) A small hard movable nodule in between or on top of a tendon or joint. This develops slowly and can sometimes be dispersed by massage. Apply a hot compress which has had 1 drop of thyme oil added. Massage the area quite firmly with the following oil:

Thyme	5 drops
Rosemary	10 drops
Tagetes	15 drops

Diluted in 2 tablespoons vegetable oil

Likely Causes: Aerobics, Athletics, Competitive sports

GROIN STRAIN An injury to the muscles or tendons in the lower abdominal groin area. Use the ice method over the tender area and afterwards use the following oil to massage gently all over the lower abdominal area, the thighs and groin, but taking care to avoid the genitals:

Hyssop	10 drops
Geranium	10 drops
Chamomile	10 drops

Diluted in 2 tablespoons vegetable oil

Do this three times a day for two days and then continue with the massage only.

Likely Causes: Competitive sports, Contact sports, Dance (male)

HAND CONTUSION Bruising of the skin and underlying tissue. Place the hand in a bowl of ice and leave it there for ten minutes. Do this three times a day over a forty-eight-hour period. Also massage as often as possible—the whole of the hand and fingers—with the following:

Peppermint	30 drops

Diluted in 2 tablespoons vegetable oil

Likely Causes: Contact sports, Falls

HAND GANGLION See Foot Ganglion, page 106.

HEAD INJURY A blow or jar to the head should always be checked by a doctor. Until then, keep the head up, apply ice and 2 drops of neat lavender to the area.

HIP STRAIN Injury to the muscles and tendons that join the hip joint to the thigh bone. Rest and take a cold sitz bath three times a day. Apply ice to the area and massage all over both hips and thighs using the following:

Ginger	10 drops
Clove	10 drops
Nutmeg	10 drops

Diluted in 2 tablespoons vegetable oil

After forty-eight hours start to take alternate cold and hot sitz baths, in which you have placed 4 drops of rosemary and 2 drops of lavender. Spend ten minutes in each bath.

Likely Causes: Contact sports, Dance, Aerobics, Running

KNEE CARTILAGE INJURY Damage to the cartilage in the knee. Apply ice to reduce swelling and inflammation. The knee should be bandaged to prevent further injury and kept elevated when the patient is sitting. Use the ice method three times a day, alternating with hot washcloths, and then massage the area with the following:

Clove	8 drops
Ginger	12 drops
Nutmeg	10 drops

Diluted in 2 tablespoons vegetable oil

Likely Causes: Contact sports, Football, Rugby, Dance, Aerobics, Jumping

KNEE SYNOVITIS (WATER ON THE KNEE) Massage four times a day with the following:

Juniper	10 drops
Marjoram	10 drops
Tagetes	10 drops

Diluted in 2 tablespoons vegetable oil

Massage from the ankle to the knee and then from the knee to the top of the thigh.

If the pain and inflammation do not subside use the ice method.

Likely Causes: Contact sports, Dance, Aerobics

LEG SPRAIN (LOWER LEG) Overstretching of the ligaments in the legs. Use an ice pack four times a day for twenty minutes at a time. Afterwards massage with the following:

Rosemary	10 drops
Eucalyptus	10 drops
Peppermint	10 drops

Diluted in 2 tablespoons vegetable oil

After forty-eight hours change to hot compresses, on which you have placed 2 drops each of rosemary and lavender. Between treatments keep the leg wrapped with an elastic bandage and periodically massage the whole of the leg from the ankle to the thigh.

Likely Causes: Dance, Jogging, Running, Jumping, Skiing, Most sports

LEG STRAIN (LOWER CALF MUSCLE) Injury to the muscles and tendons in the calf. Follow the treatment as for sprain but using this oil:

Ginger	10 drops
Clove	5 drops
Nutmeg	5 drops
Chamomile Roman	10 drops

Diluted in 2 tablespoons vegetable oil

Likely Causes: Dance, Running, Jogging, Aerobics, Most sports

NECK SPRAIN Violent overstretching of ligaments in the neck region. A collar is usually prescribed and should be worn at all times. Use an ice pack around the neck area, for at least fifteen minutes at a time. Massage the neck and shoulders three times a day using the following:

Ginger	10 drops
Rosemary	10 drops
Black pepper	5 drops
Peppermint	5 drops

Diluted in 2 tablespoons vegetable oil

The ice-cup method can be used to relieve pain. If you have headaches as a result, use 5 drops of peppermint oil in 1 teaspoon of vegetable oil and massage around the back of the neck, up to the hairline.

Likely Causes: Contact sports, Diving, Gymnastics, Motor racing

NOSE INJURY Apply an ice pack immediately. Gauze can be placed in the nostrils to stop bleeding: put 1 drop of lavender oil on the gauze before cutting it into two pieces. See a doctor. If the nose is broken, smooth the following oil gently over the forehead and cheekbones:

Chamomile	10 drops
Lavender	10 drops
Geranium	5 drops
Rosemary	5 drops

Diluted in 2 tablespoons vegetable oil

If the nose is not broken, apply ice three times a day and massage the nose area, as well as the forehead and cheekbones, with the above oil.

Likely Causes: Contact sports, Boxing, Wrestling

SHOULDER STRAIN Injury to muscles or tendons. Use the ice method for ten miutes at a time and after forty-eight hours use the heat compress or washcloth method. Three times a day massage all the arm and shoulder area with the following:

Ginger	10 drops
Chamomile	10 drops
Nutmeg	10 drops

Diluted in 2 tablespoons vegetable oil

Likely Causes: Contact sports, Boxing, Throwing

THIGH INJURY—HAMSTRINGS An injury to the hamstring tendon which connects the thigh muscle at the back and side. Use the ice method and ice packs for at least ten minutes four times per day. Also massage three times a day using the following:

Rosemary	10 drops
Eucalyptus	10 drops
Chamomile	5 drops
Lavender	5 drops

Diluted in 2 tablespoons vegetable oil

Likely Causes: Dance, Gymnastics, Running, Competitive sports

WRIST GANGLION See Foot Ganglion, page 106.

WRIST SPRAIN Overstretching of one or more ligaments in the wrist. Apply an ice pack three or four times a day. Afterwards massage with the following oil:

Ginger	20 drops
Nutmeg	17 drops
Clove	3 drops

Diluted in 2 tablespoons vegetable oil

Use an elastic bandage between the treatments.

Likely Causes: Contact sports, Pole vaulting, Skiing, Bowling

◆ CHAPTER 6 ◆

THE FRAGRANT WAY TO BEAUTY

THE HUMAN FACE is like a book—it tells a story. Each wrinkle represents a chapter in your life and each blemish tells a story of misuse. Laughter lines tell the world that your life contains humor, while a drooping mouth says there is an underlying sadness or anger to your tale. The vicissitudes of each life are written large across the front page: sadness, ill health, stress and tension, crisis, disaster, they are all there for the world to see. No face is a mask, and even if we cover our skin with camouflaging makeup, that too tells its own story—that we have something to hide.

The skin that covers our body reacts to our emotions, so that people under stress often find their skin becoming dry and taut, and in severe emotional states, dehydrated. Hormonal changes produce spots and blemishes, as well as increased oiliness with dry patches. Climate also affects face and body skin. Hot weather can produce lumps and bumps as well as dryness and wrinkles, while moist damp air has a beneficial effect and gives the skin a dewy texture. Cigarette smoke can age a face by making it gray and wrinkled, and pollution has the same effect—which is why I am seeing more and more young women with prematurely aging facial skin. We used to be able to wash our faces in soft rainwater, but who wants to do that anymore with acid rain destroying the beauty of the human face as surely as it destroys the beauty of the European forests?

Until fairly recently it was thought that skin was a waterproof coating through which nothing could be absorbed into the layers below. Now, all manner of medications are applied directly onto the skin for absorption. But those working with essential oils have always known that they are absorbed into the body, not only because their therapeutic values can be seen to be working but because oils applied directly onto the skin are excreted—through urine, feces, perspiration, and breath. This has been shown scientifically many times over, and "the sweet smell of success" is easy to observe without any scientific apparatus other than a human nose. Moreover, particular oils have their preferred methods of exit and the route they travel is a factor in deciding which oils to use. It is indeed because the skin is such an effective absorber that essential oils need not be taken orally—where in any case they only come into contact with the digestive system and all its rubbish. The natural and extremely small molecules of essential oils penetrate the dermis and get to work with their purity maintained.

Technically, the skin is an organ weighing about nine pounds which protects us from the outside world and regulates the body's natural cooling and heating systems. There are few differences between male and female skins. The epidermis is the outer layer of skin cells and the one we see, but that is the product of the lower layer of skin called the basal layer, where new plump, moist cells are produced. These travel upwards and outward and on their journey they encounter various hazards that lose them some of their moisture, making them leaner. It can take three to four months for cells to reach the epidermis, and if you are treating your skin the results may not show for that length of time (although some treatments will make you look younger in about one hour). And of course the reverse is true: damage done by eating the wrong foods, not enough vitamins, or a low immunity, can also take up to four months to show on your skin. When the skin cells reach the outer layer, they fall off and become household dust. Our skin is a living and dying, regenerating organ, forever on the move.

Skin cells are rich in a substance called keratin which also makes up nails, and skin cells, like nails, can become brittle and flaky. Skin is an excretory organ and is constantly at work to throw off toxic waste—not only under the arms, but all over. Perspiration is a method of cooling us down, and so skin regulates our inner temperature. Nerve endings are scattered throughout the skin, some registering pressure, some pain. Skin can tell us the difference between a lover's caress and the boss poking us in the shoulder with his finger! Sebaceous glands are working away to lubricate the skin, and just how hard they are working determines whether you have dry or oily skin. Skin is one big activity center, with hairs growing from their follicles, nerves sending out their messages, toxins being eliminated, temperature checks being taken out, through the capillaries, blood and lymph fluid traveling back and forth. Of vital importance to us in this chapter are the connective tissues—collagen and, to a lesser degree, elastin. These determine how spongy the skin is, or is not.

Essential oils work cosmetically and as antiaging agents in several ways. They stimulate skin cells into reproducing at a quicker rate, thus reducing the time lag between new skin growth and the elimination of old cells (and reversing the process of aging in which this time span is extended). Skin that has been treated with essential oils thus becomes more dynamic and stronger. Essential oils can prevent the congestion of toxins and expedite the elimination of toxic debris by improving the lymphatic flow and general condition of the lymph glands. They improve circulation which aids oxygenation and energizes the dermis by the rate nutrients are fed to it. Some can balance the rate at which sebum is produced by the sebaceous glands, thereby stabilizing a healthy skin condition. As bactericides they neutralize unwanted and unfriendly bacteria, preventing blemished conditions; and as antiinflammatories, they calm sensitive and damaged skin. Since some essential oils contain phyto-hormones they create an equilibrium within our endocrine system which surpasses in effectiveness that produced by any other substance. Their action on the peripheral nerve endings helps to relieve the stress and tension that so often lead directly to an aging skin—you look as worn out as you feel. Collagen and elastin are kept in good condition, and there is some basis to believe also that the nutrients and proteins contained in essential oils actually work as restorative building blocks to these all-important tissue fibers.

One of the most extraordinary aspects of working with essential oils is that a patient who comes to me for treatment of a physical condition, a backache for example, will after six weekly treatments look about ten years younger than he or she did at the beginning of treatment. Partly this is due to the relief showing as the pain lifts. But there is more to it than that. The texture of the skin all over the body, including the face, seems to go through a fundamental change, sometimes so dramatic that it looks as if the person has had a facelift. This phenomenon never ceases to amaze me and I am, again and again, reminded of how comprehensive are the benefits of the essential oils. When treatment is designed specifically for the face, results can be nothing short of miraculous.

The most expensive skin preparations in the world contain essential oils and other natural ingredients as their principal active ingredients but, because the product must be able to endure a long shelf life, they contain chemical preservatives as well. All sorts of chemicals are used in commercial cosmetic preparations and some of them, such as steroids, cause serious problems. In addition, dubious animal products are often included in commercial preparations, and with the seas now being so unhealthy that whole seal populations can be wiped out, it is true to say that when you put a store-bought product on your face, you really don't know what effect it will have. Besides bypassing all these unknown quantities, making and using your own homemade beauty products will save you a great deal of money. Advertising and packaging make store-bought products very expensive, as does the need for the manufacturer and retail outlet to make their profit. But by following the recipes here, you and your skin will be the ones to profit.

Wrinkles and the Aging Skin ◆◆◆◆◆◆◆◆◆◆◆

Age creeps up on us silently. We carry on quite happily, applying our makeup, getting dressed, going out. And then one day, perhaps after a late night, we look in the mirror and see a face that is no longer young.

The shock of growing old has driven many a tormented soul in search of the elixir of youth. Alchemists and philosophers have for centuries been trying to please their aging rulers by coming up with the secret formula that will save them from the inexorable pull of the years. Fortunes have been made by those who claim to stave off the inevitable results of living and growing older. Today, the rich and famous swap the names of cosmetic surgeons or fly to exclusive European clinics where rejuvenation is a specialty. Even stockbrokers take an active interest in wrinkles, because they know that if a company can come up with a formula that works in dispelling—or preventing—them, millions of dollars can be made as millions of people rush to snap up the product.

Behind the scenes of all this frenetic activity, nature's essential oils have been quietly playing their part. Those who fly into London for nonsurgical essential oil facelifts make up a who's who of beauty, and their secret is well kept because there's not much point in looking ten years younger if you are going to tell the whole world about it. The name of the rejuvenation game is to stay ahead of or, perhaps more accurately, stay behind the crowd.

Cellular regeneration is the key to a youthful skin, and essential oils provide a way of doing this which is far more pleasant than the most recent methods which involve using fetal cells. The nutrients and proteins in essential oils help to maintain the mattress-like bounciness of collagen, upon which the outer layers of skin rest, and encourage the regeneration of new cells. The circulation-stimulating properties of the oils oxygenate the blood which in turn energizes the cells, allowing regeneration to take place. Some oils do this particularly well. Other oils such as fennel contain hormonal-like properties, and these encourage the firming of the skin, giving it a more youthful appearance.

While treating yourself with these antiaging oils, it will obviously speed things along if you don't overload the system with yet more toxins that the skin has to work hard to eliminate. Cut out alcohol (a real ager if ever there was one), coffee, tea, sweets, red meats, and all the things that you know clog up your skin cells as well as your digestive system. Is it worth it, you ask? Undoubtedly, yes. If you can cut ten years from your appearance you'll feel ten years younger, have more energy, and even your outlook on life will change.

ANTIAGING ESSENTIAL OILS TO COMBAT WRINKLES

Violet leaf	**Frankincense**
Clary-sage	**Myrrh**
Fennel	**Lemon**
Neroli	**Hyssop**
Rose	**Carrot**
Galbanum	**Oregano**
Lavender	**Orange**
Thyme	**Vervaine**
Patchouli	**Rosemary**
Yarrow	**Palma rosa**
Chamomile German	**Lime**
	RE1*

* See appendix for list of suppliers of this ready-made product.

You can use any of these oils on their own or make combinations of two or more, to suit your needs. Use the oils in a bath, as a face oil, or body rub, and do remember to treat the bit you don't see in the mirror as often as the face—your body!

Because everyone's skin regenerates at a different rate, allow at least thirty days before expecting to see outward signs of improvement.

Later in this section you will find special formulas for face treatments for four age groups and these are combinations of many oils. But even one oil can be a great help in your personal revitalization program. Take, for example, geranium. This is an excellent oil for helping you deal with stress, tiredness, and anxiety over problems—all of which can make you look and feel much older than you are. Geranium oil won't actually get rid of the problems for you in a puff of aromatic smoke, but it will get rid of the anxiety so that you can better deal with the problems. It will also treat the various conditions that can manifest themselves on the skin as a result of difficult emotional experiences—red blotches on the chest, spots on the back, or skin that looks saggy or has flaky patches. In addition, it will reverse the apathy and body droop that often accompany the troubled mind. Use 6 drops of geranium oil in the bath; put 30 drops into 2 tablespoons light nut oil for a face oil; and 30 drops into 2 tablespoons light nut or vegetable oil for a body rub.

You can actually see an improvement after one session. Before bathing, stand naked in front of the mirror and observe the posture and look of your body. Now have a bath to which you have added 6 drops of geranium oil and lie there inhaling deeply for at least five minutes. When you get out rub the geranium body oil over your whole body and stretch in all directions for a few minutes. Now have a look in the mirror again. You'll see a marked improvement already, so imagine the difference if you used this treatment every day.

There is no getting away from the fact that we are all inexorably growing one year older each three hundred and sixty-five days, but the essential oils help to ensure that we don't give the march of time a chance to take us over. The accumulated anxieties of a busy life contribute to a general downward movement as we age. Many difficulties arise from bringing up children, maintaining good relationships, and following a career. Anxieties, however, inhibit the action of the lymphatic system. If we can eradicate anxieties and adopt a positive attitude, the lymphatic system starts to work better and accumulated toxins are cleared through the proper elimination systems of the body. Spots and blemishes disappear, the body uplifts and you find yourself saying "I feel better now." Because you feel better about yourself, both emotionally and physically, you'll look younger —and you'll feel younger because you are better able to relax and cope. Allow a little longer for the bloom to come back to your skin for the revitalization to be complete.

Forget about aging gracefully—in a way that's giving in. Fight it every step of the way. There's no time to begin or end this revitalization program. It may take you a little longer to reach peak potential when you are ninety, but even at that age the essential oils can make you feel and look younger. Clearly, being in good physical condition helps to keep the energy level up as we age and contributes to our ability to remain in control, but as far as looking better is concerned, it is as important to keep the mind young and alert. For this, bergamot is marvelous—it's a stimulating, uplifting, go-getting, forceful oil, as well as an antidepressant.

Now we come to the antiwrinkle facial treatment oils for various age groups. Use them every night on the face and, if you wish, on the neck and chest, as far as the collar bone. (See also the section on the neck, page 133; cleansers, face masks, and steaming treatments on page 119.)

WRINKLE PREVENTATIVE FOR THE OVER-TWENTIES

Neroli	8 drops
Lavender	5 drops
Fennel	5 drops
Chamomile German	3 drops
Geranium	8 drops
Carrot	1 drop

Diluted in 2 tablespoons hazelnut, almond, or apricot kernel oil

ANTIWRINKLE OIL FOR THE OVER-THIRTIES

Yarrow	10 drops
Patchouli	2 drops
Palma rosa	10 drops
Clary-sage	8 drops
Fennel	7 drops
Rose	8 drops
Carrot	5 drops
Borage seed	5 drops
Jojoba	5 drops

Diluted in 2 tablespoons hazelnut, almond, or apricot kernel oil

ANTIWRINKLE OIL FOR THE OVER-FORTIES

Neroli	10 drops
Lavender	10 drops
Frankincense	10 drops
Rosemary	2 drops
Fennel	10 drops
Lemon	3 drops
Carrot	10 drops
Evening primrose	10 drops

Diluted in 2 tablespoons hazelnut, almond, or apricot kernel oil

ANTIWRINKLE OIL FOR THE OVER-FIFTIES

Violet leaf	5 drops
Galbanum	5 drops
Rose	5 drops
Neroli	10 drops
Lavender	3 drops
Myrrh	2 drops
Carrot	10 drops
Bois de rose	10 drops
Evening primrose	10 drops
Borage seed	10 drops

Diluted in 2 tablespoons hazelnut, almond, or apricot kernel oil

Cleansers ◆◆◆◆◆◆◆◆◆◆◆◆◆

There is nothing better than a soft, pure bristle complexion brush for gently cleansing the face. This should be used with a good, gentle cleansing agent—soap, lotion, or cream—which should be rinsed off with pure water. But unfortunately pure bristle brushes take some searching out, absolutely pure and effective cleansers are not as common as they might be, and the water we rinse our faces with has probably been recycled five times, including five journeys through someone else's kidneys!

There isn't a lot we can do about tap water except make sure we use distilled or boiled and filtered water to wash in, but we can do something about the cleansing agents we use. Since the contents of any bottle of store-bought cleanser probably only costs a few pennies and what you are paying for is the packaging, advertising, and image, it makes sense to concoct your own.

The nice thing about making your own cleansers is that you can adjust them to suit your own skin type exactly, and change them as your skin changes with the seasons. In this, we are no different from many types of animal. As cleansing is concerned with the throwing off of toxins, it makes a great deal of difference whether we are cleansing to get rid of the extra perspiration and pollutants that attract to our faces on the muggy summer streets or concerned with the toxins that accumulate in the months of a sedentary life spent indoors munching fattening winter foods while huddled up to the central heating. But cleanse your face according to its seasonal requirements and you will have a skin that always looks good and ages more slowly. (See also Facial Scrubs, Face Masks, and Facial Saunas, pages 118–123.)

All vegetable and nut oils can be used for cleansing as well as for nourishing the skin, and in ancient times and in Arabian countries today, oils provide the usual way of cleansing. The ancient Romans massaged oils into their skin and then scraped them off, along with all the dirt. Use any heavy oil for dry skin, such as avocado or wheatgerm, and a light oil such as almond or sunflower for oily skins. The essential oils of clary-sage, lemon, lime, sage, or thyme are cleansing and suitable for all skin types. Other good options would be rosemary, chamomile, lavender, or geranium.

Here is a good oil-based cleansing paste which can be used for all skin types:

Almond oil	3 ounces
Ground almonds	4 ounces
Cider vinegar	2 ounces
Spring water	2 ounces
Essential oil of your choice	6 drops

Place all the ingredients in a blender and mix for a good two minutes until a smooth paste is obtained. Store in a jar.

These are the ingredients for a multipurpose cleansing oil:

Grapeseed oil	2 ounces
Sunflower oil	4 teaspoons
Sesame oil	4 teaspoons
Wheatgerm oil	1 teaspoons

Blend these oils together and then add 5 drops of the essential oil of your choice, and blend again. This can be used as a makeup remover and cleanser.

Rich Cleansing Cream

This is good for dehydrated skins:

Beeswax	½ ounce
Lanolin hydrous	1 ounce
Almond oil	2 ounces
Avocado oil	1 ounce
Grapeseed oil	1 ounce
Pure spring water	3 ounces
Clary-sage	2 drops
Lemon	2 drops

Using the bain-marie method, melt the beeswax, lanolin, and vegetable oils and stir well. Then add the essential oils and take the pot off the heat and slowly add in the water. Mix in a blender (or whisk) until the mixture is cold.

Cocoa Butter Cleanser

Cocoa butter	3 ounces
Grapeseed oil, warm	1½ ounces
Spring water, warm	1½ ounces

Using the bain-marie method, melt the cocoa butter then add in the spring water and grapeseed oil. Mix in a blender (or whisk) until cold. When the mixture is cold, add:

Rose Maroc	1 drop
Sandalwood	1 drop

Store in a jar.

Almond Face Rinse

This is suitable for all skin types:

Ground almonds	3 ounces
Cornflour	3 ounces
Grated pure vegetable soap	3 ounces

Mix these ingredients in a blender and then add the following and blend again:

Geranium	2 drops
Lemon	2 drops
Hyssop	1 drop

Store dry and use a small amount mixed with water in your hand to wash your face. Rinse well.

Soap Cleanser

Soap stew*	2 ounces
Liquid lecithin	2 ounces
Cider vinegar	1 tablespoon
Essential oil of your choice	10 drops

* See page 157.

Blend the ingredients together, preferably in a blender. Use an essential oil that suits your skin type. Bottle the mixture and store. Each time you want to use it to cleanse your face, pour a small amount into the palm of your hand, massage into your face, and rinse off very well.

Facial Scrubs ◆◆◆◆◆◆◆◆◆

Facial scrubs are used to exfoliate the skin and unplug pores, and they leave the skin looking fresh and dewy as the dead layer of cells is sloughed off. You only need about one teaspoon of the raw material and you can use many foodstuffs as your base: cereals in general make good scrubs—oatmeal, for example—or any pulse like mung beans or dried peas, as well as nuts, almonds, and hazelnuts. So use what you have in the cupboard or were going to buy anyway. Whatever you use should be ground up in a food processor or pestle and mortar so that it forms small, gritty lumps like coarse sand. The starches and enzymes in these cereals, pulses, or nuts will be activated during treatment and get to work on cleansing the face.

Oatmeal is used in many cosmetic products and combined with ground almonds makes an excellent scrub. Mix one teaspoon of each, add 1 drop of essential oil from the skin type list that relates to you on page 392, and roll the mixture over the surface of your skin with damp fingers. Rinse off with warm water.

Basil essential oil is excellent for this type of scrub, as it lifts graying cells and enlivens the skin tone. It is an important ingredient in this rejuvenating face scrub, which is best suited for normal to oily skins:

Ground almonds	1 teaspoon
Oatflakes	1 teaspoon
Salt	1 pinch
Cider vinegar	½ teaspoon
Basil	1 drop

Mix the vinegar, salt, and basil together then add the almonds and oatflakes. Use damp fingers to roll the mixture over the face. Rinse off well.

The skin really needs a spring clean after the long sunless winter months of drying central heating and pollution-laden smog, and this next formula will do a tremendous cleansing job while saving you the money it would cost at an exclusive beauty clinic.

Ground pulse or nut	1 teaspoon
Almond oil	½ teaspoon
Lemon	1 drop

Mix the ingredients together well and pat over your face; leave for thirty seconds. Roll the mixture gently over your face and then rinse away all the dirt, grime, and dead cells with the cleansing mixture. Now splash water on your face twenty times, dry, and feel that soft skin. Apply this scrub twice in one week for the full effect.

Papaya fruit contain enzymes that eat away dead cells and bacteria—just like the enzymes in biological washing powder—and provide a simple but effective treatment for open pores and blackheads. Again, you don't need a great deal so just save a bit from a papaya you would have bought anyway. You'll need one large spoonful of mashed up papaya to which you add 1 drop of bois de rose essential oil. Mix well and spread the mixture over affected areas of your face and neck, avoiding the eyes. Leave for seven minutes and wash off. Do not use on sensitive skin.

Face Masks ◆◆◆◆◆◆◆◆◆◆◆

The beneficial effects of face masks are many. They can nourish, rejuvenate, and stimulate; refine, cleanse, and peel off the outer skin layer; soothe and calm inflammation; clear acne, loosen blackheads; act as an antiwrinkle treatment and natural facelift. In all cases, a face mask improves the color and tone of a face.

The active ingredients of face masks can be contained in all sorts of materials. There are those that dry as hard as board and crack if you smile, there are gels and creams that are as soft as night cream, and a whole range of textures hot or cold. You can use practically any fruit or vegetable in a face mask, and many other edible substances. These days a popular basis of commercial face masks is made from beef, the idea being that the collagen and elastin from the meat fibers will be absorbed into the skin, although there is no proof that this method works.

Flower waters can be used to blend dry ingredients, although I much prefer to use plain spring water as the moisturizing agent plus the essential oils for their therapeutic values, all in a suitable medium. Essential oil face masks have long been used in expensive clinics and face preparations alike, and you can use any essential oil provided that it is suitable for your skin type. The merits of using just one essential oil are many, but if you use a blend of oils, make it a synergistic blend—that is, blended beforehand so that the ingredients have a chance to get together and energize each other. The following basic recipes can be adapted to accommodate your chosen essential oils, but do read the whole section before deciding which particular base mediums would be most suitable to your skin type.

Clays

There are many different types of clay, each of which has a different mineral content and a different effect on the skin. Clays have absorbed the sun and the plant and minerals of the earth over thousands of years and have rejuvenating and antiaging effects on the skin. There are red, yellow, green, white, black, and brown clays from all over the world, and each is a treatment in itself. They all combine beautifully with essential oils and the oil and clay have a synergistic effect upon each other. We will here use only the clays most commonly found in health stores and pharmacies.

WHITE KAOLIN has an astringent effect and removes impurities from the skin while cleansing, improving lymphatic flow and increasing blood circulation to the area. It is best used on normal to oily skins.

FULLER'S EARTH is a soft brown clay which is very stimulating and has a marked effect on the epidermis. It is cleansing and also has a desquamation action—that is, it removes dead cells. It is useful on oily to normal textured skin only.

GREEN CLAY can be used in all sorts of skin conditions and is the finest of the clays. It is good for treating acne and disturbed skins, and for the mature skin as it has an antiaging effect. It can also be used to balance combination skin, normalize oily skin, and revitalize dry skin. It is rich in calcium, magnesium, potassium, and sodium, and it energizes the connective tissue. It is antiseptic and healing and an emollient which leaves the skin silky smooth. It gently stimulates and is effective in increasing the lymph flow and circulation which enables oxygen to speed the elimination of waste products.

The instant face mask that you can squeeze from a tube comes full of all kinds of ingredients and may have been made in a factory under unknown conditions a year or more ago. It cannot be the fresh, pure product the manufacturers no doubt advertise. Now, however, you have another option. A homemade mask will take you no more than a few minutes to put together, and once you have the basic ingredients ready in a jar you can have your own instant face pack ready for use and tailor-made to your own skin type requirements.

Ready-for-Action Mask

This is a purifying, toning, soothing, and rejuvenating mask. The basic ingredients are:

Green clay	**2 ounces**
Cornflour	**3 teaspoons**

Mix together and keep in a jar, ready for combining in one of the formulas below. Or, use 1 tablespoon of this mixture to enough of one of the liquid ingredients below to form a paste, and add your chosen essential oils to this.

Here then are the formulas in which the ready-for-action basic ingredients can be used. Blend the ingredients together to form a smooth paste and leave on the skin for fifteen minutes. Rinse off and apply a facial treatment oil. Dab the face with a tissue.

READY-FOR-ACTION MASK FORMULAS

NORMAL SKIN

Basic mask	1 tablespoon
Egg yolk	1
Water	1 teaspoon

Combine and use 1 drop:

Geranium	2 drops
Bois de rose	1 drop

DRY SKIN

Basic mask	1 tablespoon
Egg yolk	1
Almond or evening primrose oil	1 teaspoon
Carrot oil	2 drops
Water	2 teaspoons

Combine and use 1 drop:

Chamomile	1 drop
Rose	1 drop

OILY SKIN

Basic mask	1 tablespoon
Brewer's yeast	1 tablespoon
Water	1 tablespoon

Combine and use 1 drop:

Rosemary	1 drop
Lavender	1 drop

REVITALIZING MASK
FOR DEHYDRATED SKIN

Basic mask	1 tablespoon
Egg yolk	1
Brewer's yeast	1 teaspoon
Jojoba oil	1 teaspoon
Water	1 tablespoon

Combine and use 1 drop:

Chamomile	1 drop
Carrot	2 drops

ACNE

Basic mask	1 tablespoon
Water	1 teaspoon

Combine and use 1 drop:

Chamomile	1 drop
Lavender	1 drop
Juniper	1 drop
Patchouli	1 drop

Gels

Gels are suitable for all skin types and conditions. Commercially sold gels are usually micro-emulsions—acrylic-based with a transparent look—and these are almost impossible to achieve easily in the kitchen. But there are some excellent gels you can make cheaply and quickly which are extremely effective.

TAPIOCA is a granulated starch extracted from cassava which makes a very good, nourishing face gel full of protein. It's a cooling and soothing demulcent.

Boiling water (or herbal infusion or floral water)	3 ounces
Tapioca	1½ teaspoons

Simmer the water and tapioca together until the tapioca dissolves and becomes transparent. Strain this liquid through the foot of a clean, dry pair of tights or a stocking. The way to do this is to pour the liquid into the stocking leg and then tie the stocking top around a stick which will reach to either side of a pot or bucket enabling the stocking to hang until all the liquid has drained away. When cool, the contents will set into a gel and just before they do so, stir in your essential oils. You will need 5 drops of a single oil or a blend, or for a lighter, everyday gel use 3 drops.

PECTIN is a slightly acidic powder made from the peel of apples or citrus fruits. You can make your own pectin from windfall apples by simmering the peels for thirty minutes, straining, and then continuing the simmering until the liquid forms a concentrate. This will form a gel when it is cool. You can make a floral pectin by using floral waters in the cooking, or an herbal infusion if you prefer. If using a packet of pectin powder, follow the directions until you have the gel.

For every ounce of pectin gel, add 1 teaspoon of almond oil and mix in the blender. Then add your chosen essential oils and mix well.

This makes a very good, acidic, astringent type of gel which is good for oily skins with acne. It is very soothing.

SLIPPERY ELM comes from the inner bark of the tree and is used in herbal medicines and convalescence.

Slippery elm powder	1 ounce
Water	3 ounces

Simmer the ingredients together for at least thirty minutes and then strain. The mixture will thicken on cooling, when you can add 5 drops of your chosen oil—again, choose from the lists on page 392.

This particular gel looks very pretty if you color coordinate it with the essential oil you choose, and it makes a wonderful present for friends. You can use a natural food color with, for example, rose essential oil or geranium, palma rosa, lavender, or lemon. But there's no point in doing this unless you use an absolutely natural coloring product. You can make your own rose-colored water, which you can use in the making of the gel, by infusing deep red rose petals in water, then putting the whole lot in the blender and straining the resulting liquid.

OTHER AGENTS that make gels suitable for cosmetic use are Irish moss (carrageen), agar-agar and other seaweeds, and quince seeds—which when soaked in water produce a clear gel.

Other Ingredients for Face Masks

You can substitute floral water or herbal infusions for plain water used in the making of face masks. Commercial floral waters are the by-products of distillation. If you decide to make a lavender face mask—either gel or clay—you could use a lavender infusion to make the base. Put a handful of lavender flowers in three ounces of boiling water and leave to cool, then strain and use the liquid as you would use the water in the recipe.

All the following ingredients can be incorporated into clay face masks or gels.

Rosewater: toning and soothing
Neroli/orange flower water: stimulating and toning
Witch hazel: can be drying; an astringent
Marigold infusion: moisturizing and soothing effect
Lecithin: high in natural fatty acids and good for all skin types; also moisturizing
Nettle infusion: soothing and antiseptic
Yarrow infusion: antiinflammatory
Aloe vera: contains a healing agent; soothing and calming
Chamomile infusion: antiirritant and soothing
Fennel infusion: antiwrinkle
Honey: soothing, healing, moisturizing

Icelandic Facial Sauna ♦♦♦♦♦♦♦♦♦♦

The steam machine is part of the equipment used in professional beauty treatments. Gentle puffs of steam are directed at your face, opening pores and causing you to perspire, thus releasing dirt and trapped toxins and debris from the skin. You shouldn't have a steam treatment—either professional or at home—if you have broken veins, hypersensitive skin, or inflammation of any sort including sunburn.

Steam treatments are extremely easy to do at home—all you need is a bowl of boiling water and a towel. Put your chosen essential oils on the surface of the water and cover your head with the towel, making sure that the sides are closed. You'll need to come up for air every so often, but basically plan to be under the towel for about five minutes.

This method is extremely helpful for all kinds of seborrhea and acne problem skins, as well as being regenerating for the more mature type of skin. For normal skins, a facial sauna can often increase tonality and improve the texture of the skin. These are the best oils to use for these four skin types:

NORMAL

Fennel	**Lavender**
Lemon	**Neroli**

Use 2 drops on a bowl of steaming water

DRY

Chamomile Roman or **Chamomile German**	**Rose**
	Palma rosa
	Bois de rose

Use 2 drops on a bowl of steaming water

SEBORRHEA

Clary-sage	**Juniper**
Thyme linalol	**Grapefruit**

Use 2 drops on a bowl of steaming water

ACNE

Chamomile Roman or **Chamomile German**	**Clary-sage**
	Thyme linalol
	Lavender

Use 2 drops on a bowl of steaming water

Follow the steam treatment by splashing the face with lots of cold water.

All skins benefit in terms of their tone by the ice treatment: freeze water in a Styrofoam cup and then cut the sides of the cup down by about an inch. Use this to massage in upward movements over the face. Finish the treatment by using one of the facial oils to suit your skin type.

Tonics and Astringents ♦♦♦♦♦♦♦♦♦♦♦

Tonics stimulate the circulation, reduce oiliness, and help refine open pores and unevenly textured skin. They are usually applied after cleansing to ensure complete removal of any residue left from creams or lotions. A skin tonic has a much milder effect than an astringent and should also refine the skin texture. An astringent, on the other hand, is stimulating to the whole skin system but can be drying and should only be used on oily or open-pored types of skin. Astringents should not be used on blemishes or acne as they can exacerbate the condition. Acne needs much gentler handling. Seborrhea and other skin blemish conditions need a treatment tonic that heals as well as correcting the balance of the skin.

Essential oils used in tonics and astringents are very effective, although they are not easy to blend without a dispersing agent and should always be shaken before use.

The method of making the following tonics and astringents is the same for all. Put all the ingredients in a bottle and shake well. Leave for twenty-four hours then pass through a paper coffee filter. Rebottle and use as needed after cleansing, or just to freshen up.

Cotton-wool balls can be soaked in your tonic and then separated into thinner sections before being put in a tightly sealed box with another teaspoon of tonic passed over them. Hey presto—you have your own brand of instant freshen-up, cleansing pads.

Tonics

Rosewater provides the perfect base for a skin tonic, as does any infusion of flowers or herbs. Cornflower, for example, is a decongestant and antiinflammatory that is soothing to both skin and eyelids.

NORMAL TO DRY SKIN

Rosewater	3 ounces
Sandalwood	1 drop
Palma rosa	1 drop

NORMAL TO OILY SKIN

Orange flower water	3 ounces
Neroli	1 drop
Orange	1 drop

NORMAL TO SENSITIVE SKIN

Chamomile infusion	3 ounces
Chamomile German	1 drop

BLEMISHED SKIN

Lavender water	3 ounces
Lavender	1 drop
Juniper	1 drop

Astringents

GENERAL

Witch hazel	1 ounce
Orange flower water	3 ounces
Cider vinegar	1 teaspoon
Juniper	2 drops
Lime oil	1 drop
Grapefruit	1 drop

STIMULATING

Witch hazel	1 ounce
Rose water	3 ounces
Cider vinegar	1 teaspoon
Basil	2 drops
Peppermint	1 drop
Chamomile blue	1 drop

VINEGAR

Spring water	2 ounces
Orange water	1 ounce
White wine vinegar	1 ounce
Palma rosa	2 drops
Peppermint	1 drop

Face Oils ♦♦♦♦♦♦♦♦♦♦♦♦♦

Essential oils make marvelous face oils. In this section treatments are given for three types of skin and, in general, you need 30 drops of essential oil for each 2 tablespoons base oil, unless specified. If you want a more intensive treatment, use 45 drops of essential oil.

Combination skin is a patchwork of normal, oily, and dry skin with the oily patches usually occurring on the forehead, nose, and chin, and these are often accompanied by blackheads. Treat combination skin as normal skin, and if oily patches are a problem use the face oils for oily skin on those areas. As the skin starts to balance you can adjust the treatment accordingly. Our skins can change quite rapidly, so do take notice of the changes and be ready to switch oils.

Normal Skin

Really, there is no such thing as normal skin. Or, more correctly, children have normal skin and the rest of us aspire to it!

The perfect skin of prepuberty is plump, in the sense that the cells are plump, neither dry nor oily, firm and solid, finely textured with no visible pores, spots, or blemishes, soft and velvety to the touch, and unwrinkled. Adults can only yearn for this perfection, and we call skin "normal" if it reaches somewhere near it—about halfway is good enough. The term "normal" is so inappropriate in this context that I prefer to call this type of skin "evenly balanced."

If you have skin that falls into this category you could use almost any essential oil in your skin preparations, but you should stick to the gentle or even the sensitive type of oils to ensure that your skin remains near perfect.

EVENLY BALANCED SKIN OIL BASES

Almond	**Apricot kernel**
Hazelnut	

ADDITIONS TO BASE OIL

Evening primrose	**Jojoba**
Carrot	**Borage seed**

ESSENTIAL OILS FOR EVENLY BALANCED SKIN

Chamomile German	**Lemon**
Geranium	**Fennel**
Lavender	**Jasmine**
Rose	**Bois de rose**
Neroli	**Frankincense**
Palma rosa	**Benzoin**

DAY MOISTURIZER FOR EVENLY BALANCED SKIN

Rose	15 drops
Chamomile German	5 drops
Lavender	5 drops
Lemon	5 drops

Diluted in 2 tablespoons almond or hazelnut oil

This moisturizer should be applied to damp skin. Massage it in and then dab the face with a tissue until no excess oil shows on the tissue.

NIGHT CARE OIL, FOR EVENLY BALANCED SKIN

Geranium	10 drops
Palma rosa	10 drops
Fennel	5 drops
Lemon	5 drops

Dilute in 2 tablespoons apricot kernel oil to which you have added 10 drops of evening primrose oil

If you feel that your skin needs extra nourishment, add 5 drops of carrot oil.

Dry to Normal Skin

When the sebaceous glands are not producing enough oil to keep the skin soft and supple it can become dry, prone to wrinkles, less supple, and flakiness may occur. In time it can become sensitive and prone to inflammation, and dehydrated easily by central heating, wind, and sun. This type of skin is prone to peeling and itching during periods of stress. It generally feels taut after washing. Sometimes dry skin is caused by menopause and hormonal changes.

The outer layer of skin is not hydrated from the moisture that surrounds all human cells, interstitial fluid, because there is an impervious barrier between the outer layer of skin and those layers below, and the outer layer of skin is in fact dead and without the usual interstitial fluid of all other human cells. Nor, surprisingly perhaps, is it hydrated by the action of sebaceous glands. Rather, the fat produced by the sebaceous glands acts as a trap for the imperceptible and the visible perspiration which lubricates the outer layer of skin. If there is not enough fat being produced, the perspiration evaporates too quickly, leaving the skin too dry.

DRY TO NORMAL SKIN
OIL BASES

Almond	**Olive oil**
Avocado	**Apricot kernel**
Wheatgerm	**Soya bean**

ADDITIONS TO BASE OIL

Jojoba	**Evening primrose**
Borage seed	**Carrot**

ESSENTIAL OILS FOR
DRY TO NORMAL SKIN

Chamomile German	**Hyssop**
	Benzoin
Lavender	**Calendula**
Sandalwood	**Geranium**
Patchouli	**Palma rosa**
Rose	**Rosemary**
Bois de rose	**Neroli**

DAY RE-MOISTURIZING OIL FOR
DRY TO NORMAL SKIN

Chamomile German	15 drops
Sandalwood	5 drops
Bois de rose	5 drops
Hyssop	5 drops

Dilute in 2 tablespoons of the base vegetable oil to which you have added 10 drops of evening primrose and 2 drops of carrot oil

Use in the same way as you would your usual moisturizing cream or lotion.

NIGHT OIL TREATMENT FOR
DRY TO NORMAL SKIN

Blend the base oil:

Soya bean	2 teaspoons
Avocado	2 teaspoons
Wheatgerm	2 teaspoons
Jojoba	30 drops
Borage seed	10 drops
Evening primrose	20 drops

then add

Carrot	10 drops
Hyssop	5 drops
Rosemary	5 drops
Chamomile German	10 drops
Benzoin	10 drops
Geranium	15 drops

and blend again

This makes an extremely rich night oil. Massage a small amount into the skin, leave it for a while and then wipe off the excess with a tissue.

Oily to Normal Skin

Oily skin is caused by overactive sebaceous glands. These are subject to hormonal changes which is why oily skin can become a problem during puberty. Overactive sebaceous glands can lead to seborrhea but more often the problem occurs as oily patches which leave the skin shining. Ironically, this condition often results from over-cleanliness—specifically, scrubbing the face with harsh cleansers and soaps or using astringents that contain alcohol. Many commercial lotions which are designed to degrease a skin actually cause the sebaceous glands to produce more fat to compensate for the lack of it that results. This same vicious circle can apply to hair preparations. Thankfully, the essential oils have the capacity to balance the skin without making the glands produce more sebum and can provide the perfect solution to these sometimes intractable problems.

OILY TO NORMAL SKIN OIL BASES

Almond	**Apricot kernel**
Hazelnut	**Grapeseed**

ADDITIONS TO BASE OIL

Borage seed	**Carrot**
Evening primrose	

ESSENTIAL OILS FOR
OILY TO NORMAL SKIN

Chamomile German	**Lavender**
	Geranium
Juniper	**Cypress**
Palma rosa	**Pettigraine**
Lemon	**Marjoram**
Lime	**Rosemary**
Orange	**Jasmine**
Frankincense	**Ylang-ylang**

DAY BALANCER FOR
OILY TO NORMAL SKIN

Juniper	8 drops
Geranium	10 drops
Lemon	10 drops
Rosemary	2 drops

Dilute in 2 tablespoons hazelnut oil to which you have added 10 drops of carrot oil

Massage the oil in and then dab the face with a tissue until no excess oil shows there.

NIGHT TREATMENT FOR
OILY TO NORMAL SKIN

Juniper	10 drops
Pettigraine	15 drops
Frankincense	5 drops
Marjoram	5 drops
Lemon	10 drops

Dilute in 2 tablespoons apricot kernel oil to which you have added 10 drops carrot oil

Problem Skin ♦♦♦♦♦♦♦♦♦

Broken Capillaries

The very finest branches of the blood vessel system that serve the face can sometimes become broken. Usually the problem is concentrated on the cheeks although the whole face can be affected. Broken capillaries seem to affect those with delicate and fragile skin, although this may in part be due to the fact that they just show more clearly than in thicker skin. Stimulants such as alcohol, coffee, sun, and wind are often the cause. These are the oils to use for their treatment:

BASE OILS

Almond	**Avocado**
Apricot	**Wheatgerm**

ADDITIONS TO BASE

Borage seed	**Carrot**
Evening primrose	

ESSENTIAL OILS

Parsley	**Chamomile German**
Geranium	
Cypress	

When making your own treatment oil or following the formula below, mix the essential oils together first and allow them to interact with each other to make a synergistic effect before adding to the base oil:

TREATMENT OIL FOR
BROKEN CAPILLARIES

Parsley	20 drops
Geranium	10 drops
Cypress	5 drops

Dilute in 2 tablespoons almond oil to which you have added 10 drops of evening primrose

Whiteheads (Milia)

When sebum gets trapped in a duct that has no opening on the surface a hard white lump appears. Milia usually affect dry skin and they can also appear after some damage has been done to the skin. Unfortunately, if you have had these for some time they will need to be removed by a beautician. But recently formed milia can be dispersed by massage. Use the following:

Bergamot	5 drops
Thyme linalol	5 drops

Diluted in 1 tablespoon vegetable oil

Use a very small amount of the oil to massage the milia twice a day, in the morning and at night. This will allow the milia to be reabsorbed by the body.

Blackheads (Comedones)

Blocked sebum becomes a blackhead when the surface cells develop sulphides which, in contact with the oxygen, turn the cells black. The main problem with blackheads, apart from their unsightliness, is that they can become infected when removed and the opening just gets filled up once again with more sebum. This condition is related to seborrhea, overproduction of the sebaceous glands. But even a dry-skinned person can develop blackheads, especially on the nose or chin. Blackheads can appear practically anywhere on the body, as well as on the face. A major culprit area is the back, but they can also be found on the chest, under arms, neck, and even around the pubic area. Wherever they are to be found, the treatment for blackheads is the same—they need removing.

Steaming provides an excellent way to loosen blackheads while the pores are opened. Get a bowl of hot, steaming water, put 1 drop of lavender oil on the water and cover your head with a towel, making sure the sides are closed, and steam your face for ten minutes. Rinse the face now with 1 teaspoon of cider vinegar in hot—but not boiling—water. If the blackhead is loose, gently squeeze, taking care not to damage the skin. Then splash the face with this special mix:

Mineral water	2 ounces
Cider vinegar	2 teaspoons
Witch hazel	1 teaspoon
Bergamot	2 drops
Cypress	2 drops

After dabbing the skin dry, massage the following oil into the skin. This will help prevent blackheads recurring while also loosening the ones that are already established:

Violet leaf	5 drops
Lemongrass	5 drops
Lavender	2 drops
Clary-sage	2 drops
Thyme linalol	5 drops
Jojoba oil	5 drops

Diluted in 2 tablespoons almond oil

Massage morning and night; use only pure soap; use eye makeup if you wish but avoid face makeup and powder.

Spots

Have you ever noticed how spots seem to break out when they are least wanted?

I know a woman who didn't have a single blemish on her skin until the day she married, when a big spot appeared on the end of her nose! A spot can only "know" when it will be least welcome if it's picking up signals from us, so instead of expressing negative fear—"I hope I won't get a spot on my big date"—try some positive certainty: "My skin is going to look great." If you already have a spot or one that's on its way, apply the formula below while saying, "This spot is going to go"—and try to believe it!

Just smear a little of the Spot Mix neat on the troubled area of the skin twice a day. Allow three days for the spot to clear.

SPOT MIX

Camphor	1 drop
Lemon	1 drop
Lavender	1 drop

Blend in 6 drops evening primrose oil

Small quantities of essential oil like this can be mixed in, and used from, an eggcup. If you are going to need larger quantities mix the three component oils in equal proportions in a bottle where a synergistic interaction between the molecules can take place, so that they are even more potent when you come to use them.

Acne

Beauty is more than skin deep, but it can be hard for you—and other people—to remember that when you have acne. What you more usually see is an oily skin with a profusion of blackheads and pustules (spots) and sometimes too, scarring, pitting, and inflammation. Acne occurs not only on the face, but on the neck, back, and chest as well. Secondary infection by bacteria, usually strephylococcal, causes even more problems. Not only is acne unsightly, it is painful as well. The temptation to squeeze the spots and remove the infected pus is great, and although the hope might be to improve the look of the skin, it only makes matters worse. Not only does it cause scarring, but the pus can infect other areas of the skin in the process. This is how one comes by the familiar pitted skin that invariably lasts throughout adulthood.

Although acne is very often a problem that starts with puberty, it can appear at any time. I have had patients who developed the problem in their thirties, as well as those in their twenties. Acne is often the result of seborrhea—overproduction of fat from the sebaceous glands—and this can be traced back to a hormonal imbalance. It is thought that too much of the male hormone androgen is produced. Women too experience hormonal-related acne, usually around the time of premenstrual syndrome.

Essential oil treatments combined with a sensible diet, exercise, and fresh air often clear up the problem. Lymphatic flow is increased, allowing toxic wastes to be taken away, and the circulation is improved, which allows oxygen and nutrients to reach the skin in greater quantity. The bactericide and antiinflammatory properties of essential oils are obviously extremely useful in helping the healing process. The relaxant properties of essential oils also play their part as stress is a precursor of increased sebum production.

Stimulants should be avoided. Smoking can aggravate the condition, as can alcohol, coffee, tea, and even chocolate. It is not the fattening aspect of chocolate that concerns us here but the chemical stimulants it contains, especially phenylethylamine and theobromine that imitate our hormones; and the caffeine and sugar chocolate contains make it doubly bad for acne. For some people, cutting out dairy products, especially cream and hard cheese, helps enormously. Fruits, surprisingly perhaps, do not help acne because of their high sugar content, but vegetables do. Antibiotics are often prescribed for acne but they only treat the symptoms temporarily, and as they kill off the friendly intestinal bacteria we need to digest and eliminate toxins efficiently, they can make matters worse in the long run. Retin A is used with great success, as is vitamin A. You can of course take advantage of this simply by applying carrot oil, an extremely rich source of beta carotene and a natural source of vitamin A.

The treatment that follows comes in three stages and these are the oils to use:

BASE OILS

Almond	**Borage seed**
Evening primrose	

STAGE ONE OILS

Chamomile German	**Myrrh**
	Rose
Chamomile Roman	**Palma rosa**
	Carrot
Yarrow	

STAGE TWO OILS

Bergamot	**Tea tree**
Calendula	**Clary-sage**
Lavender	**Thyme linalol**
Eucalyptus radiata	**Geranium**

STAGE THREE OILS

Neroli	**Parsley**
Fennel	**Violet leaf**
Juniper	**Galbanum**
Lemon	**Carrot**
Rose	**Lavender**
Orange	**Geranium**

STAGE ONE is to promote healing, reduce inflammation, and gently start to correct the imbalance of sebum production. This is done by using a routine over fourteen days, and it will take patience and more time for the acne to heal completely.

Use no harsh products—for cleaning the face use pure soap only and rinse at least twenty-five times with the tap running. Use warm water, not hot or cold. In the final rinse water put 2 tablespoons of cider vinegar, then pat the skin dry. During the day, wear the following oil. Do not wear any facial makeup whatsoever, nor any special coverups. Just the oil:

STAGE ONE:
DAY TREATMENT

Chamomile German	10 drops
Myrrh	3 drops
Palma rosa	10 drops
Yarrow	5 drops
Chamomile Roman	7 drops
Carrot	20 drops

Diluted in 2 tablespoons almond oil

The carrot oil is bright orange and when on the skin gives you a healthy look. Leave the oil to soak into the skin for five minutes and then dab off the excess with a tissue.

In the evening, after cleansing and rinsing, rub 5 drops of neat night oil number one over the whole of the affected area and then apply a coating of night oil number two to the area. Leave this in place for five minutes and then wipe off the excess. Do not use any other cream, lotion, or potion.

NIGHT OIL NUMBER ONE

Carrot oil	30 drops
Borage seed	60 drops
Chamomile German	5 drops

Blend together and use 5 drops each evening

NIGHT OIL NUMBER TWO

Rose	10 drops
Palma rosa	10 drops
Chamomile Roman	5 drops
Myrrh	5 drops

Diluted in 2 tablespoons base oil

During these fourteen days get into the fresh air as much as possible. Eat only "live" food—fresh vegetables, fruit in moderation, grains, pulses, carbohydrates, and fish. Drink herbal teas and plenty of mineral water. All additives and preservatives and the like must be avoided. Avoid any red meat or white that contains traces of antibiotics and hormones—which unless you have access to organically bred meats, means cut them all out. Increase your zinc with a supplement and increase your vitamins C and B intake. Use no face masks or steam treatments during this time.

STAGE TWO is to fight infection and continue the rebalancing program. Cleanse as before only this time make up a bottle that contains the following ingredients and use 1 teaspoon in the final rinse, patting dry afterwards.

Cider vinegar	4 ounces
Lavender	20 drops
Eucalyptus radiata	20 drops

Depending on the time of the day, use the appropriate oil below:

STAGE TWO:
DAY TREATMENT

Eucalyptus radiata	5 drops
Clary-sage	5 drops
Thyme linalol	5 drops
Lavender	15 drops
Carrot	5 drops

Diluted in 3 tablespoons almond oil

Leave the oil to soak into the skin for five minutes and then wipe off the excess with a tissue.

STAGE TWO:
NIGHT TREATMENT

Evening primrose	30 drops
Carrot	20 drops
Bergamot	10 drops
Lavender	5 drops
Geranium	5 drops
Eucalyptus radiata	10 drops

Diluted in 3 tablespoons almond oil

Leave the oil to soak into the skin for five minutes and then wipe off the excess.

Follow the dietary advice outlined in stage one and continue stage two treatment for fourteen days.

STAGE THREE is the last stage of the battle and by now your skin may look so much better you decide not to continue the treatment. But if you want to see further improvements, continue you must for another fourteen days. Use the cleansing rinse outlined in stage two, both morning and night, pat the face dry, and use the relevant day or night treatments below:

STAGE THREE:
DAY TREATMENT

Neroli	10 drops
Fennel	5 drops
Geranium	5 drops
Parsley	5 drops
Lemon	5 drops

Diluted in 3 tablespoons almond oil

Leave the oil to soak into the skin for five minutes and then wipe off the excess.

STAGE THREE:
NIGHT TREATMENT

Rose	10 drops
Violet leaf	8 drops
Carrot	10 drops
Galbanum	4 drops
Lemon	8 drops

Diluted in 3 tablespoons almond oil

When the six weeks are up continue to use the essential oils, choosing from those in the oily skin sections. Use only one hundred percent pure soaps and avoid harsh acne preparations.

Rosacea

Rosacea is often mistaken for acne because it is very similar and, like acne, it is associated with excessive oiliness. This condition seldom affects anyone under thirty years of age and it can be very distressing when it develops. Usually, the nose and cheeks are the worst affected areas, and these become flushed red in appearance as spots (pustules) and lumps cover the skin. The treatment is similar to that for acne, except that the essential oils used are different. Follow the dietary and vitamin intake advice in the "Acne" section and carry out the cleansing and rinsing routine given there.

Treatment comes in two stages, each of fourteen days.

ESSENTIAL OILS TO TREAT ROSACEA

STAGE ONE	STAGE TWO
Chamomile German	**Violet leaf**
Yarrow	**Cypress**
Carrot	**Geranium**
Parsley	**Hyssop**
Galbanum	**Eucalyptus radiata**

Follow the instructions for acne, stage one, but using the following formulas:

STAGE ONE:
DAY TREATMENT

Chamomile German	15 drops
Parsley	15 drops

Diluted in 3 tablespoons almond oil

STAGE ONE:
NIGHT TREATMENT

Galbanum	5 drops
Carrot	15 drops
Chamomile German	10 drops
Parsley	15 drops

Diluted in 3 tablespoons almond oil

After fourteen days, follow the instructions for acne, stage two, using the following formulas:

STAGE TWO:
DAY TREATMENT

Cypress	15 drops
Geranium	15 drops

Diluted in 3 tablespoons almond oil

STAGE TWO:
NIGHT TREATMENT

Violet leaf	10 drops
Hyssop	5 drops
Eucalyptus radiata	15 drops

Diluted in 3 tablespoons almond oil

Puffiness or Hydrated Skin

When skin has a spongy texture it usually means that it has become waterlogged. This retention of water by the body may be related to the menstrual cycle, the result of a previous illness, or a reaction to certain drugs. Allergies, hay fever, and sinus problems can all lead to puffy eyes and face. Puffiness can also be a sign of illness, and is one of the first signs of an oedemic condition. Use these oils:

BASE OILS

Almond	**Apricot**

ADDITIONS TO BASE

Carrot	**Evening primrose**

ESSENTIAL OILS
TO TREAT HYDRATED SKIN

Lemon	**Palma rosa**
Juniper	**Patchouli**
Lavender	**Fennel**
Sandalwood	**Rose**
Hyssop	**Cypress**

DAY BALANCING OIL
FOR HYDRATED SKIN

Lavender	10 drops
Sandalwood	5 drops
Fennel	10 drops
Cypress	5 drops

Diluted in 3 tablespoons almond oil

NIGHT OIL FOR HYDRATED SKIN

Carrot	5 drops
Juniper	5 drops
Patchouli	5 drops
Rose	10 drops
Sandalwood	10 drops

Diluted in 3 tablespoons apricot kernel oil

The Neck ♦♦♦♦♦♦♦♦♦♦♦♦

I once heard a cosmetician tell an audience of women that it is no good taking care of the face as if it were a rose if the stalk cannot support it. We all know what she was talking about. The neck is one of the first parts of the body to show its age, with crinkled skin and wrinkles, loss of elasticity, and double chins. All lead to an older look, no matter what effort is put into preserving the good looks of the face. And covering the problem with a scarf is not the ideal solution. Thankfully for many, the neck responds very well to essential oil treatments, cleansing and oiling especially.

ESSENTIAL OILS
FOR USE IN NECK CARE

Rose	**Lemon**
Palma rosa	**Lemongrass**
Geranium	**Black pepper**
Clary-sage	**Basil**
Pettigraine (lemon)	**Carrot**
Pettigraine (orange)	**Orange**
	Vetiver

BASE OILS

Jojoba	**Borage**
Evening primrose	**Avocado**
	Wheatgerm

The neck area is very delicate and should be cleansed with the same quality of preparation that you use on your face. You can simply add 1 drop of one of the above essential oils to each ¾ teaspoon of your usual cleansing cream. Each night apply the following oil, leave it for a few minutes and then wipe off the excess with a tissue:

NECK NIGHT OIL

Pettigraine (orange)	8 drops
Orange	3 drops

Carrot	10 drops
Palma rosa	14 drops
Lemon	5 drops
add to	
Jojoba oil	3 teaspoons
Wheatgerm oil	2 teaspoons
Avocado oil	2 teaspoons
blended well	

For special treatments use 5 drops of the following synergistic blend of oils to 1 teaspoon of evening primrose oil, as and when needed. Massage it well into the skin and leave it there for at least ten minutes before wiping off the excess:

NECK SPECIAL TREATMENT
SYNERGISTIC BLEND

Rose	10 drops
Clary-sage	7 drops
Lemon	10 drops
Carrot	20 drops
Blend together in these proportions	

Necks can get very grubby-looking, perhaps after a suntan has worn off or through wearing high-necked clothes in winter. Sloughing off the dead skin cells is an excellent way to brighten up and tone the neck and prepare it for a treatment oil. Use the following:

Ground almond	1 teaspoon
Jojoba oil	½ teaspoon

Mix the above into a paste and rub it all over the neck in upward movements. Don't forget the chest area. Rinse it off with the vinegar tonic water that follows:

Cider vinegar	¼ teaspoon
Spring water	1 tablespoon
Witch hazel	1 teaspoon
Lemon	2 drops

Mix the lemon essential oil with the witch hazel and then blend with the other ingredients, as far as is possible. Add to the final rinse water and wash the face until all trace of the almond paste has gone.

The Eyes ◆◆◆◆◆◆◆◆◆◆◆◆◆

The eyes are said to be the seat of the soul. Certainly, we spend enough on making them look attractive: at the time of writing, in the United States alone, millions of dollars are spent each year on eye makeup. But no amount of mascara or eyeliner can hide the problems that afflict the very delicate skin that surrounds the eye, and crow's feet wrinkles, creased skin, bags under the eyes, and darkening around the whole area can depress even the brightest of souls!

With regular use, essential oils applied around the eyes can diminish the creasing and smooth out the tiny cracks and crevices. The skin around the eyes, however, is extremely fragile and it is important only to use the lightest of base oils and the minimum of essential oils. Please note that if any oil gets into the eye, flush it out immediately with water.

Use the oil relevant to your age group.

OILS FOR AROUND THE EYES

EIGHTEEN TO TWENTY-FIVE YEARS

Hazelnut oil	2 teaspoons
Borage seed oil	2 drops
Chamomile German	1 drop
Carrot oil	1 drops

TWENTY-FIVE TO FORTY YEARS

Hazelnut oil	2 teaspoons
Borage seed	2 drops

Evening primrose	3 drops
Lavender	2 drops
Lemon	1 drop
Vitamin E	1 capsule*
Carrot	2 drops

*1 capsule = 250 IUs

FORTY TO FORTY-FIVE YEARS

Hazelnut oil	2 teaspoons
Evening primrose	6 drops
Borage seed	3 drops
Palma rosa	2 drops
Lavender	2 drops
Vitamin E	1 capsule*
Carrot	3 drops

*1 capsule = 250 IUs

MATURE YEARS

Hazelnut oil	2 teaspoons
Jojoba oil	5 drops
Vitamin E	2 capsules*
Lavender	1 drop
Lemon	1 drop
Bois de rose	1 drop
Carrot	3 drops

*1 capsule = 250 IUs

Mix the ingredients together well and use the lightest amount around the eye area. Weight around the eye area causes it to sag—and that applies to all oils and creams. Leave the oil for a few minutes and then very gently wipe off the excess. Apply the oil every night.

To treat puffy eyes and dark shadows around the eyes, these are the ingredients you need:

Hazelnut oil	2 teaspoons
Witch hazel	1 tablespoon
Fennel	2 drops
Chamomile German	2 drops

First, dissolve the essential oils as far as possible in ice cold witch hazel, and place it in the fridge. Wrap an ice cube in a cotton-wool ball (the shape and weight of an ice cube made in the plastic bags which you can now buy for the purpose is ideal, although "cube" is a misnomer here), dip it in the essential oil and witch hazel mixture and place it over your closed eye and the puffy area. Leave it in place for a few seconds and then, while the skin is still wet, apply a small quantity of hazelnut oil to the area.

Tired eyes benefit from a dabbing with a cold rosehip or green tea. Make up the tea and keep it in the fridge and just dab it around the eyes when they feel that they need it.

You can make up your own eye oil, bearing in mind the information that has gone before, using the following oils. It would be ideal to use this while you are giving yourself a face mask treatment, for your eyes will be closed and relaxing, and you can lie down and take it completely easy for five minutes or so. Apply the oil only around the eye area, not on the eyelids.

ESSENTIAL OILS
FOR AROUND THE EYE AREA

Chamomile German	**Carrot**
	Lemon
Lavender	**Palma rosa**
Fennel	**Rose**

BASE OILS

Hazelnut	**Almond**

ADDITIONS TO BASE

Jojoba	**Borage seed**
Evening primrose	

The Lips ◆◆◆◆◆◆◆◆◆◆◆◆◆

Lips are for kissing and should always be looking their best, ready for what they were designed for. Unfortunately, they can crack, become infected, line, and be the site of a herpes virus reaction.

A lined mouth is not particularly attractive on either a man or a woman. And it can be avoided. Nothing is more irritating than dry cracked lips, whether from ill health, too much sun, or cold. Here is an alternative to the petroleum or animal fat based products which are the generally available commercial option:

PROTECTIVE LIP GLOSS BASE

White beeswax	1 ounce
Sweet almond oil	2 tablespoons
Jojoba oil	10 drops
Carrot oil	5 drops
Vitamin E (optional)	1 capsule*

*1 capsule = 250 IUs

LIP GLOSS ESSENTIAL OILS

Geranium	**Palma rosa**
Lavender	**Lemon**
Chamomile German	**Rose**

Use the bain-marie method, melt the beeswax and then add the almond oil, stirring all the time. Then add the jojoba oil, carrot oil, and vitamin E, and stir again. Finally, mix in the 10 drops of your chosen essential oils taken from the list above, or following these recommendations:

FOR DRY, CRACKED LIPS

Geranium	5 drops
Lavender	5 drops

FOR SORE LIPS

Chamomile German	5 drops
Calendula	5 drops

If you have a cold sore around the lips, make up the following synergistic blend and add 20 drops to the lip gloss base, and use three times per day. Alternatively, dip a cotton ball into water, put 1 drop of the synergistic blend onto it and apply it directly to the cold sore once a day:

HERPES COLD SORE ON LIPS SYNERGISTIC BLEND

Geranium	8 drops
Lemon	3 drops
Chamomile German	6 drops
Tea tree	8 drops
Lavender	5 drops

Mixed together in these proportions

Teeth and Gums ◆◆◆◆◆◆

If you want to see healthy teeth and gums, go to parts of Africa where there isn't a tube of toothpaste in sight. Traditionally, certain sticks and rock salt have provided mankind with a most effective dental cleansing treatment. Today, the essential oils can provide a natural alternative to commercial products. Of course, it helps if you keep off the sweet things.

A tooth powder can be made from the following ingredients:

Clay	4 teaspoons
Salt	1 teaspoon
Peppermint	2 drops
Lemon	2 drops

Green or white clay work equally well. Mix

these together in a blender and keep in a box. Dip your toothbrush into the powder and wet with a tiny bit of water before brushing the teeth as normal.

Myrrh has been used for treating mouth problems for a very long time indeed. It is marvelous for keeping gums healthy and treating those that are not. A mouthwash can be made by adding 2 drops of essential oil of myrrh to 1 tablespoon of vodka and mixing well. Add only 2 drops of this to each glass of water you use to rinse the mouth.

Here is a recipe for a tooth powder based on a very old Swiss method. It helps to keep the teeth white:

SWISS "SNOW CAPS" TOOTH POWDER

Ground, dried orange peel	1 tablespoon
Ground, dried sage	2 teaspoons
Bicarbonate of soda	2 teaspoons
Salt	1 teaspoon
Lemon	5 drops
Peppermint	1 drop

If you are having gum problems add to the above ingredients 15 drops of tincture of myrrh (available from the pharmacist) into which you have added 1 drop of myrrh essential oil. Mix it all together well in the blender.

♦ CHAPTER 7 ♦

THE BODY BEAUTIFUL

EVER SINCE cosmetic history came to be recorded oils have featured high on the list of ingredients used. All the beauties of history used oils: first vegetable oils with a maceration of flowers and herbs and then, as distillation was invented, essential oils as these became available.

Oils leave a golden gleam on the skin which no other substance can reproduce and used regularly they give the skin a sheen which catches the light and makes heads turn. Forget about artificial body gleamers—next to the real thing they pale.

There is so much choice with both base and essential oils that you will be able to find a perfect combination that not only moisturizes your skin and makes it look and feel great, but that appeals to your nose and aesthetic judgment. The essential oils give great delight when used for pampering the body, and you can rest assured that their naturalness will be doing you nothing but good all around.

Make up your body oils using 5 drops of essential oil to 1 teaspoon of base vegetable oil. Good base oils to use are almond, grapeseed, and apricot kernel, or the rather less exotic soya bean, safflower, and sunflower. Olive oil, sesame, wheatgerm, and avocado oils have a rather strong smell and are best used as part of a base oil blend. Other good additions are evening primrose, jojoba, and carrot oil. One of my favorite body oils consists of the two base oils, almond and evening primrose, plus the essential oils of chamomile German, geranium, and lavender. You can make your body oil as simple or as complicated as you like. Wonderful oils can be made using just one essential oil or with a combination of five—the choice is yours.

It's a nice idea to aroma-coordinate the oils you use in the bath with those in your body oil, but any of the citrus oils will combine aromatically very well with most blends if you just want to add a single oil to your bath. Put 4–6 drops of essential oil in baths.

Here then are the essential oils best suited to four different skin types and a suggested synergistic blend for each type that can be used for both body oil and bath.

Baths and Bubbles ◆◆◆◆

There are four ways to use essential oils in the bath. First, of course, they can just be added neat and undiluted to the water. This gives the bath a wonderful aroma and you the therapeutic values of whichever oils you have chosen. But the oils can also be incorporated into homemade bath crystals, bath oils, and bubble baths.

Most of the prettily packaged bath crystals you can buy in the shops are nothing more than washing soda crystals with color and fragrance added. To make your own at home couldn't be easier and if you save attractive glass jars over the year, making presents for all your friends at Christmas will take about ten minutes! Simply crush washing soda crystals, add a little food coloring, and the essential oils of your choice—to each 9 ounces add 20 drops of essential oil. Tie a few ribbons around the jars, et voilà. . . .

Many people find plain tap water drying to the skin and need a bath oil to counteract its effects. There are few truly dispersable bath oils, but one that is, is a treated castor oil known as Red Turkey Oil. You can add the essential oil directly into the bottle, just as you would with any other base oil, using 5 drops to 1 teaspoon of oil; as most bottles of this oil come in 2 ounce sizes, add 50 drops of your chosen oil or blend of oils. Use about 1 teaspoon of this to each bath. Alternatively, first add your essential oil neat to the bath—4–6 drops per bath—and then put a teaspoon of Red Turkey Oil in the bath.

Nondispersable oils may also be added to baths, only in this case the oil will float on the water and then cling to your body when you get out. Any nourishing oil can be used, such as avocado, almond, apricot kernel, or grapeseed, or make a blend—again add 5 drops of essential oil per 1 teaspoon of bath oil and use a teaspoon in each bath. Here is a good proportional blend for baths:

NOURISHING OIL

Avocado	2 teaspoons
Apricot kernel	2 teaspoons
Sweet almond	2 tablespoons

Add 50 drops of essential oils of your choice

Sometimes there is nothing more appealing than lying back in a bath full of bubbles, while the aromas of the essential oils drift around you, soothing and relaxing. The following recipe is for a bubble bath that is also cleansing. Use only one hundred percent pure soap—either soap flakes or grated pure soap.

Soap flakes (or grated soap)	8 ounces
Witch hazel	2 tablespoons
Almond oil	2 cups
Spring water	2 cups

Boil the spring water and melt the soap in it. In another container, mix the witch hazel and almond oil together and shake well. (If possible, do this in a blender.) Then slowly add the soap mixture to the witch hazel and oil blend and again, shake or blend well. These amounts will make a large quantity of basic bubble bath mixture to which you can add the essential oils of your choice as and when required. For each 2 tablespoons base bubble bath use 15 drops of essential oil and mix well. Use 1–2 teaspoons of the final product in each bath.

BODY AND BATH OILS

ESSENTIAL OILS
FOR NORMAL SKIN

Palma rosa	**Carrot**
Geranium	**Jasmine**
Ylang-ylang	**Frankincense**
Sandalwood	**Patchouli**
Lavender	**Neroli**

NORMAL SKIN
SYNERGISTIC BLEND

Frankincense	3 drops
Palma rosa	10 drops
Neroli	5 drops
Lavender	12 drops

ESSENTIAL OILS
FOR DRY SKIN

Benzoin	**Palma rosa**
Patchouli	**Carrot**
Chamomile German	**Pettigraine**
Geranium	**Lavender**
Bois de rose	**Rose**

DRY SKIN
SYNERGISTIC BLEND

Palma rosa	10 drops
Chamomile German	5 drops
Carrot	5 drops
Bois de rose	10 drops

ESSENTIAL OILS
FOR GREASY SKIN

Chamomile Roman	**Ylang-ylang**
	Jasmine
Orange	**Neroli**
Lemon	**Nutmeg**
Lavender	**Cypress**
Clary-sage	**Bergamot**

GREASY SKIN
SYNERGISTIC BLEND

Lemon	15 drops
Cypress	10 drops
Ylang-ylang	5 drops

ESSENTIAL OILS
FOR BLEMISHED SKIN

Niaouli	**Chamomile Roman**
Geranium	
Clary-sage	**Chamomile German**
Eucalyptus lemon	
	Lavender
Eucalyptus peppermint	**Myrrh**
	Thyme linalol

BLEMISHED SKIN
SYNERGISTIC BLEND

Eucalyptus lemon	15 drops
Lavender	5 drops
Thyme linalol	5 drops
Chamomile Roman	5 drops

Pre-Bath Body Oils ♦♦♦

Body oils can be applied before getting in the bath, as opposed to the more usual practice of applying them after a bath, and they have a tremendously satisfying effect as the body is enveloped in an oil that is heated by water and absorbed into the body by osmosis. You can use any combination of essential oils for a variety of skin conditions; see the previous lists and formulate your own blends. This method is also particularly useful for the treatment of arthritic and rheumatoid conditions. Use 5 drops of essential oil to each 1 teaspoon of Pre-Bath Oil Base. Apply the oil all over your body before stepping into the bath (this method does not have the same effect in a shower).

PRE-BATH BASE OIL

Grapeseed	2 tablespoons
Jojoba	20 drops
Evening primrose	10 drops
Carrot	5 drops

The following formulas are designed to be diluted in 2 teaspoons of Pre-Bath Base Oil:

PURIFYING PRE-BATH OIL

Lemon	2 drops
Peppermint	3 drops
Juniper	5 drops

REFINING PRE-BATH OIL

Geranium	2 drops
Orange	3 drops
Pettigraine	5 drops

TONING PRE-BATH OIL

Ginger	2 drops
Lemongrass	5 drops
Black pepper	3 drops

Deodorizing Body Oils ◆◆◆◆◆◆◆◆◆◆◆◆

If you are prone to profuse and odorous perspiration there could be an underlying hormonal or physiological cause, but using a deodorizing body oil after a bath helps. Make up the formula below or use the oils listed to make your own massage formula. Use all over the body after a bath:

DEODORIZING BODY OIL

Sage	15 drops
Thyme	10 drops
Eucalyptus peppermint	5 drops

Diluted in 2 tablespoons vegetable oil

DEODORIZING BODY ESSENTIAL OILS

Sage	**Peppermint**
Clary-sage	**Eucalyptus peppermint**
Thyme	

Body Lotions ◆◆◆◆◆◆◆◆◆

A lotion is an amalgamation of water in oil or oil in water, both containing an emulsifying agent; and it can be very hard to achieve just the right balance using the raw materials at home. In theory essential oils can be incorporated into any lotion or cream and there are many on the market that are pure and natural and that you could use as a base. Just add a single oil or blend of essential oils to the lotion or cream and mix as thoroughly as possible. The essential oils will not be as effective as if diluted in a simple vegetable base oil, because they may not be distributed as evenly.

Body Splashes ◆◆◆◆◆◆◆◆

Body splashes are invigorating sprays or slap-on water-based lotions that have a variety of uses. They can stimulate or tone, uplift or relax—depending on what essential oils you use. They are fun to make because they are so simple, and they also make good gifts for friends. Have an array of them in your bathroom ready to use whenever the mood takes you. Splashes are a favorite with men as they do a great job of making you feel good without leaving an oily residue. They leave the skin feeling soft, and as bactericides and deodorants they are highly effective. In times past body splashes were called "les vinaigres de toilette" and we follow the same principle and use, in some cases, the same ingredients. The vinegar to use is white wine or cider, whichever you prefer. If you use vodka, the higher the proof the better. Don't use these splashes, however, if you have sensitive or dehydrated skin.

DEODORANT SPLASH

Vinegar	4 ounces
Vodka	2 teaspoons
Lavender	5 drops
Sage	5 drops
Lemon	5 drops
Rosemary	5 drops
Peppermint	3 drops
Grapefruit	5 drops

Add to 2 cups spring water

First blend the essential oils together. Add them to the vodka and shake well for as long as you can. Leave them all to settle, then add the vinegar. Pour the whole mixture into 2 cups of spring water and again, shake well. Finally, pass the liquid through a paper coffee filter. The longer you leave the essential oils in the vodka and vinegar mix before adding to the water, the stronger the scent will be.

Follow this same procedure when making all the splashes that follow. Here again are the basic ingredients:

BODY SPLASHES
BASIC INGREDIENTS

High proof vodka	2 teaspoons
White wine or cider vinegar	4 ounces
Spring water	2 cups

INVIGORATING SPLASH

Lime	10 drops
Lavender	10 drops
Peppermint	5 drops
Lemon	3 drops

SOOTHING SPLASH

Benzoin	10 drops
Nutmeg	2 drops
Sandalwood	10 drops
Geranium	5 drops

FRUITY SPLASH

Orange	10 drops
Lemon	5 drops
Mandarin	10 drops
Grapefruit	5 drops

TONING SPLASH

Lemongrass	18 drops
Basil	2 drops
Black pepper	3 drops
Sage	5 drops
Patchouli	3 drops

Body Packs and Scrubs ♦♦♦♦♦♦♦♦♦♦♦♦♦♦♦

Body packs are like face packs in that they remove impurities and improve the texture of the skin while providing a good toning treatment. Some body packs can also be slimming. They are used a great deal in European spa resorts where you can get plastered in herbal packs made of mud, clay, or seaweed. But body packs are very easy to do at home and essential oils are the perfect ingredient to use, not only because of their therapeutic values but because their aromatic qualities make lying around like a basted chicken a far more enjoyable experience! When the waiting is done and you can wash the pack off, you and your body will both feel great. If you are feeling a bit neglected and depressed, go the whole way with a body pack and essential oil bath followed by an essential oil massage. You'll feel one hundred percent better and your bank manager, if he but knew it, would be much happier than if you'd gone off to Switzerland for a bit of pampering.

Clay is wonderfully absorbent and seems to act as a magnet to all the toxins and debris lurking in our skins. Cover the place you intend to lie down on with plastic—two split black trash can liners work perfectly well. Mix about 7 ounces of green or white clay (kaolin) with enough water to make a paste that's not too stiff but resembles in consistency that of yogurt. In another dish add 10 drops of essential oil to the yolk of an egg and mix well. Use lemon to remove impurities, lavender to relax, or rosemary for stimulation. Now mix this well into the clay pack and carefully smooth it all over your body. Leave it on for fifteen minutes, then sponge off with tepid water. Soak yourself now in an essential oil bath and follow with a massage oil.

Ground, dried seaweed or algae can be bought already in powder form and makes a good alternative to the clay. Like the clay, it is also valuable in treating muscular or joint conditions. Just substitute this for the clay and follow the directions as above.

Body scrubs are designed to slough off dead skin cells, thus allowing the new skin to be exposed and giving the skin an improved texture and color. Again, they are very easy to do at home. Any ground nut or pulse can be used as the basic ingredient although lentils mixed with coarse oatmeal make an excellent base. Grind a handful of brown lentils in a blender or by pestle and mortar and then add a handful of coarse oatmeal and blend again until you have a powder. Add 4 drops of grapefruit and 4 drops of carrot essential oil and blend until you have a paste. Rub this all over the skin, paying particular attention to dry, scaling areas such as elbows, knees, and the backs of heels. Rinse off in the shower or bath and then use a body oil. Here are some other body scrubs:

FOR DRY SKIN

Ground almond	1 handful
Oatmeal	1 handful
Sandalwood	2 drops
Evening primrose	2 drops

FOR OILY SKIN

Aduki beans	1 handful
Oatmeal	1 handful
Rosemary	2 drops
Lavender	2 drops

FOR BLEMISHED BACK/CHEST

Ground almonds	1 handful
Oatmeal	1 handful
Thyme linalol	2 drops
Lemon	2 drops

The Harem Special

One of the most luxurious and sensual body preparations comes to us from the East where, reputedly, it was used when women in the harem were prepared for the sultan's pleasure. It removes dead skin cells and leaves the skin glowing, fragrant, and as soft as silk:

Ground, dried citrus fruit peel	1 teaspoon
Ground almonds	3 teaspoons
Oatmeal	2 teaspoons
Clove powder	1 pinch
Crushed, dried rose petals	1 teaspoon
Nutmeg powder	1 pinch
Almond oil	2 tablespoons
Neroli (or a citrus oil, Lemon or Orange)	2 drops
Sandalwood (or Patchouli)	2 drops

Blend all the ingredients together until you have a paste. Add more almond oil if you feel it needs it. Have a bath, dry yourself off and, standing in the bath, roll the mixture all over your body. Massage it into dry areas of skin. The idea is to cover the skin with a very fine layer, which is why you need to roll the paste over the body. (This is a technique we don't know or use very much in the West but which is employed, for example, in Morocco when making very thin pastry—the ball of dough is slapped on to a hot place so that just the thinnest layer of dough is left on its surface.) By the time you have finished rolling the paste all over your body you'll be ready to go back to the part of the body you started with and brush the fine dust off. Gently wipe any remaining areas of paste with a dry washcloth.

The Fat Attack/Cellulite ◆◆◆◆◆◆

To reduce fat you need to exercise and take in less food. There is no wonder drug or plant substance that can help you to eat less, so it's really down to self-control. But eating sensibly is important so that the body doesn't draw on muscle as fuel instead of the fat. If you do not diet correctly your scales may show a reduction of weight but it will be valuable muscle tissue that has gone and you'll be left with all the fat and cellulite. Think of a piece of meat and mentally cut and separate the lean meat from the fat and put them on either side of the chopping board. If you eat fresh fruits, vegetables, fish, and meat, your tissue will look like the lean meat, and if you eat cakes, sweets, and potatoes steeped in butter, your tissue will look like the fat.

As well as diet and exercise, good massage and using essential oils will ensure that you are not left with flabby skin and stretch marks, and that you have a good shape. Use the essential oils in the bath and—dare I say it—even if you don't diet, you'll see a vast improvement in body tissuc tonc.

Here are the essential oils to use. Many of the oils on the general list also have a diuretic effect:

GENERAL FAT ATTACK ESSENTIAL OILS

Orange	**Sage**
Basil	**Thyme**
Lavender	**Pettigraine**
Grapefruit	**Lime**
Rosemary	**Lemongrass**

DIURETIC FAT ATTACK ESSENTIAL OILS

Fennel	**Cypress**
Celery	**Lemon**
Grapefruit	**Juniper**
Oregano	

These are two synergistic blends that you can use while you are on a diet. They are designed for use in baths—the oils work by osmosis. Prepare your bottle of essential oils in these proportions and use 6 drop in each bath:

GENERAL FAT ATTACK BATHS FOR DIETERS

SYNERGISTIC BLEND 1

Lavender	4 drops
Grapefruit	8 drops
Cypress	5 drops
Juniper	3 drops
Basil	4 drops

SYNERGISTIC BLEND 2

Lemongrass	4 drops
Oregano	5 drops
Fennel	3 drops
Pettigraine	8 drops
Basil	4 drops

Here are four toning bath synergistic blends. Make up a bottle in these proportions or use these quantities for two baths:

TONING BATHS

SYNERGISTIC BLEND 1

Grapefruit	5 drops
Basil	3 drops

SYNERGISTIC BLEND 2

Rosemary	5 drops
Pettigraine	3 drops

SYNERGISTIC BLEND 3

Lemongrass	4 drops
Lavender	4 drops

SYNERGISTIC BLEND 4

Orange	6 drops
Thyme	2 drops

And here are four diuretic bath synergistic blends. Again, make up a bottle in these proportions or use these quantities for two baths:

DIURETIC BATHS

SYNERGISTIC BLEND 1

Juniper	2 drops
Lemon	6 drops

SYNERGISTIC BLEND 2

Fennel	5 drops
Cypress	3 drops

SYNERGISTIC BLEND 3

Celery	2 drops
Grapefruit	6 drops

SYNERGISTIC BLEND 4

Oregano	2 drops
Lemon	6 drops

Fat attack massage oils are made by adding 30 drops of essential oil to 2 tablespoons good almond oil to which 10 drops of carrot oil have been added. Blend the almond and carrot together before adding your essential oils:

GENERAL FAT ATTACK MASSAGE OILS FOR DIETERS

FORMULA 1

Grapefruit	8 drops
Oregano	2 drops
Rosemary	10 drops
Cypress	10 drops

FORMULA 2

Pettigraine	5 drops
Lime	10 drops
Juniper	5 drops
Basil	10 drops

TONING MASSAGE OILS

FORMULA 1

Basil	10 drops
Lemongrass	5 drops
Lavender	15 drops

FORMULA 2

Red thyme	5 drops
Rosemary	10 drops
Orange	15 drops

DIURETIC MASSAGE OILS

FORMULA 1

Juniper	8 drops
Fennel	10 drops
Grapefruit	12 drops

FORMULA 2

Cypress	15 drops
Lemon	15 drops
Juniper	5 drops

Lymphatic drainage helps both general weight loss and cellulite dispersal but it is not easy to do without the help of a therapist. However, a mild form of this can be done at home if you have a detachable showerhead. With the shower fully turned on cold (the cold contracts the blood vessels and lymph) use the impact of the water on your skin to massage up the inside of the leg, especially the thighs to the groin. Then move the water around your abdomen in circular movements, then up the inner arms to the armpit. Do this as often as you can.

Cellulite

Cellulite has a variety of causes, from poor circulation and a lack of oxygen to water retention or hormonal changes. It may be related to the menstrual cycle in some women or to poor lymph drainage in both men and women. An unbalanced endocrine system has also been identified as a possible cause of some people's cellulite problem while others can blame their allergy—to wheat and milk products particularly. Toxicity is a major cause and this could be environmental and beyond our control, or dietary and within it. The first thing to do is cut out tea, coffee, and alcohol.

Treatment to eliminate these unsightly fat deposits is not easy and cellulite can always return if you have a predisposition to it. The fight against cellulite can become a lifelong battle which is made infinitely worse by the fact that our whole environment is saturated with toxins. Not only is the air we breathe and the water we drink polluted, but vegetables now contain residues of the pesticides, herbicides, and fungicides used in modern farming methods; meat contains residues of the steroids, hormones, and antibiotics that are routinely fed to the animals; and the fish we eat swim and breed in seas awash with unnatural and dangerous contaminants. In view of all this it is hardly surprising that so many people's body tissue gets clogged up with the toxins that cause cellulite.

The first front of attack is diet. Many severe cases of cellulite can be reversed with no more than a change of diet and an increased intake of vitamins and minerals. Ideally, eat only raw vegetables including bean sprouts—all soaked and scrubbed whenever possible. Buy free-range chickens, turkeys, and eggs, organically grown wholemeal bread, pulses, and rice. Drink only spring water and fruit juices or herb teas such as rosemary to which you can add 1 drop of lemon essential oil or 1 drop each of rosemary and lemon essential oils. Most important of all, eat no dairy products from cows. Cut out any fermented foods. Eating raw cabbage is one of the best dietary steps you can take to eliminate toxic debris. Increase your vitamin C supplement to 1000mg per day until the cellulite has gone and step up your zinc and vitamin B intake too. All the B vitamins are important here, but check supplements to make sure they are not derived from yeast.

Here is a six-point plan of action against cellulite:

1) Increase blood circulation by skin brushing. Using a brush of real bristles, brush in upward movements all over the body, as in the shower lymph drainage method.

2) Do exercises that work specifically on the cellulite areas, as these are often the places that get no exercise and hence gather toxic waste like stagnant water.

3) Massage every day—not only the cellulite areas but the whole body. Cellulite may show only in certain areas but essentially it's a whole-body problem.

4) Essential oils in the bath penetrate the skin by osmosis, and while you are bathing pinch and pummel cellulite areas to help break down the fatty deposits.

5) Oxygen is vital for a healthy body so breathing deeply is important. Breathing exercises actually help to shift cellulite and their results can be very impressive.

6) Relaxation is needed to allow the body to shift the waste and fat deposits. Stress, on the other hand, can cause cellulite to stick.

ESSENTIAL OILS TO FIGHT CELLULITE

Oregano	**Celery**
Juniper	**Thyme (all)**
Grapefruit	**Rosemary**
Lemon	**Sage**
Cedarwood	**Basil**
Fennel	**Patchouli**
Cypress	

See also the Diuretic list on page 146.

SPECIAL TOXIN ELIMINATOR BATH

Place in the bath:

Epsom salts (magnesium sulphate)	2 handfuls
Rock salt	1 handful

Then run the water and add 8 drops of the synergistic blend.

Oregano	6 drops
Juniper	6 drops
Lemon	10 drops
Grapefruit	10 drops
Basil	8 drops

Blend together

Massage the cellulite areas while they are under the water.

These anticellulite bath synergistic blends can be made up in the following proportions for future use; or use these quantities for two baths. In either case use 6 drops per bath:

ANTICELLULITE BATHS

BLEND 1

Thyme	8 drops
Lemon	4 drops

BLEND 2

Sage	8 drops
Patchouli	4 drops

BLEND 3

Rosemary	6 drops
Juniper	6 drops

BLEND 4

Oregano	6 drops
Lemon	6 drops

The base oil for cellulite massage oils is important. Use as your base 2 tablespoons of almond oil and add to this 5 drops each of jojoba and carrot oils. Blend these together well before adding your essential oils:

ANTICELLULITE MASSAGE OIL FORMULAS

FORMULA 1

Juniper	14 drops
Lemon	10 drops
Oregano	6 drops

FORMULA 2

Fennel	8 drops
Lemon	10 drops
Grapefruit	12 drops

FORMULA 3

Basil	10 drops
Thyme	8 drops
Grapefruit	12 drops

The full anticellulite program is as follows. Before bathing brush the skin as described in point one of the anticellulite program. Baths should be taken once a day using one of the formulas in warm to hot water. Afterwards use the cold shower drainage system as described on page 147. Then massage over the entire body with one of the massage formulas. In addition, massage the body once again each day—preferably use the massage oil twice, in the morning and at night. Twice a week take a toxin eliminator bath, having the water as hot as you can comfortably lie in. You will sweat, so shower or sponge yourself down afterwards.

Seaweed and cabbage are both excellent in the treatment of cellulite. Poultices can be made of chopped up seaweed or cabbage placed between two pieces of fine material such as gauze or muslin and ironed (yes, ironed). Wrap this all around the area and leave for fifteen minutes. This is very beneficial if done after the eliminator bath and before using the massage oil.

Breasts ♦♦♦♦♦♦♦♦♦♦♦♦♦♦♦♦

Whether we are trying to increase our breast size or decrease it, the matter is generally beyond our control and dependent upon the adipose fatty tissue that gives our breasts their shape. Keeping the upright, firm breast line of the teenage years involves hard work and patience and needs to be started at a very early age. Pectoral muscles that are underworked show up in signs of sagging, or as droopy bustlines. Breast stroke in the water—and out—is a good pectoral exercise, as is pushing your hands against each other when placed at chin level with the elbows stuck out on either side. Essential oils can help, together with exercise and cold water and ice treatments—the cold contracts the tissues. Splash the breasts or apply an ice-cup, in outward, circular movements around the breasts and follow by applying a massage oil. Massage is the best way to help prevent stretch marks, caused by fluctuation in breast weight.

ESSENTIAL OILS TO INCREASE AND FIRM BREASTS

Fennel	**Cypress**
Clary-sage	**Carrot**
Sage	**Hop**
Angelica	**Parsley**
Lemongrass	**Spearmint**
Geranium	

The best base vegetable oils to use on breasts are grapeseed or almond. To make massage oils use 5 drops of essential oil to each 1 teaspoon of base oil.

TREATMENT 1 Dilute 3 drops of cypress oil as well as you possibly can in 1 teaspoon of witch hazel. Add this to a bowl of cold water, or cold water in a basin, and splash the breasts alternately—at least ten times each. This is done alternately to allow for contraction and dilation. Then massage the breasts in outward, circular movements with this formula:

BREAST MASSAGE OIL 1

Clary-sage	3 drops
Geranium	5 drops

Fennel	12 drops
Lemongrass	10 drops

Diluted in 2 tablespoons base oil

This firming treatment must be done every day after exercise.

TREATMENT 2 While you are having a warm bath use the ice-cup over the breasts in outward, circular movements. Massage afterwards using this formula:

BREAST MASSAGE OIL 2

Lemongrass	10 drops
Cypress	10 drops
Spearmint	8 drops
Black pepper	2 drops

Diluted in 2 tablespoons base oil

If you really cannot bear the ice-cup method, use cold water from a showerhead.

Arms ◆◆◆◆◆◆◆◆◆◆◆◆◆◆◆◆

The upper arms are as prone to sagging as are the breasts and neck. Cellulite also tends to affect this area. Sensible arm exercise helps keep the arms toned and firm, and if this is your only problem area then use the following formula and treatment. The underside of the upper arm is very near the lymph gland in the armpit and this makes treating the underarms very easy with a form of lymphatic drainage. First make up your synergistic blend:

UNDERARM SYNERGISTIC BLEND

Cypress	5 drops
Lavender	10 drops
Fennel	8 drops
Juniper	7 drops

Make up a synergistic blend using the above proportions and then make a massage oil using 5 drops of the blend to each 1 teaspoon of base vegetable oil; use 8 drops to a bottle containing 4 ounces of water for the splash.

Hold one arm straight in the air above your head and with the other stroke it firmly downward towards the armpit, as if trying to push the flesh under your arm. Do this at least ten times with each arm. Now repeat the whole procedure but this time using a washcloth which has been soaked in the essential oil and water splash. Dry, then massage the whole of one arm towards the armpit, and then the other arm.

Hands ◆◆◆◆◆◆◆◆◆◆◆◆◆◆◆

We can look after our faces and work out at the gym but if we don't take care of our hands it can all be a bit of a waste of time, because the hands reflect our age very well and give the game away in an instant. Age spots make their first appearance on the hands and one of the first signs of departed youth is when the skin on the back of the hands becomes loose and wrinkled. Unfortunately, if you work with your hands a great deal this stretches the skin more than ever, and everyone's hands are exposed to pollutants more than any other part of the body—just think of how much dirt, grease, grime, and heavy detergents a pair of hands has to handle every day. Although the skin on the palm of the hands is thicker than on other parts of the body, except for the soles of the feet, we should really wear rubber gloves for many of the jobs we do—but how many people bother?

Thankfully, essential oils can help to keep hands looking their best. If you have a favorite hand cream you can simply blend the essential oils into that, although it is always better to make a cream from scratch. Don't be surprised if you find that you are supplying the whole family—essential oil hand creams tend to disappear very quickly!

ESSENTIAL OILS FOR HANDS

Rose	Rosemary
Geranium	Lemon
Sandalwood	Lime
Patchouli	Carrot
Lavender	Neroli

ANTISEPTIC OILS

Rosemary	Lavender
Lemon	Lime
Eucalyptus lemon	

OILS FOR DRY HANDS

Rose	Patchouli
Geranium	Carrot
Sandalwood	

OILS FOR NEGLECTED HANDS

Rose	Geranium
Neroli	Patchouli
Lemon	

Choose from these lists the essential oils you require and add them to the following lotions: basic hand cream (10 drops), barrier cream (20 drops), and jelly barrier (10 drops).

Basic Hand Cream

Cocoa butter	½ ounce
Almond oil	2 tablespoons
Beeswax	½ ounce
Evening primrose oil	5 drops
Carrot oil	5 drops

Melt the cocoa butter and the beeswax in a bain-marie, then add the almond, evening primrose, and carrot oils. You now have a basic hand cream that can be made thinner by adding more almond oil, or thicker by putting less almond oil in to begin with. Finally, add your chosen 10 drops of essential oil.

Luxurious Hand Oil

Carrot oil	10 drops
Avocado oil	2 teaspoons
Jojoba oil	10 drops
Evening primrose oil	10 drops
Vitamin E capsules	2*

Blend well then add

Rose	5 drops
Lemon	2 drops
Geranium	1 drop
Sandalwood	2 drops

*1 capsule = 250 IUs

You need only a tiny amount of this oil each time. Massage it well into the hands.

Barrier Cream

Lanolin	1 ounce
Beeswax	½ ounce
Mineral oil	3 ounces
Lavender floral water*	4 ounces
Borax	1 good pinch (approx. ¼ teaspoon)

*See page 325.

Mix the lanolin and beeswax, then add the mineral oil. In another container mix the lavender water and borax. Combine both mixtures thoroughly in a blender. Add the essential oils of your choice. Rosemary, lavender, and thyme are very good choices for use in a barrier cream because they have antibacterial properties. Use a total of 20 drops of essential oil.

Jelly Barrier

Arrowroot	1 tablespoon
Glycerine	1 tablespoon
Floral water*	5 ounces
Essential oil of your choice	10 drops

*See page 325.

Put the glycerine in a small pot and heat very slowly. Add the arrowroot and then the floral water (I like the rose best, but use whichever you prefer). Blend this mixture in a blender, then add the essential oils.

Nails ♦♦♦♦♦♦♦♦♦♦♦♦♦♦♦♦♦

To have good strong healthy nails you have to attend not only to the part of the nail that we cut, but to the nail bed, or cuticle. Many physical conditions show up in the nails as ridges or thickening, including arthritic and rheumatoid conditions in which the nails thicken and become distorted. All therapists involved in body work must keep their nails short, and for aromatherapists this is a full-time job because their hands are constantly in good essential oil blends and these make the nails grow furiously. I'm not exaggerating when I tell you that after a week's holiday, those of us working with essential oils will have beautiful strong, long nails. All we have to do is watch them grow.

ESSENTIAL OILS TO STIMULATE STRONG HEALTHY NAIL GROWTH

Lemon	**Carrot**
Lavender	**Grapefruit**
Eucalyptus peppermint	**Rosemary**
	Cypress

VEGETABLE OILS

Jojoba	**Evening primrose**
Borage	

BASE OILS

Apricot kernel	**Almond**
Grapeseed	**Avocado**

Here is a general strengthening synergistic blend of oils. Make up the blend and store it in a bottle ready for use. When you want to use it, add 10 drops of the synergistic blend to 1 teaspoon of avocado oil and massage it well into the fingers and nails, or toes and nails. Do this after your manicure, but don't put nail polish on afterwards.

NAIL STRENGTHENER SYNERGISTIC BLEND

Grapeseed oil	2 teaspoons
Jojoba oil	5 drops
Carrot oil	3 drops
Lemon	8 drops
Rosemary	2 drops

Cuticle Softener

Jojoba oil	1 teaspoon
Carrot oil	5 drops
Eucalyptus peppermint	2 drops

Massage well into the cuticle.

If you are unfortunate enough to have a fungal infection of the nails cut the 2 drops of eucalyptus peppermint oil from the formula above and substitute all the oils below:

Lavender	2 drops
Oregano	1 drop
Tea tree	2 drops

ESSENTIAL OILS TO TREAT NAIL INFECTIONS

Tea tree	**Thyme (all)**
Eucalyptus radiata	**Ravensara**
	Myrrh
Lavender	**Patchouli**
Oregano	**Calendula**

GENERAL NAIL INFECTION OIL

Tea tree	10 drops
Eucalyptus radiata	5 drops
Patchouli	5 drops
Tagetes	10 drops

Diluted in 2 tablespoons vegetable oil

Apply around the nail bed three times a day. Massage in well.

ONYCHIA is an inflammation of the nail bed that usually affects women, due to the long periods of time their hands spend in water and detergent. Treat as above, but add 10 drops of chamomile German and 5 drops of lavender to the General Nail Infection Oil.

Feet ◆◆◆◆◆◆◆◆◆◆◆◆◆◆◆◆◆◆

Feet are often the most neglected area of the body, particularly when it comes to beauty care. And yet our feet are our most faithful friends, plodding on day after day carrying our weight, constantly under pressure, running for buses, walking up and over the dales, and generally making our active lives possible. It is only when they begin to hurt that we look down and notice them.

Feet are very undemanding when you think of all they have to do, and they are modest too. You wouldn't think it to look at them, but they actually contain 72,000 nerve endings—which is why a foot massage makes the entire body feel so wonderfully relaxed. If we do something even as simple as paddling in the sea or putting our feet in a bowl of warm water, the results are more rewarding than we might expect. Feet also act as the electrical interface between us and the earth, and it is through them that we are able to discharge and "ground" the static that builds up within us. You know how pent-up you feel after a week of walking on concrete and how marvelous it feels to throw off the shoes at the weekend and walk on the grass. This affords an actual electrical release, an "earthing" which gives us a relief that seems out of proportion to the act itself.

Some people think that feet are ugly, and when you consider how neglected and put upon they are, who is surprised? Silently they suffer as we squeeze them into ill-fitting shoes, until one day they just can't take any more and they develop a problem. Then they cry for help. But why wait until then? They deserve more, and the essential oils provide a fabulous and effective way to give them a treat. Even if we have let things go too far, the oils can do much to right the balance.

Hard skin that is allowed to build up on the feet can cause pain later on in life and should be tackled as soon as it starts to appear—or, better still, prevent it from appearing at all. Pumice stone, a natural volcanic rock, is a wonder for smoothing away hard skin and preventing buildup.

HARD SKIN PREVENTATIVE

Base oil	1 teaspoon
Salt	1 teaspoon
Calendula (or tagetes)	5 drops

Rub the pumice stone all over the foot, paying particular attention to the sides of the feet, the ball, and heel. This is easier to do after a bath. Then rub salt all over the foot, massaging it in well. Finally, massage with the essential oil blended in the base oil—again, rubbing it in well. If you already have a heavy buildup of dead skin get a chiropodist to slough it off for you and then follow the treatment above.

Feet benefit from the following essential oils: Peppermint: refreshing—great before a party or after a long day out shopping. Calendula or Tagetes: good for hard skin and corns. Lavender, chamomile, fennel: a great help to tired, swollen feet; use them alone or mix in equal parts. Geranium: strengthens the skin and improves elasticity; helps prevent blistering and improves circulation in the feet.

All feet will benefit from a soak in a bowl of warm water in which a dozen or so small, round pebbles have been placed, along with a tablespoon of salt and 4 drops of your favorite essential oils. You can inhale the gorgeous aroma while you sensuously rub the soles of your feet back and forth over the pebbles. Do it slowly—and enjoy it.

After dabbing dry, massage the following oil well into the whole of the foot, taking time to massage the toes:

SPECIAL FOOT TREATMENT
SYNERGISTIC BLEND

Palma rosa	6 drops
Lemon	4 drops
Thyme linalol	3 drops
Benzoin	2 drops

Blend together in these proportions and use 5 drops in 1 teaspoon jojoba oil

A few special treatments are all you will need to get your neglected feet back into shape.

♦ CHAPTER 8 ♦ ESSENTIAL CARE FOR YOUR HAIR

THE CONDITION OF your hair can make or break your looks. It might be your "crowning glory" or an unruly tangle that refuses to do what it's told. A fortune is spent on hair products, and yet many people, having gone through shelves of expensive preparations, are still dissatisfied with the results.

The color of hair is invariably the first identifying feature we mention when describing someone. Three very different images are conjured up by saying "She was the one with the long red hair," "... the mousy one with greasy hair," or "... the blonde with the bob-cut." In some countries everyone has the same hair color and few go out of their way to dye it, while some women in the West dye their hair a different color every month. There is nothing new in this. The Egyptians were using henna some four thousand years ago, and slave prostitutes in Ancient Greece had their hair dyed blonde with saffron, a fact perhaps not related to the Ancient Romans' association of yellow hair with immorality. Respectable Roman ladies, however, must have thought that blondes were having more fun because dyeing their hair blonde or red soon became the vogue among them. Many centuries later in Europe, red hair was associated with witches. Gray hair is, of course, associated with old age and for many ages people have been trying to cover it up. One of the oldest preparations for doing this was made from the membrane that covers walnuts and lines the walnut shell.

Essential oils do not alter your natural hair color but they can help to enhance it. Chamomile is effective in lightening blonde hair, sage is good for black or brunette hair, while carrot, not surprisingly, enhances ginger hair. If you want to obtain color from natural products, dyes are available from some stores and may be made from henna, turmeric, rhubarb, radishes, green privet, chamomile, alfalfa, tomatoes, oranges, or cucumber.

Regardless of the cut and style hair should be thick and shining, but more often than not it is either greasy or dry, lifeless and with split ends, a straw-like mass from bleaching and tinting, or thinning away.

The basic substance of hair is keratin, a strong protein that also makes nails, and in animals, claws, feathers, horns, and fur. Humans don't moult in the seasonal way that animals do, but we still lose our hair as each one comes to the end of its natural life—from between two and seven years. When this happens, the hair becomes detached from the follicle—a tiny pit in the surface of the skin—and a new hair begins to grow in its place. This should happen almost instantaneously, but with ill-health, malnutrition, tension, or stress, the time between a hair being lost and a new one starting to grow can extend so that our hair begins to thin.

At the side of each follicle there is a sebaceous gland which secretes sebum, necessary for lubricating the hair.

The condition of hair is affected by what we eat, and by what we put on our hair. We all know that animals that are ill or badly fed soon lose the sheen on their coats and can become mangy if their condition deteriorates. This is one of the ways we know an animal is not thriving. We are pretty much the same, and if the blood supply is not delivering the seventeen amino acids which make up the keratin, the hair becomes dry or greasy, the ends split, and it loses its bounce. What we need for hair is the same as what we need for the skin, the outer layer of which is also keratin. If you eat plenty of fresh food, cut down on stimulants such as coffee, tea, and alcohol, increase your dosage of vitamin B, stick with cold pressed oils and unsaturated fatty acids, and get enough sleep, you'll be on your way to a glorious head of hair.

What we put on our hair is usually a chemical cocktail. Even so-called natural products contain synthetics which are dubious. Take, for example, Lauramide dea, part natural but also part synthetic, which is used to build up a lather and which is not only drying to the hair but can cause scalp itching and dermatitis. Oleyl betaine is a synthetic much used to reduce static but it causes dandruff, dry hair and scalp, and is toxic when absorbed through the skin. Other commonly used toxins are Sodium C 14-16 and Olefin sulfate, petroleum derivatives used as wetting agents. Look out, too, for Sodium lauryl sulfate, Sodium cetyl sulfate, and Sodium laureth sulfate—synthetics that can cause all manner of allergic reactions, hair loss, dry flaky scalp, or skin rashes, but which often appear under the banner of "natural" products. Remember, too, that what you put on your hair may also be causing harm in other parts of your body.

When taking a truly natural approach to hair it makes sense to avoid using the harsh detergent-based shampoos, although many, unfortunately, do not list their ingredients. But go for a shampoo that claims to be mild, as this will be less likely to strip the hair of its acid mantle. Conditioners should be rich in proteins. To these store-bought products you can simply add the essential oils listed under the category that best suits the present condition of your hair. Better still, make your own hair preparations using the information in this chapter. There are basic recipes to which you can add the appropriate essential oils and specific recipes under different types of hair. In this way you can be sure of what you are putting on your hair, and save yourself a great deal of money at the same time. Essential oils penetrate deeply into the hair shaft and follicle and produce healthy, shining hair. There are even essential oils that encourage new hair growth.

Before we look at the basic recipes for shampoos, rinses, and conditioners, let me first explain the "bain-marie" method which often applies in the making of these natural products. Keen cooks may have their own bain-marie, which is a cooking utensil for heating ingredients on the stove without them coming into contact with water or oils. The way to copy this effect is to place a heat-proof bowl in a partly filled pot of water. As the water in the pot will need to be boiled to generate the heat required to transform your ingredients into fabulous hair products, the bowl must be large enough not to tip over when the boiling water starts to jump around. You don't need much water in the pot—just enough to maintain the required temperature and not so much that the water will flood over the edge of the bowl and ruin your blend.

Shampoo Base

There are three variations here which will give you a basic "soap stew." Make whichever you find most convenient. Once made, the soap stew will keep forever.

PURE SOAP FLAKES can be obtained from some health food stores and pharmacies.

Soap flakes	4 ounces
Spring water	1 quart

Simmer the water, add the soap flakes, stir until the soap dissolves. Cool and bottle in an old coffee jar or similar container. The mixture may gel or appear lumpy after being left for a while but don't worry, just beat it up in the blender when you make up your shampoos.

CASTILE SOAP should be pure and white.

Castile, grated finely	4 ounces
Spring water	1 quart

Simmer the water, add the soap and bring to a boil until the soap has dissolved. Pour into a jar and store until needed.

SOAPWORT ROOT is so named because it is the original raw material of soaps and other cleaning products. You will need to crush the root, which may be bought from herbalists and health food stores.

Soapwort root, crushed	½ ounce
Spring water	2 pints

Boil the water and pour it over the soapwort in a bowl. Leave to infuse for at least an hour and then filter it through muslin or a coffee filter or fine strainer, and bottle. You will need larger quantities of this base when you shampoo—at least 2 tablespoons of the finished mixture.

Rinses

Many types of natural rinse can be used but the best is simple cider vinegar. To this you can add the essential oils of your choice—2 drops per tablespoon of vinegar, added to your final rinse water.

Conditioners

Lecithin, which is included in the two conditioner bases given here, is an extremely important protein that plays a very important role within the human body. The lecithin we use here, however, has been extracted from soya beans. Health food stores sell this product in two forms, liquid and granule; we use the liquid one which resembles thick orange tar but which nevertheless emulsifies beautifully.

LECITHIN BASE 1

Liquid lecithin	2 ounces
Almond oil	2 ounces
Jojoba oil	2 teaspoons
Cocoa butter	¼ ounce

Using the bain-marie method, mix all the ingredients until well melted and blended together. Pour into a jar and use as directed for the different hair types in the following pages.

LECITHIN BASE 2

Soap stew	2 ounces
Liquid lecithin	1 ounce

Using the bain-marie method, warm the soap solution and then drip the lecithin in slowly, stirring all the time. When the mixture is well blended, bottle and keep to use as directed.

Normal Hair ◆◆◆◆◆◆◆◆◆

"Normal hair" could perhaps better be called "healthy hair" because it is hair that is neither dry nor greasy, is easy to manage and always shining. But so-called normal hair can easily become dry or greasy, or dandruff may develop, especially if you are on long-term medication or antibiotics. So try to keep your hair healthy by using gentle shampoos and treatments.

ESSENTIAL OILS FOR NORMAL HAIR

Lavender	**Parsley**
Lemon	**Geranium**
Eucalyptus lemon	**Carrot**
	Rosemary

VEGETABLE OILS FOR NORMAL HAIR

Almond	**Evening primrose**
Peach kernel	
Borage	

SHAMPOOS

STIMULATING

Soap stew	4 ounces
Rosemary	2 drops
Lemon	4 drops
Eucalyptus lemon	7 drops

Mix in blender

MOISTURIZING

Soap stew	4 ounces
Geranium	3 drops
Carrot	4 drops
Lemon	2 drops
Borage	4 drops

Conditioning Treatment

Using the bain-marie method, mix together:

Lecithin base	1 tablespoon
Almond oil	1 tablespoon
Peach kernel oil	2 teaspoons

then add

Carrot	3 drops
Geranium	2 drops

Apply all over the hair and leave for at least ten minutes before rinsing off.

Vinegar Rinse

Water	1 ounce
Cider vinegar	2 teaspoons
Lemon	3 drops

Mix the cider vinegar and lemon essential oil together, then add to the water. Use in final water to rinse hair; rinse well.

Beer Rinse

This is an additive to the vinegar rinse above. The beer coats hair and contains proteins which will help protect the hair from damage. The beer doesn't need to be "real ale" just pulled from the oaken cask —any old stale beer will do.

Beer	1 ounce
Lemon	4 drops
Rosemary	5 drops

Mix together, add to the vinegar rinse above, and use in the final water to rinse hair; rinse well.

Scalp Stimulator

Here is a lotion that stimulates the scalp and is extremely effective for men's hair growth.

Vodka	1 teaspoon
Rosemary	3 drops
Lavender	5 drops

Mix, then add to 1 tablespoon water

Dip the fingertips into the mixture and massage well into the scalp. It smells nice and can be put onto the hair any time that is convenient for you, not necessarily before or after washing the hair.

Dry Hair ♦♦♦♦♦♦♦♦♦♦♦♦♦♦

When you have dry hair, not enough sebum is being produced by the sebaceous gland to provide the hair with a protective lubricant. As a result the hair can become damaged, tangled, split, and broken. The bad condition of such hair is easily aggravated by chlorine in swimming pools, too much sun and sea, and, of course, continual bleaching and tinting. Overexposure to sun and sea frequently leads to a greasy scalp with dry brittle ends.

ESSENTIAL OILS FOR DRY HAIR

Lavender	**Carrot**
Rosemary	**Parsley**
Geranium	**Yarrow**
Birch	**Sandalwood**

VEGETABLE OILS AND WAXES FOR DRY HAIR

Sesame	**Peach kernel**
Jojoba	**Almond**
Evening primrose	**Cocoa butter**
	Sunflower
Borage	**Avocado**

SHAMPOOS

STIMULATING

Soap stew	1 cup
Almond oil	1 teaspoon
Lavender	2 drops
Carrot	5 drops
Parsley	1 drop

Mix in blender

MOISTURIZING

Soap stew	1 cup
Peach kernel oil	2 teaspoons
Jojoba oil	5 drops
Carrot oil	5 drops
Sandalwood	2 drops

Mix in blender

Conditioning Treatment

Using the bain-marie method, mix well together:

Lecithin base	1 teaspoon
Sesame oil	1 teaspoon
Cold pressed almond oil (sweet)	1 tablespoon
Peach kernel oil	1 tablespoon
Avocado oil	2 drops
Borage oil (or Evening primrose oil)	2 drops
Carrot oil	2 drops
Parsley oil	4 drops
Geranium	3 drops

Apply all over the scalp while the oil is still warm, but not hot. Leave for ten minutes and then shampoo off. This conditioning treatment works especially well if you can sit in the sun while it's on the hair.

Conditioning Treatment for Sun-Damaged or Bleached Hair

Using the bain-marie method, mix well together:

Lecithin base	2 tablespoons
Jojoba oil	1 teaspoon
Evening primrose oil	6 drops
Sesame oil	1 teaspoon
Carrot oil	2 drops
Lemon juice	1 teaspoon
Eucalyptus lemon	5 drops

Apply all over the scalp while the oil is still warm, not hot. Massage in well, then cover your hair with a plastic bag. Leave for at least ten minutes then rinse thoroughly. Finish off with the vinegar rinse that follows, leaving a small amount on the hair.

Vinegar Rinse for Dry Hair

Add 1 drop of sandalwood essential oil to 1 teaspoon of cider vinegar and mix together well. Add to a cup of boiled water and then add this to a bowl of water you will be using as your final rinse. Rinse your hair thoroughly in this water, repeatedly pouring over those parts of the hair not immersed in the water.

Greasy Hair ◆◆◆◆◆◆◆◆◆◆

Greasy hair is caused by overactivity of the grease-producing sebaceous glands, one of which lies beside each individual hair follicle. This hair is characteristically lanky and often looks unwashed. Too frequent shampooing with harsh shampoos often exacerbates this condition and then you're on a merry-go-round—the more you wash your hair, the more you need to. As with lifeless hair, greasy hair is often a sign of ill-health. And as it is often accompanied by dandruff, greasy hair can make quite an unattractive picture.

ESSENTIAL OILS FOR GREASY HAIR

Rosemary	**Pimento berry**
Lavender	**Birch**
Cypress	**Basil**
Lemon	**Sage**
Eucalyptus lemon	**Thyme**
	Yarrow

VEGETABLE OILS FOR GREASY HAIR

Evening primrose	**Borage seed**
Sesame seed	**Peach kernel**

SHAMPOOS

STIMULATING

Soap stew	4 ounces
Rosemary	3 drops
Basil	1 drop
Lemon	15 drops
Cypress	2 drops

Mix together well, in a blender, if possible; shake before use

TO MAKE THE HAIR SHINE

Soap stew	4 ounces
Thyme	6 drops
Eucalyptus peppermint	7 drops
Lavender	3 drops
Rosemary	4 drops

Mix together well, in a blender, if possible; shake before use

Dry Shampoo

The following ingredients need to be mixed together thoroughly, and although this can be done by hand it is worth borrowing a blender if you don't have one. Most blenders have a tiny hole in the lid which could almost have been designed for adding essential oils, drop by drop, to blends. Make sure the lid is on tightly otherwise you could end up giving the entire kitchen a dry shampoo! Purified talc is the basis of many pharmaceutical drugs and most pharmacists stock the loose powder.

Purified talc	1 ounce
Lemon	10 drops
Rosemary	2 drops

Blend together well

Use about a teaspoon on a real bristle brush and brush through the hair on the days you don't wet-shampoo but when your hair still needs some attention.

Conditioning Pack

Greasy hair needs conditioning as much as any other type of hair. Mix the following ingredients together in a bain-marie:

Lecithin base	1 tablespoon
Sunflower oil	1 teaspoon
Green clay	1 tablespoon
Vodka	1 teaspoon

Put the lecithin in the bowl first, then add the sunflower oil, vodka, and green clay. Frankly, you will now have a yucky mess, but carry on—it will be worth it! Now add your essential oils and mix them in well:

Birch (or Rosemary)	3 drops
Lavender	3 drops
Yarrow	2 drops

Smear the mixture over your hair, leave on for ten minutes, then shampoo off.

Vinegar Rinse for Greasy Hair

Add 3 drops of thyme essential oil to 1 tablespoon of cider vinegar and mix to dissolve the thyme as much as possible. Then add to half a pint of spring water. Add this to the final rinse water in a bowl, after shampooing, and run it through the hair several times to ensure effective coverage.

Fragile Hair ◆◆◆◆◆◆◆◆◆◆

Fragile hair has often been abused so much by perms, colors, mousses, and gels that there is not much left that isn't thin, split, or that doesn't break on touching. It has to be treated very gently to avoid further breaking and the scalp needs stimulating to encourage new and stronger growth. Until that new growth is at the length you want it, the fragile hair needs to be treated with great care. These are the oils to use:

ESSENTIAL OILS FOR FRAGILE HAIR

Parsley	**Calendula**
Lavender	**Carrot**
Chamomile	**Sandalwood**
Birch	**Clary-sage**
Thyme	

VEGETABLE OILS AND WAXES FOR FRAGILE HAIR

Jojoba nut	**Peach kernel**
Borage seed	**Almond**
Evening primrose	**Cocoa butter**

SHAMPOOS

STIMULATING

Soapwort shampoo base	4 ounces
Lavender	2 drops
Yarrow	2 drops

Mix together well, in a blender if possible

Use once a week.

CONDITIONING

Soapwort shampoo base	4 ounces
Lecithin base	1 teaspoon
Borage seed oil	3 drops
Lavender	2 drops

Mix together well, in a blender if possible

Use as needed.

Fragile Hair Conditioner

Cocoa butter	1 ounce
Lecithin base	1 tablespoon
Almond oil	2 ounces
Borage seed oil	4 drops
Evening primrose oil	10 drops
Birch oil	5 drops
Chamomile Roman	3 drops

Using the bain-marie method, first melt the cocoa butter and lecithin. Then add the almond oil, stirring all the time, add the other ingredients and blend together well. Pour into a storage jar until needed. (The volumes here will provide two or three treatments.) After shampooing, leave on the hair for at least ten minutes before rinsing off. Gradually this treatment will build up the remaining cells and help prevent breakage.

Protein Gel

This you use rather like a face pack, but on the hair:

Plain gelatin	½ ounce
Mineral water	1 cup
Cider vinegar	1 teaspoon
Carrot oil	3 drops
Clary-sage	3 drops

Mix the gelatin and water together until you have a smooth liquid. Stir and leave it until it forms a gel type of substance, but don't leave it to set. Now add the vinegar, carrot, and clary-sage—this will prevent it from becoming solid. Use as a hair pack, covering the whole of the hair. Leave on for ten minutes, then rinse off thoroughly. Use once a week.

Falling Hair ◆◆◆◆◆◆◆◆◆◆

When you start to notice that more hairs are coming away in your hairbrush than normal, it's time to treat your falling hair. This is not as serious as hair loss, which is covered in the next section, but when hairs start to come away from the scalp and you find them on the furniture and all over the place, use the following treatments.

Shampoos

There are two recipes here. Use whichever you prefer but not more than once a week—washing too often does nothing to help the problem. Blend the ingredients together:

SHAMPOO 1

Soap stew	4 ounces
Jojoba oil	4 drops
Chamomile	2 drops
Palma rosa	3 drops

SHAMPOO 2

Soap stew	4 ounces
Jojoba oil	5 drops
Rosemary	3 drops
Lemon	2 drops

Conditioners

Use these conditioners before shampooing, and leave on the hair for ten minutes before rinsing off. Blend them using the bain-marie method.

CONDITIONER 1

Cocoa butter	½ ounce
Almond oil	2 tablespoons
Clary-sage	5 drops

CONDITIONER 2

Lecithin base	2 teaspoons
Jojoba oil	5 drops
Evening primrose oil	10 drops
Almond oil	2 tablespoons

Rinses

There are again two options for the rinse. Blend the ingredients of the rinse you choose then add to 1 pint of boiled or filtered water and put in the final rinse after you've shampooed your hair:

RINSE 1

Cider vinegar	1 ounce
Spring water	4 ounces
Lemon	10 drops

RINSE 2

Cider vinegar	1 ounce
Spring water	4 ounces
Rosemary	3 drops
Lavender	3 drops

Hair Loss ◆◆◆◆◆◆◆◆◆◆◆◆

When hair starts coming out in handfuls and bald patches appear, you have a serious problem of hair loss. Balding is a separate subject and is discussed on page 275, but for those who suddenly start to lose their hair in a more haphazard way, and without the reassuring knowledge that their hair loss is hereditary, the sight of a clump of hair in the comb can be a really frightening experience.

The first thing to do is to see your doctor and make sure that you are not suffering from a deficiency of the thyroid or pituitary gland, especially if you have other symptoms. Scarlet fever and syphilis can also cause bald patches. Hair loss is something of a mystery once these medical conditions have been ruled out, and the medical profession does not know the basic physiological reasons for the hair follicles suddenly refusing to do their job. Other known causes include severe mental strain, radiation treatment, certain prolonged medical treatments, ill-health, and wrong hair care, but these do not apply to all the unfortunate sufferers of this very distressing condition.

In this section the treatments recommended are for alopecia, and those with a less serious case of hair loss can apply the essential oils for reducing hair loss listed below to those treatments. Essential oils, and indeed many nut oils, can stimulate the hair follicle and increase circulation and oxidization sufficiently to bring about regrowth of hair, although in some cases this may resemble vellus, or baby hair. While encouraging growth with the essential oil treatments, use only purified water (boiled or filtered) to wash your hair. Avoid chlorinated swimming pools and do not swim in polluted seas. Eat correctly and take vitamin B supplements. Shampooing too often can increase hair loss, so cut down on that, and avoid heavy conditioning treatments which can stretch weakened hair, causing it to break. Chemical products may leave a residue which if it builds up can lead to hair loss. So turn to the natural option: first, the oils.

ESSENTIAL OILS
FOR TREATING ALOPECIA

Thyme	**Carrot**
Rosemary	**Sage**
Lavender	

ESSENTIAL OILS
THAT REDUCE HAIR LOSS

Chamomile Roman	**Rose**
	Yarrow
Cypress	**Carrot**
Lemon	**Sage**
Birch	**Clary-sage**
Palma rosa	**Rosemary**
Thyme	**Calendula**

VEGETABLE OILS
FOR TREATING ALOPECIA

Jojoba	**Evening primrose**
Borage seed	

Alopecia Shampoo

Blend the ingredients together in a bain-marie and use the shampoo once a week. Don't shampoo in between but instead get adventurous with the scarves—or

ALOPECIA SHAMPOO

Soap stew	4 ounces
Jojoba oil	12 drops
Carrot oil	6 drops
Rosemary	6 drops
Lavender	10 drops

See also the following conditioner which should be applied beforehand.

Alopecia Conditioner

Before shampooing, apply the following conditioner. Blend the ingredients together and massage into the scalp. Leave on the hair for at least thirty minutes before washing off.

ALOPECIA CONDITIONER

Jojoba oil	½ teaspoon
Evening primrose oil	10 drops
Palma rosa	3 drops

Nighttime Treatment for Alopecia

Every night apply the following treatment all over the scalp. Mix the ingredients together and store in a clean bottle. Use 1 teaspoon for each application, diluted in 1 tablespoon of cold water, preferably ice-cold.

Cider vinegar	4 ounces
Carrot oil	20 drops
Rosemary	10 drops

Dandruff ♦♦♦♦♦♦♦♦♦♦♦♦

The tell-tale flakes of dead skin cells scattered on shoulders proclaim that someone's head and hair are in bad condition. Even if you brush your hair thoroughly in the morning and brush your shoulders before leaving the house, by lunchtime those horrid little white flakes are back again, making a mess of your appearance and even, sometimes, your life. The manufacturers of dandruff shampoos are not in the business of clearing up the condition permanently, or who would there be to buy their product? But with essential oils you can get to the root of the problem and banish this scourge once and for all.

ESSENTIAL OILS
TO TREAT DANDRUFF

Rosemary	**Cypress**
Lemon	**Lavender**
Lime	**Eucalyptus peppermint**
Birch	
Basil	**Sage**
Thyme	**Carrot**
Pimento berry	

VEGETABLE OILS
TO TREAT DANDRUFF

Evening primrose	**Borage**
	Jojoba

Shampoos

This first shampoo loosens the crusty layer of dead skin cells and, in the washing, these are taken off. Also, it stimulates the healing mechanisms of the skin to prevent a further buildup of dandruff scales. Use this shampoo only, avoiding the harsh shampoos on the market.

Soap stew	4 ounces
Rosemary	18 drops
Thyme	10 drops
Sage	8 drops

Blend together well

This next shampoo stimulates a healthy scalp and thick, shining hair:

Soap stew	4 ounces
Sage	10 drops
Lemon	10 drops
Basil	5 drops
Eucalyptus peppermint	15 drops

Blend together well

Vinegar Rinse

Dandruff responds very well to treatment with the vinegar rinse. These are the basic ingredients:

Cider vinegar	1 tablespoon
Thyme	5 drops
Eucalyptus peppermint	5 drops
Sage	3 drops
Carrot	5 drops

Mix these together and put them into 1 ounce of spring water. Using about a teaspoon each time, massage into the scalp (not the hair) every night before going to bed.

Here is another overnight treatment that works very well. Again, this is a scalp conditioner so don't rub it into the hair. Blend the ingredients together, dip your fingertips into the mixture, and massage the scalp:

Carrot oil	5 drops
Jojoba oil	15 drops
Evening primrose oil	15 drops
Cypress	3 drops

♦ CHAPTER 9 ♦
THE GENTLE TOUCH FOR BABIES AND CHILDREN

FROM TINY BEGINNINGS, children grow with amazing speed, as many mothers will vouch for, having watched in amazement as their little ones shoot right past their shoulder and by adolescence tower above them! When treating children with essential oils we have to employ a sliding scale of dosage to mirror their growth, so this chapter is broken down into sections for newborn babies, babies between two and twelve months old, children between one and five years, five and seven, and so forth. Refer to the main chart of essential oils for children to see which oils you can use and at what age. Not all oils are suitable until full growth has been reached and others must only be given in reduced dosages.

Newborn Babies ♦♦♦♦♦♦

As soon as you know you are pregnant, start looking around for suitable pots and bottles to store your baby's various creams and potions in. The pharmacy will sell you small brown, glass bottles, but you will also need tiny little pots or pillboxes which should all be washed and then sterilized in the baby's sterilizing unit. When the time comes to make a remedy you won't want to be running around looking for a suitable container for the absolutely tiny quantities you will be using.

These are the only essential oils that I recommend you use on babies up to two months unless specifically directed in a formula in this section:

NEWBORN BABIES' ESSENTIAL OILS

Chamomile Roman	**Lavender**
Chamomile German	**Yarrow**
	Dill

One of the gentlest and yet most effective ways to treat various common ailments involves allowing the molecules of essential oil to evaporate and circulate throughout the baby's room. This can be done in two ways. First, you can place a bowl of steaming water on the floor, away from your baby's head, and add the essential oil so that it rises with the steam and permeates the atmosphere. Just 1 drop of essential oil to 1 pint of water will be quite adequate for small babies.

The second method involves using a diffuser. Make certain that it has a glazed surface, so that it can be thoroughly cleaned. Avoid the natural-looking porous clay type of diffuser for use with babies and children.

Do not use essential oil neat on a diffuser in a baby's room. Even one drop on a diffuser is too powerful because all the molecules will eventually be released by the heat, whereas with the bowl method not all the molecules will be released into the atmosphere before the water goes cold. So add 1 drop of essential oil to 2 teaspoons of water, mix well, and add a little of this water to the cupped area of the glazed diffuser bowl.

If the baby is suffering from any kind of digestive problem—colic, indigestion, constipation, diarrhea, or regurgitation—use dill essential oil in one of the room methods just outlined. You will recognize the smell because it is the active ingredient in many infant digestive preparations.

If your baby isn't sleeping well, use chamomile Roman.

To clean up the air in your baby's room and make it smell delightful, use lavender essential oil for its antibiotic, antiseptic, disinfectant, and slightly antiviral properties. Even using the tiny quantity of essential oil recommended, the aroma will be lovely and infinitely better for your baby than the chemical air fresheners that you can now buy for a baby's room.

Your Baby's Skin

When the baby is first born he or she is often partly covered in a greasy substance which is thought to protect the skin as it floats in the amniotic fluid. Appropriately enough, this makes the baby look as if it's just swum the Channel! This vernix caseosa, as it is called, can't be removed with water, so oil is used instead. The more natural this oil is, the better for your baby, so you could make up your own and take it into the hospital and ask the staff to use that. Some hospitals will automatically use olive oil BP, which is a better option than a mineral-based oil but still has the disadvantage of having gone through a great deal of processing and a long storage period. An ideal oil for your baby's first clean would be made by mixing 2 tablespoons almond oil with 5 drops evening primrose (or borage) oil, plus 3 drops of jojoba oil and 10 drops of wheatgerm oil. This is a bland, nonaromatic oil which the staff should not have any objection to and which can be used as a massage oil for you or the baby later on.

You shouldn't think about using an essential oil on a baby until it is at least twenty-four hours old, and then there has to be a good reason. One such reason is dry and wrinkled skin, which is quite common in babies that are overdue or induced. It can be off-putting to find you have a dry-skinned and wrinkled baby instead of the dewy-soft little angel you had expected, but the problem is easily solved. When my little girl arrived, long overdue, she had red flaking skin on her ankles, wrists, and in all the small delicate folds. I was given a bottle of olive oil BP by the hospital staff and told to rub that in but instead phoned my mother and asked her to make up a 2 tablespoon bottle containing 80 percent hazelnut oil, 10 percent wheatgerm oil, and 10 percent pure virgin olive oil (which is quite different from olive oil BP). I already had with me a set of baby oils ready for any eventuality and made up a synergistic blend of the essential oils below in a spare bottle with a dropper:

WRINKLED SKIN SYNERGISTIC BLEND

Chamomile German	8 drops
Lavender	1 drop

Use 3 drops only to 2 tablespoons skin oil, as above

Don't be surprised when the skin oil turns a blue-green as you make it up—that is due to the azulane content of the chamomile German essential oil.

The point about making a synergistic blend is that it enables you to get the proportions correct, and therefore you have the exact remedy you need to solve the problem. Often, too, there is no waste—as in this case because the remaining 6 drops may be used, 1 drop at a time, in your baby's next baths. Within a day, my daughter's skin was beautiful and the doctor was suitably impressed. My daughter and I meanwhile had established the habit of daily massages, which we both enjoyed.

The oil for wrinkled skin may be used to treat two other skin problems that can occur in babies. Small, red, mottled spots which form, especially around the neck and eye area, will disappear without treatment but their dispersal can be aided by massaging the wrinkled skin oil very gently into the baby's back. Negroid babies can have blue spots which resemble bruises. These are caused by a concentration of pigmentation and they fade quite rapidly. To help the process along, massage the affected area once a day with the wrinkled skin oil. Do this for fifteen days, break for a week, and start again if necessary.

There is no treatment for birthmarks known as "port wine stains." These generally disappear or fade in a year or so, but large birthmarks can be removed by surgery later in life if they are found to be disfiguring.

Diaper rash is, of course, the most common of baby problems and although thought of as a minor inconvenience it is actually very painful for the baby and worrying for the mother. Essential oils provide an easy solution to the problem. There are two combinations that work equally well—make your choice according to which oils you happen to have in the home:

FOR DIAPER RASH

Chamomile German **Lavender**

or

Yarrow **Lavender**

In equal proportions

When you wash your baby's bottom, use cotton wool dipped in a bowl of warm water to which you have added 1 drop each of your chosen two-part combination of essential oils per pint of water (swish the water around well first). Use clean cotton wool each time and avoid chemically perfumed "baby wipes." Now dry the baby thoroughly and apply a mixture of zinc and castor oil cream to which you have added your chosen combination of essential oils: 1 drop of each to 4 teaspoons of

ESSENTIAL OILS FOR BABIES AND CHILDREN

Essential Oils	Base Oils	Base Oil Additives (maximum 10% of base unless otherwise stated)
NEWBORN BABIES		
Chamomile Roman	**Hazelnut**	**Jojoba**
Chamomile German	**Sweet almond***	**Borage**
Yarrow		**Wheatgerm**
Dill		
Lavender		
Dosage: 1–3 drops diluted in 2 tablespoons Base Oil		
*Not bitter almond which is used in confectionery.		
2–6 MONTHS OLD		
As above, plus:	As above	As above
Mandarin		
Eucalyptus		
Coriander		
Neroli		
Dosage: 3–5 drops diluted in 2 tablespoons Base Oil		
6–12 MONTHS OLD		
As above, plus:	As above	As above
Palma rosa		
Calendula		
Grapefruit		
Aniseed		
Tea tree		
Dosage: 3–5 drops diluted in 2 tablespoons Base Oil		
1–5 YEARS OLD		
All the above, plus:	As above	As above
Ginger BUT only use ⅓ the dosage directed for other oils		**Carrot**
Dosage: 5–10 drops diluted in 2 tablespoons Base Oil		

ESSENTIAL OILS FOR BABIES AND CHILDREN (cont.)

Essential Oils	Base Oils	Base Oil Additives
5–7 YEARS OLD		
All the above, plus the following used in ⅓ the dosage directed for other oils	**Hazelnut** **Sweet almond** **Apricot*** **Soya bean*** **Grapeseed***	As above
Ginger **Peppermint** **Rosemary** **Nutmeg** **Benzoin** **Thyme** **Hyssop** **Clary-sage** **Geranium**		

Dosage: 5–12 dreops diluted in 2 tablespoons Base Oil

*These are slightly thicker and heavier than the previous base oils but if the baby or child needs treating and you don't have a recommended base oil in the house, use whatever you have—even cooking oil—until you can get to a pharmacist or store to purchase something better.

7–12 YEARS OLD		
All those to 7 years; plus the following at ⅓ dosage directed for other oils: **Fennel** **Frankincense** **Cypress** **Basil**	As above	As above

Dosage: 5–15 drops diluted in 2 tablespoons Base Oil

PUBERTY		
All the above at full dose, plus:	As above	As above

FEMALE	MALE
Rose	**Marjoram**
Geranium	**Bergamot**
Marjoram	

Dosage: 10–20 drops diluted in 2 tablespoons Base Oil

cream. This is when your prepared baby pots will come in handy. If you make up a synergistic blend using equal proportions of your two essential oils, you can mix just 1 drop in with 2 teaspoons of cream because you really won't need much more than this. Do make sure that you blend the essential oils in well with the cream before applying to the baby's bottom.

Cradle cap is an unsightly crusting on the scalp which can come off in rather big lumps. Olive oil is usually recommended, but I find that too heavy for a baby's delicate scalp. Almond oil is much better. Use the following formula to make a massage oil and very gently apply to the scalp with your fingertips, avoiding the fontanelle. Don't even think of substituting lavender oil because that makes the skin grow too quickly—the opposite of the result wanted here. Use the following formula once a day until the cradle cap goes.

CRADLE CAP REMEDY

Eucalyptus lemon	1 drop
Geranium	1 drop

Dilute in 2 tablespoons almond oil, and mix very well

The Umbilical Cord

At birth, the umbilical cord will be cut and tied, leaving a rather ugly stump. This shrivels up and falls off on its own accord around the sixth or seventh day. Generally, you want to do as little as possible to this area and leave it all to Mother Nature; simply keep the area clean and dry to help avoid infection. If any discharge or redness occurs an antiseptic powder may be prescribed or you can make your own by blending one ounce of pure talc BP (available from your pharmacist) and adding 5 drops of lavender oil. See the section on page 160–161 on how to make your own dry powders. In Europe they use pure powdered thyme, which is available from herbalists. Apply your chosen antiseptic powder once a day after the bath with a new powder-puff or cotton-wool ball. Alternatively get a cotton ball, dip it in the bottle of lavender oil, then immediately dip it in a cup of water and squeeze it with clean fingers to release the excess liquid. Now gently rub around the umbilical area. Do this twice a day.

If your baby develops a hernia, or swelling, simply leave it alone and point it out to your doctor or midwife. Indeed, you should report any inflammation or redness if and when it occurs.

Other Early Problems

All young babies sweat slightly and occasionally throw up their food and have runny stools. However, excessive sweating, diarrhea, and vomiting must all be taken seriously as they can affect a baby's health very quickly and lead to dehydration. See a doctor at once. Of course, deciding what is excessive is the tricky part but err on the side of caution secure in the knowledge that doctors have a great tolerance of overcautious parents, however impatient and dismissive they may be with you as the patient. Also, have confidence in—and develop—your own intuition. That will be your greatest asset in child care.

Babies from Two to Twelve Months ◆◆◆◆◆

Babies are difficult to care for because they can't tell us what is making them cry. It is very important to establish contact between the mother and the baby, to repair the shock caused to the baby when he or she came out of mother's womb. The newborn baby responds well to touch, which is an important part of the bonding system, and massage should start straight away.

Commercial baby products are usually petroleum based, which makes them good for protecting the baby's skin from water and urine but not necessarily intrinsically good for the baby's skin. In this formula, however, we use a base oil which *is* good for skin and essential oils which are good for a great deal more besides. The amount of essential oil used here is about one-tenth that of an adult's massage oil. Even so, this formula treats eczema and cradle cap, inflammation, and teething problems, while boosting the immune system and acting as a general strengthener. It also has a marvelously calming effect on the nervous system, and babies become more contented—appreciating as well, no doubt, the loving touch they receive. Massage over the whole of the baby's body but avoid the eyes and genitals:

BABY'S MASSAGE OIL FORMULA

Chamomile Roman	1 drop
Lavender	1 drop
Geranium	1 drop

Diluted in 2 tablespoons sweet almond oil

This massage oil is the only baby remedy that I recommend to be used on a continual or daily basis. All other remedies should be used on alternate days, or as directed, or when immediately needed. There is no need to use any treatment "just in case." Wait until the baby actually develops a problem and then deal with it.

Colic

Crying is a baby's way of letting us know that something is wrong. All mothers know that a hungry baby will cry relentlessly until the breast or bottle is presented. The red-faced, bawling baby is transformed into a preoccupied angel. But if your baby is crying and hunger isn't the reason, don't ignore it. Most probably the reason is colic, and this usually can be helped by rubbing the baby's tummy gently with the massage oil. Then turn the baby over and rub the middle portion of the back in gentle, circular movements.

If the colic is more severe, use the following formula in the same way. It smells like gripe water because gripe water is made of dill!

SEVERE COLIC REMEDY

Dill	1 drop

Diluted in 1 tablespoon sweet almond oil

Cartoonists have had a heyday with the classic image of mother or father walking up and down with baby up against a shoulder, their hand patting and rubbing in the attempt to elicit wind from the usually half-asleep baby. And it's certainly a time-consuming business. Wind can be caused by a baby taking in air during feeding or by crying. Whatever the cause, the treatment is the same.

Fretfulness in babies and children is a subject for which there are as many theories as there are mothers. One of the most interesting of these comes from Jean Liedloff in her book *The Continuum Concept* (Addison-Wesley), in which she discusses the differences between Western baby care practices and those of the Yequana, with whom she spent several years in the South American jungle. Her theory is that over the millions of years man has been developing, babies have evolved to expect to arrive into the world and straight into their mother's arms. A cot in the other room will not do. Missing the closeness which "instinct" has led them to expect, they cry, trying to draw our attention to the matter and put it right. We, meanwhile, are reading baby care books in an attempt to drown out our instinct to pick them up. But perhaps picking them up more often would make them less fretful.

Fretfulness as a frequent occurrence in a baby is an upsetting business for all concerned, but it also makes it difficult to know when the baby has wind, teething troubles, or a condition which needs seeing by the doctor. Happy, healthy babies do not cry a lot, go red in the face and whimper, sweat or fail to sleep; those who do are anxious, need some care and attention from their mother or father, or they are ill.

Fretfulness

Occasional fretfulness affects us all. Babies have frustration to deal with, and aggravation too—imagine what a baby makes of a blaring TV in the corner, complete with gun battles and car chases. Touch works wonders for any anxiety condition, and baby massage is soothing for mother and baby alike. The following massage oils may be applied a couple of times a week or when your baby seems fretful:

FRETFUL BABY MASSAGE FORMULAS

FORMULA 1

Chamomile Roman	3 drops
Lavender	4 drops

Diluted in 2 tablespoons of sweet almond oil

FORMULA 2

Chamomile Roman	4 drops
Geranium	3 drops

Diluted in 2 tablespoons of sweet almond oil

FORMULA 3

Tangerine	7 drops
Chamomile Roman	2 drops

Diluted in 2 tablespoons of sweet almond oil

FORMULA 4

Mandarin	7 drops
Chamomile Roman	2 drops

Diluted in 2 tablespoons of sweet almond oil

One very effective way to bring comfort to a fretful baby is to massage its feet in the following way: doing both feet at the same time, rub your thumbs from the center of the sole of the foot towards the bottom of the toes, over the ball of the foot, in gentle rhythmic movements. You can do this with the massage oil or simply over the baby's cloth footwear. At first the infant may wiggle around but you can hold both feet firmly between thumb and fingers and the baby will soon settle down. This is an ancient Chinese method which is now much in use by nannies all over the world, and you'll be amazed by the calming response this foot massage elicits from an apparently inconsolable baby.

Sickness and Vomiting

If your baby is constantly being sick it could be that he or she is allergic to cow's milk. Try changing the brand of milk, but if the condition continues consult your doctor who will usually prescribe soya-product milk. Babies who are not allergic but consistently throw up a large portion of their feed can, however, be treated effectively with peppermint oil which calms the stomach and makes digestion easier. Put one drop on a cotton-wool ball and place this in the baby's cot at the opposite end to the baby's head.

Projectile vomiting, when the baby throws up the food with such force that it lands several feet away, is a medical condition caused by a muscular abnormality and must be attended to. Don't be put off; insist on a thorough examination.

Sleeping

If your baby isn't sleeping, here is a remedy that can be used on alternate nights until he or she has learned to sleep through the night. There is no need to use the remedy every night, yet slowly the baby's sleeping pattern will change—for the better all around. When you put your baby to bed, place beneath the cot on the floor, not directly under the child's head, a bowl of boiling water. Add 1 drop of chamomile Roman and 1 drop of geranium oil. Keep the door almost closed to retain the aroma molecules in baby's room. A few alternate days of this and your baby will soon learn to conserve his energies during the night and save them for another demanding day!

Teething

By the time a child is two or three years old it will have developed twenty milk teeth. Teething usually begins at around six months, but there is a wide variation in this, as in all aspects of child development: some may not have started by the time they are one, others begin very early indeed, and it has even been known for a baby to be born with teeth. Teething may cause inflammation and soreness of the gums and, if there is discomfort, fever. Rashes are often associated with teething but they are more likely to be caused by saliva; if left wet the skin becomes sore. Some babies seem to suffer more than others and many sleepless nights are caused by teething, starting a cycle of discomfort and tiredness which makes the baby more irritable.

Giving your baby something to chew on is important at this time. Teeth need to be used. The Chinese give their children bones to chew on, but if you do that make sure there are no small pieces which could be broken off. Apples are great for teeth but even little pieces can become stuck in a baby's throat.

Teething can also cause runny stools or a runny nose. Some babies get constipated, and the best thing for them is fruit juice.

Teething can get wrongly blamed for causing just about every problem a small baby might present so a greater awareness of your baby's condition is important at this stage. Here are the oils to use for teething problems:

TEETHING ESSENTIAL OILS

Chamomile Roman	**Chamomile German**
Lavender	**Yarrow**

And here are several remedies that help the teeth and gums and also calm the baby. You can use one of three essential oils for this first treatment, singly or in an equal mix (if using two oils, 6 drops each; if three, 3 drops each). Their effect is equally good:

Chamomile Roman	6 drops
or	
Chamomile German	6 drops
or	
Yarrow	6 drops

Dilute in 5 teaspoons vegetable oil and mix well

then

Take 1 teaspoon oil mix and put in an eggcup. Fill with ice-cold water. STIR VERY WELL.

You now have two mixtures for this two-part treatment. First, dip a cotton-wool ball into the mixture in the eggcup and wipe it very gently around the baby's gums. Then, using just the oil mix, massage around the outside of the face along the line of the jaw. You only need a couple of drops each time; rub it a little between your fingers before applying.

A simpler alternative which quickly takes what the French call the "heating element" out of the gum involves adding 1 drop of chamomile essential oil to an eggcupful of cold water and stirring well. Dip a cotton-wool ball in this mixture and rub gently around the baby's gums. Store the mixture in the fridge for whenever you need it.

One of the components of chamomile is azulene, an antiinflammatory that is extracted from the flowers. Aloe vera is also very soothing and may be used in liquid form as an alternative to the water and oil in the first remedy above and instead of the water in the second.

Lavender may also be used for teething problems. Put 5 drops of lavender into 1 tablespoon of vegetable oil. Mix well. Using only about 2 drops of this dilution, massage around the baby's exterior jaw and up the neck area.

Homeopathic chamomile teething grains are also very useful in conjunction with all the above.

Colds and Coughs

Protecting a baby from colds, especially during winter in a house full of other children, is a matter many mothers have had to worry about. But don't use essential oil treatments on babies and children as a precaution because another member of the family has a cold or flu. If that's the case and you want to protect the baby, use essential oils diluted in water in a plant-spray around the house—spray the corridor outside the baby's room but not inside the room.

We all know how miserable it is to have a cold, and it must be twice as bad for a baby who doesn't know what's happening and can't blow his or her little nose. Feeding becomes a struggle as the poor baby gasps for breath between sucks and even the process of breathing is difficult. Although it is distressing, however, a cold is not a serious problem. But colds are often forerunners of something more serious, and so if your baby also has a temperature, is feverish, off food, or crying a lot, have him checked by the doctor. If a baby under three weeks old has a cough he should be seen by a doctor.

A simple solution to baby colds involves placing on the floor under the baby's cot, but not directly under the head, a small bowl of boiling water to which you have added 3 drops of eucalyptus oil. The steam will rise, releasing the molecules of aroma into the room.

Or here is an excellent synergistic blend treatment:

SNIFF AND SNUFFLES
SYNERGISTIC BLEND

Eucalyptus	10 drops
Tea tree	10 drops
Lavender	10 drops

Mix together in these proportions

Place 3 drops on an infuser in the bedroom for overnight, and again during the day. If breathing is very difficult, place 2 drops on a piece of cotton and place it under the edge of the pillow as well.

When you bathe the baby add 1 drop of the synergistic blend to the water and swish it around. (For babies and children between one year and five, add 2 drops to the bath.)

Also, you can make a massage oil using 3 drops of the synergistic blend to 2 teaspoons vegetable oil; massage this over the baby's back and chest. This three-part treatment should not be given for more than a week at a time.

If the baby has a severe cough, whooping cough, severe bronchitis, or other respiratory problems, use the following formula in a small bowl of boiling water left in baby's room overnight or in a diffuser. Use the remedy for three consecutive nights, take a break of two nights and, if necessary, continue on this three on–two off basis:

SEVERE RESPIRATORY PROBLEMS
BABY FORMULA

Eucalyptus	3 drops
Hyssop	1 drop
Thyme	1 drop

Use 2 drops

Whenever using essential oils in a diffuser, dilute them in a small amount of water beforehand.

Allergies

Eczema can often be treated successfully simply by massaging the baby with the massage oil formula given on page 12. However, the root cause of the problem may be an allergy—the most common being allergies to cow's milk or eggs. Your doctor should be able to check for allergies. Also, although it has not been proved conclusively, there does seem to be a correlation between allergies in the family and eczema on a baby. If either parent or even grandparent has a history of eczema, hay fever, asthma, or psoriasis it is possible that the baby's eczema is related to this. If the mother has food allergies she may have passed these to the baby and so, as solid foods are introduced, the baby manifests these in developing eczema.

Children ♦♦♦♦♦♦♦♦♦♦♦♦♦

If we are what we eat, our children are what we feed them. Recent research in Britain and America has shown that an absence of wholesome food because of the preference for junk food affects negatively both behavior and intellectual development. It is not simply that junk food does you no good, rather that an absence of the nutrients found in good food causes potential to be eroded. As it is so difficult to persuade children not to fill their tummies with Coca-Cola and chips, both at home and when they are out of sight, perhaps vitamin supplements are a good idea. If the research proves right, your children should become better behaved and produce better report cards. It must be worth a try!

The nutritional status of children has also been shown to affect their health. This is a complex subject and an important one, because diet can affect almost every medical ailment from recurrent coughs and colds to cancer. For more information on this subject write to the British College of Naturopathy and Osteopathy in London.

Cuts, Grazes, Bruises, and Burns

Children are constantly getting into scrapes of one sort or another. As far as they are concerned, trees are for climbing. In learning what "hot" is, they burn themselves. Running around, they fall over. And you can tell your youngster a hundred times not to run on the gravel—he will get so excited playing cowboys and Indians that he'll simply forget. All one can do is be prepared for the inevitable knocks he is going to have to take in this action packed period of his life. Often children don't even realize they have damaged themselves because they get so elated while having their fun. How often have you asked, "What have you done?" to be answered with, "I don't know, it just came"?

SCRAPES AND CUTS ESSENTIAL OILS

Lavender	**Tea tree**
Eucalyptus	**Niaouli**
Lemon	**Pine**

The essential oils fight infection and promote healing, thus providing parents with an excellent helpmate in caring for their child. Remember, too, to use them in the healing stage, because for some unknown reason children love picking off their scabs. The appeal of this activity escapes me—perhaps they are trying to discover what lies beneath or perhaps they just find the scabs aggravating. But trying to stop them is almost impossible and so the essential oils come in handy just to keep the damage to a minimum.

The danger in children getting into scrapes is infection. Make absolutely sure that splinters are taken out and that all the dirt is thoroughly bathed away from any cut, graze, or scratch. As your bathing solution, add 10 drops of lavender or one of the above to a pint of warm water in a bowl. This doesn't sting as much as disinfectant and the aroma does both of you more good. It gives strength to the faint-hearted—you—and has a calming effect on your child. Allow the damaged skin to heal in the fresh air if at all possible, for it will heal quicker. Obviously cover it if there is danger of reinfection—if, for example, playtime has just begun. And repeat the bathing with essential oil a few hours later, whether the cut has been covered or not. If you apply a plaster, put a drop of neat lavender oil on the plaster beforehand. This will heal the wound quickly and in most instances there will be no scar.

BRUISES ESSENTIAL OILS

Hyssop	**Geranium**
Lavender	

Bruises need another sort of care. First, wrap some ice cubes in a towel and hold this against the area that has received the blow. Then apply an oil made with 30 drops of hyssop diluted in 2 tablespoons vegetable oil. The homeopathic tincture of arnica is also extremely good. Treat the bruise twice a day.

Burns

Burns need the heat taken out of them immediately. Invisible to the eye, a process known as denaturation is taking place in the tissues (see page 72).

BURNS ESSENTIAL OILS

Lavender	**Chamomile German**
Eucalyptus	**Yarrow**
Geranium	

Run the area of the burn under cold water and if that part of the body can't reach the tap, apply a cold compress. Prepare a bowl of cold water, and add ice cubes; put 2 neat drops of lavender on a clean washcloth and wring it out in the water; apply. This usually prevents blistering.

Insomnia

To provide the energy to run around getting into scrapes, children need their sleep. And so, come to that, do you. Insomnia in children can have many causes, ranging from overanxiety at school to tummy ache. And then there are the numerous monsters of the night, fears and phobias that can prevent a healthy child from sleeping. Apart from the usual reassurance that a parent can give, help can come in many ways with the essential oils. They have been used by countless families over the centuries for just this situation.

A warm bath that becomes a part of winding down to bedtime, relaxing before the head hits the pillows, is one of the best ways to overcome sleeplessness in children. After all, if we went to bed with a head full of the day's problems and the expected ones of tomorrow, would we sleep? There's a lot to be said for a warm drink, a cuddle, and a story—but while still up, not in bed. Try not to allow your child to come in late from playing and go straight to bed. An interlude of rock music on the headphones doesn't count. The idea is to calm and soothe the growing nerves and brain cells.

CHILDREN'S INSOMNIA ESSENTIAL OILS

FROM TWELVE MONTHS TO FIVE YEARS

Mandarin	**Lavender**
Chamomile Roman	**Palma rosa**

IN BATHS:

1 drop per year old to a maximum of three

FROM FIVE TO TWELVE YEARS

As before, plus:

Geranium	**Clary-sage**
Nutmeg	

IN BATHS:

3 drops until seven years
4 drops between seven and ten
5 drops when eleven and twelve

And here are a couple of excellent synergistic blends you might like to try:

INSOMNIA SYNERGISTIC BLEND
FROM TWELVE MONTHS TO FIVE YEARS

Palma rosa	10 drops
Chamomile Roman	7 drops
Mandarin	5 drops

INSOMNIA SYNERGISTIC BLEND
FROM FIVE TO TWELVE YEARS

Chamomile Roman	10 drops
Geranium	8 drops
Nutmeg	4 drops

Make up a blend of essential oils using these proportions and use as many drops as recommended above for each age. Or you could make up a blend using any combination from the main list—utilize what you have in the cupboard, again maintaining the dosage above. Or use oils singly.

A foot massage is very relaxing, and after a bath and before bed it's a real soporific. Make up a massage oil with the synergistic blend, or by making your own blend from the list or using one oil on the list. Do bear in mind that certain oils can become stimulants rather than relaxants if used in high dosage. Always under-dose, rather than overdose. Use 10 drops of essential oil to 2 tablespoons vegetable oil for the foot massage oil.

Aches and Pains

Children have so many aches and pains, the cause of which is often a mystery, that the term "growing pains" has been coined to explain them. Often they come at night and go by morning, especially aches in the arms and legs. Sometimes these are just due to too much exercise at school, swimming perhaps. But if a child complains of a pain continuing in the same place for a long time you should take him to the doctor.

Massage helps all sorts of aches and pains. Make up an oil for your child's particular need. If the legs ache, for example, use a little lavender and if your child is over five years old, rosemary. Each ache will be as individual as each child, so experiment to find the solution, using the information in this section and the list of oils for children of your child's age.

OVEREXERCISED CHILD MASSAGE OIL

Peppermint	5 drops
Rosemary	5 drops
Lavender	5 drops

Diluted in 2 tablespoons vegetable oil

Tummy aches can have many root causes, from overexercise and overeating to anxiety. But they may also indicate more serious problems—an appendicitis often starts as a mild stomachache, for example—so do refer to your doctor to be on the safe side.

TUMMY ACHE ESSENTIAL OILS

Peppermint	**Geranium**
Dill	**Rosemary**
Eucalyptus	**Lavender**
Coriander	

Make up a massage oil using 15 drops of one of these essential oils to 2 tablespoons vegetable oil

Massage the child's abdomen in a clockwise direction, more or less around the belly button. It often helps to massage the back as well—again, in a clockwise direction. Here's a formula that works well:

GENERAL TUMMY ACHE FORMULA

Dill	9 drops
Geranium	6 drops

Diluted in 2 tablespoons vegetable oil

Fevers

When a child develops a fever it is very distressing for child and parents alike. It's worrying, too, because in extreme cases fever can lead to a seizure. Don't mistake shivering as a sign that the child is cold—the body will use all the methods at its disposal to try to get rid of the fever. A child who has a fever and is shivering should not be made extra warm; that will only make things worse. What you need to do is cool the body down, and as it cools, the shaking will go.

Remove all extra clothing and bedding and cover the child with a sheet—this is quite sufficient. Wipe the head and body continuously with a cool cloth—not cold as this will be a shock to their body. Cold water applied to the skin will only keep the heat in as the blood vessels contract in their usual way in response to a cold temperature. Also sponge down occasionally using lukewarm water to which you have added the essential oil (2 drops oil to 1 quart water).

COOLING ESSENTIAL OILS

Eucalyptus	**Peppermint** (in a room diffuser only)
Tea tree	**Lavender**
Camomile Roman	

Use whatever oils you have in the cupboard. Eucalyptus and lavender in equal proportions make an excellent cooling oil.

If the fever has become acute, make up a large bowl of lukewarm water to which you have added 10 drops of essential oil. Swish it around. Make a compress with any old material you have (see page 96), soak it in the solution and wring out. Put a rubber sheet or piece of plastic underneath the child and apply the oiled water to the armpits, groin (but not the genitals), forehead, and lower back. As soon as the compresses are warm, change them for cool ones. Repeat until the fever subsides. A treatment frequently used for severe feverish conditions involves wrapping the whole baby in a cool sheet that has been soaked in the essential oil water.

If the glands are swollen, apply the following formula:

SWOLLEN GLANDS/FEVER
SYNERGISTIC BLEND OIL

Eucalyptus	5 drops
Lavender	5 drops
Tea tree	5 drops

Make up a synergistic blend using these proportions. Put 5 drops in a teaspoon of vegetable oil, mix well. Rub gently into the glands, neck, and groin (avoid the genitals), once every hour.

And continue with the other methods given above.

If the child goes into a fit, remove his clothing and lie him on his side. Keep him cool and get someone to call a doctor. Make sure the child can't hurt himself—don't leave him on his own.

Impetigo

Impetigo is an infection of the outer layers of the skin which can be caused by an infected scratch or insect bite. It starts as tiny red spots, turns into blisters, and can change into a sore pus-filled area that gets bigger and spreads. Not only is impetigo contagious from person to person but infection can be spread from one area of skin to another on the same person. It is quite a common complaint, and if one child in the school has it you can be pretty sure that others will too.

Sores do not just go away and they must be treated as soon as they are noticed. It is important to get all the infected pus out of the sore. To clean it out, prepare a small bowl of cooled, boiled water (about 4 ounces), add 10 drops of lavender and, using clean cotton wool, wash the sores out thoroughly. Now apply a compress.

First, prepare your essential oils—equal amounts of tagetes and myrrh in a synergistic blend. You will also need a piece of cotton cut in a rectangle large enough to cover the area of the sore twice. Soak the cotton in water and then put 2 drops of the synergistic blend in the center. Fold over the two ends of the cotton so that the essential oil will not be directly on the sore. Bandage the cotton to the body, or if the sores are on an awkward part of the body attach it with plaster. Leave the cotton there for an hour and then remove it so that the sore can be exposed to the air. If the sores do not clear, repeat the treatment until they do.

Constipation

Constipation in children can be caused by several factors, from a change in food habits to stress, and even by toilet training in the toddler. The stools become dehydrated and rabbit-like. The problem can usually be quickly relieved with a combination of essential oil massage and plenty of fruit juice and water.

ESSENTIAL OILS
TO TREAT CONSTIPATION

Geranium	**Patchouli**
Rosemary	**Mandarin**
Chamomile Roman	**Tangerine**

Use any of the oils singly or in combination, or use my formula:

CHILDREN'S CONSTIPATION
MASSAGE OIL FORMULA

Geranium	4 drops
Patchouli	6 drops
Mandarin	15 drops

Diluted in 2 tablespoons vegetable oil

At bedtime give the child a large glass of natural fruit juice and water, and massage the whole of his abdomen in gentle movements, working around the belly button in a clockwise direction—the direction in which the intestines go.

Diarrhea

Diarrhea in a child has many causes. It could be a physical problem, such as bacteria, viruses, ear infections, and flu. It could be that the child has an allergic reaction to a food, or is suffering side effects from a medication. Nervous tension and stress could also be the culprits: has your child been upset by bullying at school, worried about exams, or even made anxious by parental arguments?

With a case of diarrhea it is important that the lost fluid is replaced so that dehydration does not occur. If it continues for more than twenty-four hours you should call a doctor. Don't urge the child to eat, but do give him lots of liquid. Feed him diluted soups and drinks with honey dissolved in them. Don't give the child dairy products as they will only make matters worse.

The following oils can be included in a massage oil to rub gently on the abdomen:

ESSENTIAL OILS TO TREAT DIARRHEA

Chamomile Roman	**Sandalwood**
Geranium	**Ginger**

Or use my formula:

CHILDREN'S DIARRHEA MASSAGE OIL FORMULA

Ginger	5 drops
Sandalwood	8 drops
Chamomile Roman	8 drops

Diluted in 2 tablespoons vegetable oil

If the child has a sore bottom, make up a chamomile ointment (see page 96) and apply around the anal area to reduce soreness and burning.

Keep your child off cow dairy products for at least a week following a bout of diarrhea and serve gentle foods such as banana, scrambled egg, stewed apple, rice, and oats.

Teeth/Gums

It is important to establish a routine of thorough teeth cleaning right from the word go. Stand behind a small child when you clean his teeth and encourage him to "help" from about the age of three.

Gum disease seems to be on the increase, and tincture of myrrh used as a mouthwash can help prevent this. Tincture of myrrh is available at a pharmacy.

If your child already has a problem with gum disease or tooth decay, the following oils can help:

ESSENTIAL OILS FOR GUMS

Myrrh	**Chamomile Roman**
Lavender	
Calendula	

Use 1 drop only in a tumbler of warm water and rinse around the mouth. *Do not swallow.* Do this once a day until there are signs of improvement.

Tonsillitis

In tonsillitis, the tonsils become enlarged and infected. The swelling may be painful and the throat is red and sore. Small yellow spots are often seen on the tonsils. The child feels unwell, could be running a temperature, or have an earache, headache, neck ache, or tummy ache.

Give the child plenty of drinks, and add honey to soothe and help heal the throat.

Rose syrup, marigold syrup, and geranium syrup are all extremely useful. (See page 334, for how to make these.) They can be used in two ways. If the child likes the taste, simply slide a teaspoon of syrup down the throat. If not, or in addition, dilute a teaspoon of syrup in a small glass of warm water and have the child gargle with it. Do this three times a day to promote healing.

The essential oils can be used in several ways. Use the oils singly, in a blend, or follow the synergistic formula:

TONSILLITIS OILS

Lavender	**Ginger**
Tea tree	**Chamomile Roman**
Lemon	

TONSILLITIS SYNERGISTIC BLEND

Lavender	10 drops
Tea tree	15 drops
Ginger	5 drops
Lemon	2 drops

Use 4 drops on a warm compress twice a day over the throat area. Also, make up a massage oil using 5 drops of essential oil to 2 teaspoons vegetable oil and apply over the upper abdomen and back. The essential oils can also be used in a diffuser.

An excellent remedy for tonsillitis follows. It can be used as a gargle or a mouthwash if the child cannot gargle:

TONSILLITIS REMEDY

Cider vinegar	3 tablespoons
Honey	1 tablespoon
Ginger	3 drops
Lemon	5 drops

Blend the ingredients together until well amalgamated and put 1 teaspoon in a tumbler of warm water

Get your child to gargle twice a day, and follow with a teaspoon of rose honey (see page 355) which should be swallowed.

Sore Throats

Sore throats range from the mild, tickly type to the unable to swallow type—all irritating and unpleasant. They are usually caused by a virus or by bacteria. Follow the tonsillitis treatments.

Ears

Ear infections can have such diverse causes as a cold, blowing extra hard through both nostrils, or poking a pencil in the ear! Earache should always be checked to see if there is infection, because if left in babies and children it could lead in later life to deafness and the infection may even spread to the brain. Earache that doesn't clear up with antibiotics and has doctors baffled can often be helped by such old-fashioned remedies as putting a piece of cotton wool soaked in olive oil into the ear. The cotton wool must be large enough to prevent it being pushed down into the ear. To improve this old remedy, add 1 drop of lavender essential oil to a teaspoon of olive oil, mix well and soak a piece of cotton wool in it. Leave this in the ear, changing it twice a day. If the child insists on pulling the cotton wool out, put it there while you have the opportunity to keep an eye on it—while you read him a story, for example, or in some other way distract his attention. Do make sure you use pure, virgin, first pressing olive oil, and squeeze the excess oil out before putting the cotton wool in the ear.

Earache can make a child very miserable and in babies can lead to diarrhea and vomiting. You may see a watery discharge or pus coming from the ear, and if so you must change the ear plug every hour until it stops. If the ear is inflamed, use one of the chamomile essential oils—preferably chamomile German—as well as the lavender (1 drop of each).

If a virus is causing the trouble, follow the procedure above using either lavender or one of the antiviral oils: tea tree or red thyme. Make an oil by combining 5 drops of one of these essential oils to 1 teaspoon vegetable oil and apply, using only a few drops, on both sides in a line from the back of the ear down the neck, crossing the collarbone and into the armpit. Then put some along the panty line at the front—from the side hips to the groin along the tops of the legs, making absolutely sure not to get any near the genitals. As you only need to wipe a thin layer of the oil on the skin, this shouldn't be difficult. Do this twice a day until the infection goes.

Bronchiolitis and Bronchitis

These are both conditions affecting the bronchioles, the air tubes. Bronchiolitis usually affects babies under eighteen months. In both conditions, the air tubes become filled with mucus and the infection spreads into the lungs, causing shortness of breath. A baby's breathing can become frighteningly rapid and labored. Coughs and colds can start these conditions off; they are caused by many different types of viruses.

Essential oils help in all cases of bronchial congestion. Their antiviral and antibacterial properties are very useful and they are inhaled right to the site of the trouble. Children respond well to essential oil treatments of the respiratory tract, and you can use them secure in the knowledge that they are compatible with any medicine the doctor will prescribe if used in the correct dosage.

If a baby has bronchiolitis keep him warm and try to stop him crying. Cuddles are the order of the day as he will be restless, distressed, and irritable. Feeding should be in small rather than large quantities, and often. Call your doctor if you have not already done so. If things get bad, the baby might need hospitalization and oxygen.

BRONCHIOLITIS ESSENTIAL OILS

Tea tree	**Eucalyptus***
Chamomile Roman	**Lavender**

*The best eucalyptus to get if you can find it is eucalyptus radiata.

BRONCHITIS ESSENTIAL OILS FOR CHILDREN OVER FIVE YEARS

As listed above plus:

Rosemary	**Thyme***
Hyssop	

*I particularly recommend a thyme called thymus vulgaris linololiferum for this treatment as it works well on children. It is slightly more expensive than other species of thyme but is well worth the investment because it is excellent for many children's conditions.

As an alternative to any of the formulas below, substitute Bronchotect—a specially formulated preparation for respiratory tract problems. Use the same number of drops as in the formulas.

These are two-part treatments:

INHALATIONS

UNDER FIVE YEARS

Tea tree	8 drops
Chamomile Roman	7 drops
Eucalyptus	10 drops

OVER FIVE YEARS

Tea tree	8 drops
Red thyme	10 drops
Chamomile Roman	7 drops

Make into a synergistic blend. Use 3 drops in a diffuser or in the water-bowl method, three times a day.

AND MASSAGE

UNDER FIVE YEARS

Tea tree	10 drops
Eucalyptus	10 drops
Lavender	10 drops

OVER FIVE YEARS

Red thyme	15 drops
Tea tree	15 drops

Add the amounts above to 2 tablespoons base vegetable oil. Massage three times a day over chest and back, concentrating on the back and lung area.

Childhood Asthma

The helplessness that parents so often feel in relation to a sick child is very pronounced in the case of the asthmatic child. To have to watch your child wheezing and fighting for breath must be heartbreaking and frightening at the same time. These parents are sometimes asthmatic themselves and so can identify closely with the suffering the child is going through, aware too of how this illness is keeping the child from enjoying fully life with his peers. It is encouraging to know that asthma often stops at puberty.

But parents can help in many ways. Keep a diary and write down everything that affects your child—what he eats, what exercise he has taken, what illnesses and complaints he has had, and the pollen count. How far you go with this depends upon how much time you have to spare, because asthmatic children have been found to be allergic to hairspray, deodorant, perfume, polish, dust, grass, animal fur, feathers—not to mention heat, cold, and damp. This diary could keep you so busy you don't have time to spray your hair, polish the furniture, or cut the grass! Also record when attacks occur and their severity, look for a pattern and adapt diet and lifestyle accordingly.

Many children respond well to the naturopathic approach. No dairy products. No wheat. No fizzy drinks (you'd be surprised by how many children get better after having stopped drinking them). No additives or preservatives. Nothing out of a tin or packet. Hard? Yes. But worth it? Most definitely yes, yes, yes.

Children with asthma have a very highly developed intuition and they know when you are anxious and this just makes them worry more—which can exacerbate an attack. During an attack, *don't fuss.*

Don't discourage the child from taking exercise but make sure that it is not over-strenuous. An asthmatic child needs strong lungs to cope with an attack. Yoga breathing methods are very good for strengthening the lungs and diaphragm. Your child may need a bronchodilator which helps the muscles of the lungs, thereby making breathing easier.

Many of the flower essential oils help in diluted form. They are best used in massage, which in itself is enormously beneficial. Combined and used as a preventative measure, they may prevent attacks occurring so frequently. Massage the back in long sweeping movements. Start at the base of the spine, your hands on either side of the vertebrae, and move in upward strokes to the shoulder, over the shoulder and down the sides of the body. The massage will also be very reassuring to the child. Use the following formulas:

ASTHMA MASSAGE FORMULAS

BABIES UP TO TWO YEARS

Lavender	5 drops
or	
Geranium	5 drops

TWO TO SEVEN YEARS

Lavender	5 drops
Geranium	3 drops
Frankincense	3 drops

SEVEN TO TWELVE YEARS

Geranium	5 drops
Cypress	5 drops
Frankincense	5 drops

All diluted in 2 tablespoons vegetable oil

Allergies

Why people develop allergies remains a medical mystery. Allergies are a very complicated subject, and finding a cure often proves difficult. The best line of defense, until we know more about them, is to remove the offending allergic agent. But finding the cause of the trouble may take some time because almost any substance in the world can trigger an allergic reaction, from the air we breathe to the water we drink; from the people we love to the clothes we wear. As well as the distressing physical results of an allergy there is the inconvenience of having to change lifestyle, sometimes drastically.

For children, it is often the common, everyday things that produce a reaction. Cow products, grass, house dust, pets, wheat, colorants, additives, and preservatives are often the cause. An allergy can manifest itself as asthma, eczema, hyperactivity, fatigue, itching, runny nose, sneezing, headaches, lumps, and bumps.

Allergic reactions to essential oils are rare if used correctly. A child with hay fever or eczema may be slightly more at risk. In the case of an allergy to one oil, don't lump similar-seeming oils together and assume there will be an allergy to them too. Allergy to orange, for example, does not necessarily mean there will be a reaction to lemon essential oil.

ECZEMA is very itchy and here is a remedy for that. Apply to the affected area twice a day:

Chamomile German	10 drops
Yarrow	5 drops
Tagetes	5 drops

Diluted in

Vegetable oil	2 tablespoons
Jojoba oil	30 drops
Evening primrose oil	10 drops

HIVES are usually white lumps or weals that look as if the child has been hit. They are very itchy. Use the same treatment as for eczema. Also, put 2 drops of chamomile German into a quarter of a cup of baking soda and add to the bath.

HAY FEVER needs to be treated with a special formula. Consult your local aromatherapist.

BEE STINGS produce an allergic reaction in a small percentage of children: the body can swell up and breathing becomes labored. Try to remove the stinger and treat with 1 drop of a synergistic blend of equal proportions of lavender and chamomile German. Lavender contains antivenom properties and often acts as an antidote to the poison, so stopping the reaction.

MIGRAINE is covered in full in the following section, but as migraine in children is often caused by an allergic reaction to certain foods it is worth considering it in relation to your child's diet. Remove from the diet all foods that are not fresh. As well as all the obvious items packed with artificial colorants, flavorants, additives, and preservatives, cut out all tinned and packaged goods no matter what promises of purity are made on the label. It is absolutely crucial to cut out dairy products. The child can have grains, but no wheat. Cut out tea and fizzy drinks. No red meat.

You might begin to think that there's nothing left to feed the child! Give him plenty of fish and chicken, fresh vegetables and fruit, mineral waters and natural fruit juices diluted with mineral water. Breakfast can consist of real oats, puffed rice with soya milk, or follow the recipe for real muesli on page 356. Popsicles should be made with natural fruit juices. Give herb teas at bedtime—chamomile sweetened with a little honey is good. If the child has had sick migraines, give peppermint herb tea during the day.

This new regime could provoke withdrawal symptoms such as headache or stomach ache in the first few days. These soon go.

Grapefruit essential oil is excellent in the treatment of this debilitating condition. Use 4 drops in a nice warm bath or soak a compress in 1 pint of water to which you have added 2 drops of grapefruit oil and apply it to the head. Also, make a massage oil using 15 drops of grapefruit to 2 tablespoons vegetable oil.

Migraine

Essential oil massages over a period of time often alleviate migraine. Most aromatherapists are trained how to deal with this problem but you can also help your child at home. Set a time when you can both be relaxed and take the phone off the hook—you are acting as therapist. Get the child to lie face-down on the bed and massage following the general instructions on page 410. Do this for at least fifteen minutes once a week, or if under stress. Use the following oils either singly or in combination:

CHILDREN'S MIGRAINE ESSENTIAL OILS

Grapefruit	**Neroli**
Lavender	**Peppermint**
Chamomile Roman	**Rosemary**

Or use my formula:

CHILDREN'S MIGRAINE FORMULA

Chamomile Roman	5 drops
Grapefruit	10 drops
Peppermint	5 drops
Rosemary	3 drops

Children under seven: Diluted in 4 ounces vegetable oil

Children over seven: Diluted in 2 ounces vegetable oil

The essential oils can be a great help to children who suffer migraine and many cases which came to me for treatment have been cleaned up by the parent following the directions above. You might also follow the diet outlined in the allergy section above. Common causes of migraine in children are insufficient breakfast and lunch, stress, allergies, and television. Sleep is one of the best remedies.

Mumps

Mumps is a common airborne viral disease whose target is the parotid salivary glands. Two or three weeks after infection the symptoms appear, the most characteristic of these being large, egg-like swellings on either side of the neck just below the ears. Sometimes only one side is affected. Other symptoms are mild fever, earache, pain when eating, and headache. Usually mumps is a fairly harmless condition and the symptoms go after a couple of days. Sometimes, however, the infection can spread to other glands, and in bad cases the testes, ovaries, and pancreas become involved. There is usually no danger unless the child is around puberty or older when the ovaries become painful and the testes swollen and sore, and male sterility can occur. Permanent deafness may occasionally follow an attack of mumps. Treatment for mumps is therefore advised to make sure that your child doesn't become one of the unfortunate few. Adult males who haven't had mumps should avoid contact with the child, as the virus is passed through saliva and nasal droplets and through the air.

The child should rest in bed and not be given acid drinks such as orange juice. Dryness of the mouth can be helped by using a mouthwash.

Use the following oils sprayed in the air with a plant-spray (new or clean) so that the essential oil molecules are inhaled by the child:

ESSENTIAL OILS FOR MUMPS

Tea tree	**Niaouli**
Coriander	**Lavender**

5 drops to 2½ cups water

Or mix a synergistic blend:

MUMPS SYNERGISTIC BLEND

Tea tree	10 drops
Lavender	10 drops
Coriander	10 drops
Lemon	10 drops

Blend together

Make up a blend of oil using 30 drops of essential oil to 2 tablespoons vegetable oil and apply gently around the sore area, the back of the neck, and the abdominal area. Use three times a day for ten days. The remaining 10 drops can be used in a room spray—5 drops to ½ pint of water.

Measles

Measles is a highly contagious disease that is often dismissed as part of growing up. It is, in fact, a killer. The major problem is that during the infectious stage the child is especially vulnerable to bacterial infection including bronchitis, pneumonia, and ear infections which can lead to deafness.

Like many childhood illnesses, measles can start as nothing more than a runny nose and a sore throat and you think your irritable patient has just got a cold. Other early symptoms are sore and runny eyes, fever, and enlarged glands in the neck, but symptoms are numerous and vary from child to child. The most telling symptom is spots—small red ones with white centers on the lining of the mouth, followed by spots on the cheeks which turn into a rash around the fourth day, spreading down the body.

Keep the child in bed and away from other children. The virus is spread by airborne droplets and saliva. Use a blend of antiviral oils as an air freshener through the house so that other members of the family can inhale it. Spray the child's room too, and keep it warm.

Make a synergistic blend of equal proportions chamomile German and lavender essential oils and use 5 drops of this in a pint of tepid water for a wash-down solution. The water should be warm. Add the oils to the water in a bowl, swish them around, soak your sponge or cloth, wring it out and gently wash the child. Do the whole body. This will soothe the spots and aid recovery.

If you wish to cover the spots in calamine lotion, add 5 drops each of chamomile German and lavender essential oil to a 4 ounce bottle of calamine and shake well.

Rubella (German Measles)

German measles is a very mild version of measles that isn't much of a problem unless contracted during the first four months of pregnancy. It can cause serious defects in the unborn child and so young women are vaccinated against it if they haven't had German measles during childhood. Epidemics of this viral infection seem to occur every three or four years. It is another rash condition, which this time starts behind the ears and spreads to the rest of the body. In some cases no rash appears and the child is only feverish and generally feeling under the weather.

Treat in the same way as all viral infections by spraying an antiviral oil or using diffusers to clear the atmosphere.

Also, add 4 drops of one of the oils below or 4 drops of the synergistic blend to a pint of warm water and use this to sponge the child down once a day:

RUBELLA SPONGE-DOWN

ESSENTIAL OILS

Lavender	**Chamomile Roman**
Chamomile German	**Tea tree**

SYNERGISTIC BLEND

Lavender	15 drops
Chamomile Roman	15 drops
Tea tree	5 drops

Chicken Pox

Chicken pox is yet another viral infection, and highly contagious. It is commonly believed that once you have had chicken pox you never get it again but I know children who have had it several times, including myself. The virus can lie dormant and return as shingles later in life.

After the incubation period of two weeks the child's temperature will rise and almost immediately a rash will appear. This is made up of small spots which may turn into blisters which burst and crust over. Trying to stop your child scratching and picking off the scabs is a full-time occupation. The spots start on the trunk of the body and then appear on the face and limbs. The child should be isolated until the last scab has fallen off.

Bed rest may prevent fever, and the child should be encouraged to sleep as this is one of the best things for chicken pox. Treatment involves trying to stop the very irritating itching. Add 10 drops of lavender and 10 of chamomile German to a 4 ounce bottle of calamine lotion and shake the bottle. Apply all over the body twice a day. Baths can also relieve the itching: add 2 drops of lavender to 1 cup of bicarbonate of soda and put in the bath. Also, spray the air with an antiviral mixture.

Whooping Cough

Pertussis is called whooping cough because a "whoop" sound is made as the child draws in air against the resistance of the glottis which is usually closed by the cough reflex. Before he learns to do this, the child appears to be suffocating because he cannot take in air while he is coughing. Basically, the pertussis cough comes on too suddenly for the usual taking in of air before a cough. The coughing is violent and uncontrolled and there can be as many as fifty coughing fits during a twenty-four hour period. You can forget about having a peaceful night's sleep—whooping cough will keep you and the child up for three or four weeks if you are lucky, twelve if you are not. This is a very serious disease indeed, especially to babies and the under-fives. It can cause brain damage, convulsions, ear infections, pneumonia, bronchitis, hernia, and a collapsed lung. It also makes the child susceptible to other serious infections.

Whooping cough is an extremely distressing disease, not only because the coughing and vomiting are so obviously painful and uncomfortable for the child but because the complications it can cause are worrying for you. The treatment below isn't simple but it is well worth making the effort it entails to try to keep the condition to a minimum. Results will be evident after a few days and will reward your perseverance.

First of all, keep your child away from other children for at least two weeks. Even if a child has been immunized he can still catch a mild form of the disease and will still be highly infectious. Whooping cough is more common than one would like to think and sometimes a child with a mild case of it appears simply to have a bad cold. Such a child can easily infect many classmates before anyone realizes what is happening.

In the treatment of whooping cough we use oils which are not on the main list for children and introduce more vital and aggressive essential oils. You will perhaps already have some of them in the house:

ESSENTIAL OILS
FOR TREATING WHOOPING COUGH

Cinnamon	**Niaouli**
Lavender	**Grapefruit**
Hyssop	**AV1 (Dermatect)**
Red thyme	**Thyme linalol**
Cypress	

Change the child's diet to one that is light and nutritious. Cut out milk products which can cause excess mucus in the body. Give the child chicken, fish, eggs, wholemeal bread, vegetables, fruit juices, mineral water, and herb teas. Sorbets and Popsicles made at home with diluted natural fruit juices will be soothing. Make soups and liquidize vegetables to make them easier to swallow. Cod liver oil helps, as does vitamin C (get the water soluble variety which can be sipped as a drink). Multivitamin and mineral tablets and a zinc supplement are particularly helpful at this time. As during any disease, the body will be working very hard to rid itself of the offending organism. One should try to help the body now, not hinder it: so no sweets, additives, or preservatives of any kind. That means no fizzy drinks. Give only mineral water and pure fruit juices.

Do not keep the child in hot stuffy rooms which dehydrate the body, but let him have plenty of fresh air. Open the windows during the day, ensuring that the child is well wrapped up. Steam also helps. Put bowls of hot steaming water in the child's room at night to keep the atmosphere as humid as possible and thus avoid dehydration of the bronchial tract. Make a synergistic blend of the following oils and use them in the room—in the hot water bowls, in a diffuser, or on a source of heat. Use 3 drops each time, three times a day.

ROOM METHOD SYNERGISTIC BLEND

Hyssop	10 drops
Thyme vulgaris	10 drops
Cinnamon	10 drops

Make into a synergistic blend using these proportions *or* substitute Dermatect

Make up another formula for use in the bath (4 drops each time) and also put 3 drops of this on a piece of cotton and leave it tucked under the edge of the child's pillow overnight:

BATH AND PILLOW
SYNERGISTIC BLEND

Cypress	10 drops
Niaouli	5 drops
Lavender	2 drops
Thyme vulgaris	3 drops

Make into a synergistic blend using these proportions

Also make up a massage oil and massage the chest night and day:

MASSAGE OIL FORMULA

Red thyme	5 drops
Niaouli	5 drops
Lavender	5 drops
Hyssop	5 drops

Dilute in 2 tablespoons vegetable oil
or
Substitute 20 drops of Dermatect in 2 tablespoons vegetable oil

If your child is under one year old, halve the dosages in all treatments above.

Verrucas and Warts

Viruses are responsible for both verrucas and warts. Warts look like little lumps and although they can grow anywhere, they are most common on the fingers or hands. Verrucas are foot warts but instead of growing outward, they grow inward. They can be extremely painful. You can spot them by the tell-tale black spot in the center of the painful area. Warts will often go away without any help, but in many cases nothing seems to shift them.

There are several essential oils which can be a real boon to sufferers of verrucas and warts, and although I always use the formula AV1 many good reports have been given for these:

VERRUCA AND WART ESSENTIAL OILS

Lemon	**Lavender**
Cypress	

When treating a child under twelve years of age for verrucas or warts it is crucial to dilute the essential oils beforehand. You can use any oil above singly or in combination, diluted in cider vinegar, or follow my suggestion:

Lemon	10 drops
Cypress	5 drops

per 2 teaspoons cider vinegar. Put all three ingredients in a clean bottle and shake well. If you are using Dermatect concentrate, dilute 5 drops to 2 teaspoons vinegar. Using a cotton-wool ball apply twice a day to the infected area only, avoiding the surrounding skin.

The essential oils can be applied neat if the child is over twelve. Again, use a cotton-wool ball and be careful not to get the oil on the uninfected skin. Apply twice a day.

Athlete's Foot

Little athletes are just as likely as big ones to get athlete's foot. All they have to do is walk barefoot where someone with the infection has walked before. Swimming pools and gymnasiums are excellent breeding grounds for this infectious fungi which causes the skin to flake and become itchy. The skin between the toes becomes white and sponge-like.

ATHLETE'S FOOT ESSENTIAL OILS

Tea tree	**Tagetes**
Lavender	**Cypress**

Of these oils, tea tree and tagetes are the better options. Give the child a foot bath once a day: add 5 drops of tea tree to a cup of salt and put into a large bowl of water. Get the child to soak his feet for at least five minutes daily.

Make up a foot powder by adding 10 drops of tea tree to a cup of dry green clay, or talc if you can't find clay (usually available in health food stores). You need to mix this really well, and an electric blender is perfect for the job: it usually has a tiny hole in the lid which enables you to add the essential oil at intervals to ensure a thorough mix. Powder the feet every day. It is very important to keep the skin between the toes dry. Avoid nylon socks—use only pure cotton or wool.

Also make a massage oil using 30 drops of tagetes to 2 tablespoons vegetable oil and massage the child's feet before bed. (See Foot Massage, page 411.)

Ringworm

"Ringworm" is a generic term used to describe many species of fungi which cause diseases of the outer layer of skin. Strictly speaking, athlete's foot is ringworm. Here we are concerned with other forms that affect the skin, anywhere on the body but especially the scalp. The name "ringworm" comes from the ring shape that appears on the skin and which is formed as the disease spreads outward in a circular shape. This outer ring marks the active area of the disease while the center heals as the fungi move outward. Ringworm is very itchy. If it appears on the scalp it can cause small patches of hair to be lost temporarily. Sometimes an allergic reaction causes small itchy blisters to appear on parts of the body that can be far removed from the ringworm itself. Ringworm is infectious and can be caught from people and domestic animals. Use these oils to treat it:

ESSENTIAL OILS TO TREAT RINGWORM

Tea tree	**Thyme linalol**
Lavender	

Tea tree essential oil provides an extremely effective treatment for ringworm. Apply 1 neat drop over the infected area three times a day until it's clear. This should take no more than ten days. After that, apply an oil composed of 30 drops of tea tree diluted in 2 tablespoons vegetable oil. Rub over the area daily.

Worms

The human body is an attractive home for many a tiny creature, intestinal parasites among them. In this section I shall be largely concerned with the most common of these, threadworms, but treatment is the same for all worms. Follow the general directions outlined here but substitute a more relevant treatment or oil if mentioned at the end of this section.

Worms inhabit all types of children—the good, the bad, and the naughty. It doesn't much matter whether your child goes to a private school or public school, the chances are that at some time he or she may contract worms. Worms can be passed from person to person, direct from feces or, recent discoveries seem to indicate, simply from breathing in the eggs as they cruise in the air. Wherever the eggs happen to be, on toilets, on the people's hands, on objects handled by an infected person, or even an object that eggs happen to have been laid upon, they can very easily be picked up and transferred to the mouth. Once inside a person, the eggs move through the stomach to the intestine where they develop into a worm. At night, the female worms wiggle their way down to the anus and lay their eggs. This causes the main symptom—itching. Although some would say this is indeed the only symptom, worms could be the cause of your child always being a bit under the weather. Worms are responsible for weight loss, swollen abdomen, irritability, inability to concentrate, lethargy, headaches, and teeth-grinding. Although none of these may be dreadfully serious, there seems little point in allowing the little creatures to live off your child when they can be got rid of so easily.

Threadworms resemble little pieces of white sewing cotton, about half an inch long. They come out of the bowel in stools and can be seen around the anal area or on toilet paper. As small children have an insatiable curiosity about all things that come out of their bodies it's quite useful to ask the child to look out for "threads." Don't frighten the child like the mother who asked her four-year-old daughter to look "in case the cotton came out"; her child went about terrified that her tummy would fall out because the stitches had come out.

The first line of defense against worms is to teach your children good personal hygiene habits—always to wash their hands after going to the toilet and before eating. All members of the household should have and use their own towel and facecloth. Any medication for worms given by the doctor or pharmacist will not conflict with essential oil treatment.

The following essential oils are effective used as a tummy rub:

ESSENTIAL OILS FOR WORMS

BLEND 1

Niaouli	**Ecalyptus**
Chamomile Roman	**Lemon**
	Lavender

Use 30 drops to 2 tablespoons vegetable oil

BLEND 2

Red thyme	**Cinnamon**
Fennel	

Use 15 drops to 2 tablespoons vegetable oil

Children in French villages used to wear necklaces made of garlic to prevent them getting worms; nowadays garlic bread or garlic soup is given instead. Certainly worms hate garlic, and a good garlic soup is by far one of the best natural remedies for children. Garlic pills can also help. To counteract the smell of garlic on the breath, chew parsley.

The life cycle of a threadworm is two weeks, so treatment should be at least that long. If one member of the family has threadworms, all members should be treated. Make up an essential oil tummy rub using the quantities above and rub over the whole of the abdominal area for at least two weeks. Double the dose for adults.

Inhaling the oils helps too, so make up this synergistic blend and add 2 drops in warm baths and 3 drops in a diffuser in the child's room, or in the hot water bowl method:

WORMS SYNERGISTIC BLEND

Niaouli	10 drops
Lavender	14 drops
Red thyme	5 drops

Tapeworms, which do look like small pieces of tape, are paralyzed by pomegranates and can then be flushed out of the body with a good purge. You can treat your children without their even knowing it provided you can get them to eat pomegranates, followed by the prunes, dried apricots, apples, bananas, or whatever for the purge. Dried fruits are more effective than the fresh variety for this purpose. Pomegranates contain an alkaloid drug, pelletierine, which stuns the worms so effectively that it seems a good idea to make a point of doing this procedure once a year when the pomegranates are in season just to ensure that your child is clear of this particular parasite. Certainly, if you hear that there is an outbreak of tapeworms at school, this treatment would be a good precaution. If you have pets, of course, your child is more likely to contract worms and you can make a pomegranate syrup (see page 354) which can be given daily to the child or give one pomegranate three times on the day you worm your pet.

Roundworm and hookworm respond particularly well to chenopodium essential oil which contains ascaridole.

Head Lice

Lice are tiny, six-legged insects that live in hair. They aren't fussy—blondes, brunettes, people with kinky hair and straight are all at risk. All lice want is a nice warm home to lay their eggs. Lice are smaller than a match head but visible to the eye. They are brownish-gray and lay their cream-colored eggs close to the skin. When the baby lice are hatched they leave behind the empty shells which are white and minuscule; they look like dandruff and are found further away from the scalp than the lice. The empty shells are called nits.

Lice obtain their food by biting and sucking out the blood. They may bite as often as a thousand times a day and in their saliva is a type of antiseptic which can, over a very long period of time, cause dullness in the host. This is possibly the origin of the term "nitwit."

A lice-infected head doesn't start itching until the little creatures have been present in some numbers for a couple of months. Because of this, it is important to keep an eye on the condition of your child's head. It makes no difference if the child goes to the best school and only mixes with the nicest of people, he or she is still vulnerable to this extremely common little parasite—as, indeed, are you. Infection does not denote a lack of personal hygiene, for lice can jump from one head to another and an overcrowded subway, for example, provides every opportunity for catching them.

The dandruff-like nits provide the easiest method of detecting the presence of lice, because the lice themselves are light-sensitive and scuttle away very quickly if you part the hair looking for them. The nits, however, attach themselves firmly to the hair or clothing and will not brush out like dandruff. Look for signs of this little monster under bangs, by the nape of the neck, and above the ears. When combing the hair, work in layers: you will need all your ingenuity to catch sight of a louse, but the eggs and nits are easier to spot. Also examine the water after shampooing your child's hair, for lice float on the surface.

It is possible to prevent lice taking a hold in your family. First, teach your child (and the adults) to brush or comb the hair very thoroughly, morning and night. Lice are not so strong that they can survive a vigorous brushing. Use the following essential oils in a lotion or as an addition to the rinsing water when washing the hair:

LICE DETERRENT ESSENTIAL OILS

Rosemary	**Eucalyptus**
Geranium	**Lemon**
Lavender	

These are the most suitable oils for children.

An excellent preventative synergistic blend would comprise equal parts of rosemary, lavender, and lemon. Add 2 drops to the final rinse after shampooing. Rosemary is used in many Asian hair preparations as it discourages all manner of small creepy-crawlies from making their home in the hair. Lavender, of course, is a well-established insect repellant. Only use the oils in this way spasmodically.

If you suspect the presence of lice, here is a remedy that should be rubbed well into the scalp and left overnight:

LICE SYNERGISTIC BLEND

Rosemary	**Lavender**
Geranium	

Make into a synergistic blend using equal proportions, and use 27 drops of each

add to

White beeswax	1 ounce
Castor oil	2 ounces

Melt the beeswax in a bain-marie (or a dish over a pot of boiling water) and add the castor oil until a creamy consistency is achieved. Cool, then add the essential oils while stirring well.

If your child has already got lice and has scratched his head so much that he has caused an inflammatory reaction through breaking the skin, use one of the following oils or the synergistic blend. These oils are antiseptic and have cooling and calming properties:

ANTISEPTIC COOLING AND CALMING ESSENTIAL OILS

Geranium	**Chamomile German**
Chamomile Roman	**Lavender**

SYNERGISTIC BLEND

Chamomile German	20 drops
Lavender	10 drops
Lemon	5 drops

The essential oils can be used as a rinse, added to the beeswax and castor oil cream, as above, and left overnight, or in an oil made by adding 30 drops of essential oil to 2 tablespoons vegetable oil; again, leave overnight.

When treating your child for lice, don't make him feel like a dirty pariah. As we have seen, lice can attach themselves to anyone.

The Teenage Years ♦♦♦♦

As well as peer pressure and the awakening of sexual awareness, prepubescent children have to contend with bodily changes, school exams, and the parting from lifelong friends as they begin a new school elsewhere. They are no longer top dogs at elementary school but the new boy or girl in a place where they must learn to cope with an increasingly competitive atmosphere. Unlike adults who only have to compete in one area—the one for which they have already shown an aptitude and which is their profession—the young adult at school is under pressure to succeed in many diverse areas.

Meanwhile, the teenager's body is going through profound changes. This transition also brings its particular problems. Boys sometimes suffer from gynecomastia, when the breasts swell as the male and female sex hormones adjust and find their new balance. This usually clears up by itself in time but any accompanying pain can meanwhile be eased by a rub of 15 drops of lavender in 2 tablespoons vegetable oil. Other problems of puberty for boys can be swollen scrotum, involuntary erection, and emission of semen. Girls may suffer from irregular or painful periods and premenstrual syndrome.

Skin Problems

Skin disorders are common in teenagers and can be most distressing. They are caused by the increase in sex hormones which in turn cause an increase in sebum production of the sebaceous glands. As the outer epidermis becomes thicker the pores have a tendency to dilate and if they become blocked by dead skin cells, sebum can become blocked and infected by the bacteria that live on all human skin. Cleansing the skin to clear away the dead skin cells is crucial to avoid skin breakouts, especially during the hormonally active teens. Here then is a facial scrub which is equally good for those with or trying to avoid skin problems, and which will not damage the skin:

THE ESSENTIAL TEENAGE FACIAL SCRUB

Ground almonds	2 tablespoons
Raw egg white	1 teaspoon
Lemon essential oil	4 drops

Mix the ingredients together well, put a small amount into the palm of your hand and apply to a previously wetted face. Rub the mixture all over the face in a rolling movement; wash with a good allergenic soap; rinse off with plenty of water. Now dab the face with a lavender splash made by adding 5 drops of lavender essential oil to 2 tablespoons spring water. Shake the bottle before each use and just dab the liquid over the face and leave it. Repeat this treatment each day.

Acne sufferers have been shown to have markedly lower zinc levels in their bodies than nonsufferers and it would seem only sensible to increase your zinc level, by diet or supplements. Other skin treatments can be found in Chapter 6, as can shampoos which will alleviate the problem of greasy hair which is also caused by overproduction of sebum.

School can be as stressful to a child as the office is to an adult and the essential oils are just as useful in alleviating this. So run a bath for your child and give her a favorite comic and send her off to the bathroom with instructions to take it easy for half an hour. It is best to do this after you have spent some time lending an ear to any problems she may have so they are off the chest. Use 4 drops of one of the following oils:

BATH OILS FOR CLASSROOM STRESS

Chamomile Roman	**Nutmeg**
Geranium	**Marjoram**
Lavender	**Lemon**
	Bergamot

Or follow one of these formulas which are designed to help your child cope with classroom stress:

Bergamot	2 drops
Lavender	2 drops
Marjoram	2 drops
Lemon	2 drops

Enough for 2 baths

Geranium	3 drops
Mandarin	3 drops
Clary-sage	3 drops

Enough for 3 baths

Once again, lavender provides a solution to the problem. Add 2 drops only to the bath (more will act as a stimulant rather than a relaxant); afterwards give the child a big mug of something warm, and a foot rub. No child can remain uptight after that!

Teenagers need to touch "home base" as much as anyone else does, despite the fact that they are forever extending their sights outward—or perhaps more so because of that. Touch is extremely important for everyone, but parents tend to touch their children less as they grow older and some children will have years during which nobody touches them closely at all. Cuddles may seem childish to a teenager and so massage, which is very grown up, is a good way to get in touch with your child, literally and figuratively. You can massage the hands or feet as well as the shoulders, back, or legs or, indeed, the whole body. The following are particularly good for this purpose:

BOYS	GIRLS
Cypress	**Rose**
Marjoram	**Geranium**
Bergamot	**Marjoram**

Lavender	**Eucalyptus lemon**
Chamomile Roman	**Orange**
Valerian	

Drug Abuse

Unfortunately drugs feature prominently in modern life and we cannot expect our children never to come into contact with them. Some will inevitably be sucked into the negative vortex created by "heavy" drugs, and aromatherapists, like practitioners in all fields of complementary medicine, have been asked for help by many a desperate parent. Withdrawal from heroin, cocaine, or speed-type drugs is never easy and the essential oils cannot offer a magical panacea. Someone who has gone down this road can only expect a period of difficult emotional and physical transition back to normality. However, the essential oils can help the process in two ways: as a general strengthener to both the emotional and physical system as the addict tries to withstand the pull of the drug; and in specific treatments of the many side effects of withdrawal. These include insomnia, acute anxiety, night sweats, palpitations, nausea, cramps, headaches, loss of appetite, and trembling. The following essential oils are very useful in baths and massage oils and can give addicts tremendous help as they struggle to overcome their problem:

ESSENTIAL OILS FOR USE
IN DRUG WITHDRAWAL

Rose	**Grapefruit**
Sandalwood	**Marjoram**
Fennel	**Bergamot**
Birch	**Basil**
Parsley	**Eucalyptus peppermint**
Nutmeg	

The Handicapped Child ♦♦♦♦♦♦♦♦♦♦♦♦♦♦♦♦♦

People who live or work with handicapped children often say things which surprise and stimulate the rest of us. One very old and rather ill couple I know have over the forty-two years that they have been caring for their Down's syndrome son come to see him as a blessing. Today he fetches and carries for them good-humoredly and regularly appears at their side holding the very object they were thinking of asking him to get. He cannot discuss with them an article in the newspaper but he can read their minds. And theirs is a very active and happy home. Another woman who works with the handicapped points out that we are all handicapped. According to one dictionary definition of the word, "Anything that lessens one's chance of success or makes progress difficult," this is certainly true for those of us who are no good with figures or cannot change a car tire. She pointed out that we all interact daily in a way that makes us all connected, and that every member of the huge web called society has a contribution to make. While some contribute in an obvious way in terms of the commercial system, others do so by teaching about caring, love, compassion, and understanding—all the important things. Perhaps it is because handicapped children fall into this last category that they bring their parents and others such tremendous joy.

It is wrong for handicapped people to be segregated from the community at large, not only because it prevents the able-bodied from learning valuable lessons about the real nature of being human, but because it makes those who have the physical or mental disability feel like pariahs. It is vital therefore that the parents of a handicapped child should make all attempts to have their child integrated as much as possible into the wider world. They would be helped in this if the rest of us stopped looking at and treating the handicapped as aliens from outer space who have wrongly invaded our cozy little world, and city planners and architects designed the environment so that the handicapped could get around it. In the present situation of segregation encouraging your child into the wider world is, of course, easier said than done. Nevertheless, do make all efforts at integration so that your child will have a better chance of independence when you are no longer around to shelter him from the realities of life.

The attitude of the able-bodied is one of the most difficult things to handle when you have a child with a disability. But the day-to-day caring job is already quite enough hard work as it is. It can be exhausting, physically and emotionally, and it is important for everyone concerned that the parents ensure that they themselves relax fully occasionally. Essential oil baths and massages are marvelous after a long day of bending the back, straining the arms, and generally reaching out. Get your partner to massage your arms, shoulders, and back or, if it is possible, get your child to do this. It will be a great pleasure for him to be able to return your caring if he can. And by offering the child the opportunity to expand his repertoire of activities you will be adding greatly to his confidence.

Much of the advice in the following pages applies equally to the handicapped adult.

Spina Bifida

Spina bifida is a congenital defect of the backbone, usually of the lower vertebrae. The seriousness of the condition varies enormously, from a small area of numbness to full paralysis from the waist down, and the degree will depend upon how many vertebrae arches have failed to develop, leaving a gap into which the spinal cord pushes. As the spinal cord is, in fact, an extension of the brain, mental handicap can occur and pressure can be put on the brain because cerebrospinal fluid drainage is affected.

There are no magical cures for spina bifida, either from the allopathic medical tradition or from complementary systems. There is, however, much that can be done to increase the child's general health and ease any pain by working on the nervous system. The essential oils may also be used to calm or stimulate the child, as necessary. The spina bifida child benefits from an increased intake of vitamins, including all vitamin B groups and lethicin.

Massage is beneficial for both the physically and mentally handicapped child. It can also create a marvelous bond between parent and child or carer and child. Use gentle stroking movements and work upwards, toward the head. Follow the general directions for massaging the physically handicapped (see "Aromassage") or do a three-point massage: starting at the feet, move to the hands and then the scalp.

Use the following essential oils to make your massage oil, to a total of 15 drops essential oil to 2 tablespoons vegetable oil, either singly or in any combination you choose:

SPINA BIFIDA ESSENTIAL OILS FOR CHILDREN

Lavender	**Eucalyptus peppermint**
Chamomile (both)	**Rosemary**
Calendula	**Sweet orange**
Parsley	**Lemon**
Nutmeg	

RELAXING/CALMING MASSAGE OIL

Lavender	5 drops
Sweet orange	5 drops
Chamomile Roman	5 drops

Diluted in 2 tablespoons vegetable oil

STIMULATING MASSAGE OIL

Rosemary	5 drops
Lemon	6 drops
Eucalyptus peppermint	4 drops

Diluted in 2 tablespoons vegetable oil

Paraplegia

The term paraplegia refers to paralysis of the lower half of the body. Quadriplegia means that all four limbs have lost their sensation; monoplegia, that only one limb is affected; and with hemiplegia, the paralysis affects one side of the body. I am here addressing myself to the paraplegic, but the treatment can be adjusted to suit all categories.

The most usual cause of paraplegia is an injury to the spinal cord, although disease can also be responsible. Incontinence is often the most difficult aspect of the condition to manage. Each child has special needs but all would benefit very greatly from daily massages, and not only for the benefit of those areas of the body not affected by paralysis. Kirlian photography has shown that all living matter retains its magnetic energy whether its parts are functional, paralyzed, or amputated. That applies equally to human limbs and plant leaves. The essential oils are, like ourselves, thoroughly natural and have the ability to influence living matter on a level that chemical-based medications cannot do.

Somehow, you will have to find the time in your already busy day to give your child the daily essential oil massages that will be of such benefit. And if you are an adult paraplegic, massage yourself or start a massage group where you can give and receive the vital massage.

Essential oils are divided into two groups, hot and cold, for certain purposes. The treatment of paraplegia is one such purpose. We use so-called "hot" oils on cold parts of the body and vice versa. But when we say a part of the body is hot or cold, we don't mean literally, to the touch, but in muscle value. A part of the body which is paralyzed or has some loss of sensation is "cold" and needs a "hot" oil to treat it. By the same token, if the torso is unaffected by paralysis it is "hot" and needs a "cold" oil. Muscle wastage is inevitable with a paralyzed limb, but manual exercise and massage will greatly improve its overall tone. Make two massage oils—one "hot" and one "cold"—by blending up to three essential oils from each list. Make your choice dependent upon availability and personal aroma preference. Use 30 drops of essential oil to 2 tablespoons vegetable oil:

"HOT" ESSENTIAL OILS

Benzoin	**Rosemary**
Black pepper	**Cardamom**
Ginger	**Red thyme**
Basil	

"COLD" ESSENTIAL OILS

Chamomile (both)	**Eucalyptus blue mallee**
Eucalyptus peppermint	**Green mint**
	Geranium
Eucalyptus lemon	**Thyme linalol**

You can also make a massage oil with oils that are "hot" *and* "cold":

"HOT" AND "COLD"

Lavender	**Lemon**
Neroli	**Grapefruit**
Orange	

To give your child a full body massage start on the back, moving in firm but loving upward strokes on either side of the vertebrae. Gently stimulate in this way for at least ten minutes. Move now to the back of the legs, changing oils from "hot" to "cold" as needed. Do the feet now—these are very important. Then massage from the front—starting on the head (but not the face) and ending at the feet again. This time, finish by holding the feet firmly in both hands and sending your love into them, and the child's whole body. Many parents report that this is a special time of exchange between them and the child.

You can try the combination of benzoin and black pepper recommended by Madame Maury, a pioneer in the use of massage and essential oils. Or follow my suggested formulas:

"HOT" FORMULAS
FOR COLD LIMBS AND BODY

FORMULA 1

Ginger	10 drops
Benzoin	10 drops
Cardamom	5 drops
Basil	5 drops

Diluted in 2 tablespoons vegetable oil

FORMULA 2

Red thyme	5 drops
Lavender	5 drops
Grapefruit	10 drops
Black pepper	10 drops

Diluted in 2 tablespoons vegetable oil

"COLD" FORMULAS
FOR HOT LIMBS AND BODY

FORMULA 1

Eucalyptus peppermint	8 drops
Geranium	9 drops
Lavender	9 drops
Lemon	4 drops

Diluted in 2 tablespoons vegetable oil

FORMULA 2

Eucalyptus blue mallee	5 drops
Lemon	10 drops
Eucalyptus lemon	5 drops
Geranium	10 drops

Diluted in 2 tablespoons vegetable oil

Atrophy

Atrophy refers to the shrinkage of a part of the body. In the West the word is generally used to describe limbs that do not use their muscles because of paralysis or because they have been fractured and kept in a splint, and in which the muscle has wasted away. An impaired blood supply because of disease also causes atrophy to tissue or organs. In the Third World the term atrophy is also used to describe organ degeneration due to lack of nutrition. Use the "hot" essential oils for this cold condition (see under Paraplegia, earlier).

Muscular Dystrophy

Muscular dystrophy is a very mysterious disease. The nerves supplying the muscles appear normal but do not work. This affects the efficient working of the muscles, to varying degrees in different people. It is a progressive disease and there is no allopathic (conventional medical) cure. That is why it is crucial to slow down the progression as much as possible by fighting all the way, in every way. The disease can strike previously perfectly normal, active children. Suddenly the child finds difficulty climbing the stairs, getting out of a chair, walking or running. This weakness of the limbs obviously makes life very difficult.

The battle begins with diet. Buy the best food you can afford—all fresh, no tins, no preservatives or additives. Avoid excessive fats, dairy and wheat products, and cut out all processed foods. Increase vitamin and mineral intake and consult a nutritional therapist. If your child needs any teeth filled avoid the use of mercury fillings.

Bring as much laughter into your lives as you can, and turn off aggression on TV and put away books with morbid stories.

Remember, your child may always have had a tendency towards this disease but he didn't always have it. The fight continues with massage and movement. When the muscles get tired, massage and try again.

MUSCULAR DYSTROPHY ESSENTIAL OILS

Lavender	**Geranium**
Immortelle	**Rosemary**
Eucalyptus peppermint	**Basil**
	Ginger
Eucalyptus viridiflora	**Lemon**
	Orange
Eucalyptus blue mallee	**Rose**
	Palma rosa

The essential oils can be broken down into those that are stimulating and those that are relaxing:

STIMULATING ESSENTIAL OILS FOR MUSCULAR DYSTROPHY

Immortelle	**Eucalyptus peppermint**
Eucalyptus blue mallee	**Rosemary**
Eucalyptus viridiflora	**Basil**
	Ginger

RELAXING ESSENTIAL OILS FOR MUSCULAR DYSTROPHY

Lavender	**Lemon**
Geranium	**Orange**
Palma rosa	

It is nice to have something that smells pleasant as well as being medicinal, so I suggest this is a formula for a relaxing bath:

RELAXING BATH FORMULA

Palma rosa	5 drops
Geranium	6 drops
Orange	7 drops

Mix together in these proportions and add 4 drops to baths

Massage must become part of the daily routine for anyone from four years onwards suffering from muscular dystrophy. Put your hands on either side of the spine and work in upward strokes. If for some reason it is not possible to do the back, do the FHH massage—feet, hands, and head. Each day, alternate between a brisk, stimulating massage and a gentle, relaxing one. You might like to follow these formulas:

STIMULATING MASSAGE OIL

Eucalyptus blue mallee	10 drops
Basil	10 drops
Lemon	10 drops

Diluted in 2 tablespoons vegetable oil

RELAXING MASSAGE OIL

Immortelle	5 drops
Geranium	10 drops
Lemon	8 drops
Lavender	7 drops

Diluted in 2 tablespoons vegetable oil

Spasticity

Spasticity means that the muscles are held in a permanent position. Massage greatly eases the pain and tenderness which is associated with the affected areas and also facilitates the release of toxins which have built up in the muscle. Unless you are a trained therapist, massage should consist of gentle, repetitive stroking movements that become one continuous flow.

ESSENTIAL OILS FOR SPASTICITY

Benzoin	**Lemon**
Ginger	**Sandalwood**
Rosemary	**Juniper**
Cypress	**Lavender**

All the above essential oils on their own are effective as a massage oil for spastic limbs. Dilute 30 drops in 2 tablespoons vegetable oil. Or make a formula to a total of 30 drops with a combination of oils from the list above. The following formula works well:

MASSAGE OIL FOR SPASTICITY

Ginger	10 drops
Lemon	16 drops
Cypress	4 drops

Diluted in 2 tablespoons vegetable oil

And here are two formulas that are highly successful in getting the muscles to excrete the toxins:

FORMULA 1

Benzoin	10 drops
Lemon	15 drops
Sandalwood	5 drops

Diluted in 2 tablespoons vegetable oil

FORMULA 2

Rosemary	12 drops
Lavender	10 drops
Ginger	5 drops
Juniper	3 drops

Diluted in 2 tablespoons vegetable oil

Cerebral Palsy

Spastic paralysis from birth is called cerebral palsy. Again, the degree of difficulty the child encounters varies widely among those suffering from this disorder, which is caused when groups of nerve cells in the brain fail to operate. This in turn causes several types of movement disorder: lack of coordination, spasm and movement which is uncontrolled and without purpose. Sometimes mental ability is impaired, sometimes the child merely appears to be retarded because he has such difficulty in making his responses clearly, and in speaking.

Muscle weakness is common to all sufferers of cerebral palsy and massage with the essential oils certainly helps in this respect. Include massage of the limbs and spine in any developmental program your child is involved in, and teach him to do it for himself as he gets older. The essential oils have such a lovely aroma and massage is in itself so relaxing that this should be a time of enjoyment for your child, as well as being therapeutic.

ESSENTIAL OILS
FOR MUSCULAR SPASM

Coriander	**Marjoram**
Eucalyptus lemon	**Geranium**
	Cypress
Ginger	**Lavender**
Nutmeg	

ESSENTIAL OILS
FOR MUSCULAR WEAKNESS

Immortelle	**Orange**
Eucalyptus peppermint	**Basil**
	Neroli
Eucalyptus viridiflora	**Lemon**
	Rosemary

CEREBRAL PALSY
MUSCULAR SPASM FORMULA

Ginger	10 drops
Marjoram	10 drops
Lavender	5 drops
Eucalyptus lemon	5 drops

Diluted in 2 tablespoons vegetable oil

CEREBRAL PALSY
MUSCULAR WEAKNESS FORMULA

Basil	5 drops
Lemon	8 drops
Eucalyptus peppermint	9 drops
Immortelle	8 drops

Diluted in 2 tablespoons vegetable oil

Pressure Sores

Pressure sores occur at points of the body that are constantly resting in a certain position. The bedridden are particularly liable to develop these sores but they can also develop on those confined to a wheelchair for long periods. Buttocks, heels, and other parts of the body in constant touch with the bed or chair become dry and irritable and crack. Constantly turning the body around helps relieve the pressure and so avoids the buildup of sores, but unfortunately, in spite of all precautions, they do still occur.

If a sore has developed, put 3 cups warm water in a bowl, add 10 drops of lavender and bathe the whole area. Then put 5 drops of neat lavender on a sterile piece of muslin and apply to the sore once a day.

As a preventative, calendula makes a very useful body rub. Add 30 drops of calendula essential oil to 2 tablespoons vegetable oil and apply with friction all over the suspect pressure areas. Do this at least once a week.

Geranium may be used in the same way as lavender, and as a preventative measure in the same way as calendula.

Increased levels of vitamin C and calcium also help.

Diabetes

Diabetes causes all manner of symptoms and can even be a killer. It is still something of a mystery, and current theories as to why childhood diabetes develops range from viral infection to genetic causes. All parts of a child's body can be affected by diabetes in one way or another. One common problem is that the legs become cold and numb at times and there is pain when walking. For this, make a foot bath by adding 5 drops of geranium and 2 drops of ginger to a bowl of warm water and get the child to rest his or her feet there for at least fifteen minutes. Also massage the feet, legs, hands, and arms with the following formula:

FEET, LEGS, HANDS, AND ARMS MASSAGE FORMULA

Geranium	10 drops
Ginger	10 drops
Cypress	10 drops

Diluted in 2 tablespoons vegetable oil

A twice-weekly full body massage does in some cases help to prevent some of the complications caused by diabetes in children. Choose from the list below and make your own formula, or follow mine:

DIABETES ESSENTIAL OILS

Eucalyptus peppermint	**Eucalyptus blue mallee**
Eucalyptus viridiflora	**Geranium**
	Cypress
Eucalyptus lemon	**Lavender**
	Hyssop
Eucalyptus australiana	**Ginger**

DIABETES BODY MASSAGE

Lavender	3 drops
Geranium	12 drops
Eucalyptus peppermint	5 drops
Eucalyptus blue mallee	5 drops
Ginger	5 drops

Diluted in 2 tablespoons vegetable oil

Down's Syndrome

Because of the distinctive physical characteristics of children with Down's syndrome it is easy to think that they are all the same in physical or mental ability. But, like all children, they have their own unique personalities and their degree of handicap varies greatly. Generally speaking, though, Down's syndrome children are a diligent, happy, and joyous group with an infectious sense of humor. As they get older they are very willing to help at home and at the workplace and can pull their weight just like anyone else. Problems may sometimes arise during puberty for both male and female children with Down's syndrome as they become sexually aware. These should be discussed with the social group or center attended by your child.

Down's syndrome children have an inborn sense pulling them towards the pleasure of smell and touch and they respond to the essential oils accordingly. Why not make it a family routine? The child will be only too pleased to massage his mother's or father's aching feet and hands using such lovely oils. It also teaches the child sensitivity and gives him a chance to give back.

Following the "Aromassage" section you can use any oils you like on Down's syndrome children. Experiment with the oils and have fun making different massage oils for the whole family. Let them all choose their own. And, pleasure apart, use the oils for specific medicinal problems as you would for any child.

Arthritis

Chronic inflammation of the joints which causes pain is called arthritis. Strictly speaking, gout is a form of the disease but here we are considering the two other forms—rheumatoid arthritis and osteoarthritis. Rheumatoid arthritis affects the connective tissues, and it is thought to be a condition brought about when the autoimmune system turns on itself and attacks healthy cells. Joints can become useless and muscle wasting occurs. Symptoms are acute or chronic pain, headaches, and swollen and tender lymph nodes. Arthritis attacks young children and those in the prime of life, as well as the elderly.

The method of treatment we use for both rheumatoid and osteoarthritis is the same, but the essential oils are different. In osteoarthritis the cartilage of the joints wears away and the bones form rough deposits. There is no inflammation as such but the cellular changes cause pain and difficulty in movement.

In the treatment of both forms of arthritis nutritional factors are very important. Cut from the diet all dairy and wheat products, red meat, salt, sugar, acidic fruits, and soft drinks. Feed vegetarian foods or white fish and poultry, with lots of raw vegetables and salads and cabbage in any way, shape, or form. Carrot juice and plenty of water should be drunk. Increase any vitamin and mineral supplement, concentrating on the intake of calcium, vitamins C, B, and D, and zinc.

RHEUMATOID ARTHRITIS ESSENTIAL OILS

Eucalyptus peppermint	**Geranium**
Chamomile Roman	**Rosemary**
Chamomile German	**Lemon**
	Thyme linalol
	Lavender

OSTEOARTHRITIS ESSENTIAL OILS

Ginger	**Coriander**
Eucalyptus viridiflora	**Marjoram**
Thyme linalol	**Lemon**
	Basil

The essential oils are used in baths and massage oils. But first the toxins must be drawn out. In the case of rheumatoid arthritis, clay poultices work well. Add the essential oils to green clay which is available from health food stores:

RHEUMATOID POULTICE

Eucalyptus peppermint	3 drops
Chamomile Roman	3 drops
Lavender	1 drop

Make a stiff paste by adding water to 1 tablespoon dry clay. Add the essential oils and mix well.

Smear the mixture over the affected joints and painful areas, cover with muslin (which you can buy by the yard), and rest. Follow this procedure twice a day.

For osteoarthritis try the cabbage treatment which is very effective. Iron the leaf to release the active properties and wrap it, warm, around the affected joint.

Whether you are using the clay poultice or cabbage methods of detoxifying, get your child to rest with her joints covered for an hour and then give her a bath to which you have added 4 drops of an essential oil or mix of oils from lists above and one cup Epsom salts. Afterwards massage the affected areas with the relevant massage formula—again, twice a day:

RHEUMATOID ARTHRITIS MASSAGE OIL

Lavender	10 drops
Eucalyptus peppermint	10 drops
Thyme linalol	5 drops

Diluted in 2 tablespoons vegetable oil

OSTEOARTHRITIS MASSAGE OIL

Ginger	10 drops
Basil	5 drops
Marjoram	10 drops

Diluted in 2 tablespoons vegetable oil

See page 293 for further advice on the treatment of arthritis.

Club Foot

When a deformed foot is noticed at birth much can be achieved by starting massage right away, or as soon as possible. While other mothers are playing with their babies' fingers, you will be gently but firmly massaging the foot straight. It can seem a daunting task to transform the tiny inward and downward pointing foot into the usual form and place but you will not be wasting your time, and any move in the right direction will be worth all the trouble. Use the essential oils below and see a therapist who can advise you on ways to massage the foot and legs. In some cases your doctor may prescribe physiotherapy for your child and in severe cases of club foot an orthopedic surgeon should be consulted.

ESSENTIAL OILS
FOR CLUB FOOT MASSAGE

Lavender	**Rosemary***
Chamomile (both)	**Ginger***

*These oils are not to be used on babies except in specific cases such as this.

FORMULA FOR CLUB FOOT MASSAGE

Lavender	3 drops
Chamomile Roman	3 drops
Ginger	3 drops

Diluted in 2 tablespoons vegetable oil

Massage the leg from the knee to the ankle in firm but gentle downward strokes. Hold the foot for a few moments and gently ease it slightly towards the straight position. Then massage the whole leg to the foot and once again take a fractional step further towards the straight position by gently manipulating your child's foot. The more times during the day you can repeat this gentle easing in the right direction the better, but make it twice a day at least. Use only the oils listed above or the formula diluted in vegetable oil.

Blindness

Loss of sight is something that a sighted person can only imagine. Children born blind never know what they have missed and yet will sometimes describe the world around them with an accuracy that can only fill us with wonder and remind us of how little we perceive and know. Certainly the blind develop other senses to compensate for their lack of sight; one of those senses is touch, and another is smell. Blind children show great delight when you touch as they do, using your fingers as if they were your tools of sight and feeling the contours of their face and body. Add to this the wonderful aromas of the essential oils and you have at your fingertips a wealth of communication between you and the child.

The sensitivity that the nonsighted develop in their hands is a wonderful bonus that family and friends can enjoy, so don't be surprised if your child becomes the family therapist. Nine times out of ten the child will be able to identify the essential oils by smell and touch, if not ten times out of ten with a little practice. In China there are schools where the blind learn the skills of manipulative therapists, and let's hope that one day we in the West will have similar institutions where our unsighted children can learn to play a full and active part in this rewarding area of work. Aromatherapy is one profession in which the senses of touch and smell override in importance that of sight, so perhaps in years to come your child will be leading a fulfilling life helping others by this means.

The Autistic Child

If ever there was a handicap which puts the sufferer apart from the rest of society, autism is it. The autistic child lives in a world inside himself, trapped in the shadows of the mind, unable to communicate, touch, respond, give or take, paralyzed not in body but in the ability to form relationships with other human beings. These children are wrapped in fear and often turn their frustration and bewilderment, anxiety and distress upon themselves with a destructive tendency to screaming, violence, and self-mutilation. The parents of autistic children have the hardest task of all because their efforts to help the child are met with indifference or open hostility.

Nothing can prepare the parents of an autistic child for the rejection they are bound to face. Babies turn away from their mother's gaze or scream incessantly. Children go cold and rigid when touched and break up their environment when left alone. Fear has frozen these children's ability to communicate and they are held within a cage of despair. Not to be able to reach in there and help the child is excruciating—a profound problem besides which the other difficulties of getting the child to eat or be toilet trained may seem insignificant.

Yet autistic children are capable of generating enormous love and affection in their families and those who care for them. They have a special quality of other-worldliness which mystifies and at the same time attracts. They are souls who despite their apparent disinclination to take any part in life can be brought back into the fold of humanity. But whichever route proves successful, the way is very, very long and labor-intensive.

A major problem is that nobody really knows what causes autism and how best to cure it. Theories abound, of course, and there are some successful approaches. Your child may benefit very greatly from the regime devised by Dr. Kitahara and taught at the Higashi School in Boston. "Holding therapy" has also shown some very good results and this is something you can do at home. For an hour each morning and evening hold the child tight, despite its wriggling and desperate efforts to escape, and attempt to make eye contact. Until eye contact can be made, there is no way in to your child, so however long it may take—and it may take years—and however difficult, the word has to be persevere. Patience and perseverance are absolutely essential in every form of treatment, and it does pay off. Changes do come.

DIET A wholefood diet not only helps the child but the whole family as well. Use only fresh produce—no processed foods at all—and keep the carbohydrate level low. Fresh fruits and vegetables should be the order of the day with whole grains in small amounts and fresh eggs. Check to see whether your child has any food allergies, especially if he is hyperactive. Use your imagination to create bright, colorful dishes to stimulate your child's interest in food. Vitamin and mineral supplements have also been prescribed, such as vitamins B1, B2, B3, and B6, and magnesium and zinc. A hair analysis may be useful to assess your child's levels by means of these important building blocks. It has been suggested that autism is in some cases partly due to having too high levels of copper, iron, mercury, and lead in the body.

EXERCISE Many autistic children are weak, with atrophied muscles. But such wasting away should not be allowed to happen because these children are not physically handicapped and have enough problems without becoming so. A crucial cornerstone of the therapy devised by Dr. Kitahara is intense physical exercise—not only because, as she says, "building up of physical powers fosters a strong spirit with a power of endurance" but because it releases the child's fear. Intense physical activity, as joggers know, gives a "high" caused by the release of endorphins, and it is these brain chemicals which calm a person down. It will be very difficult to goad your child into a heavy routine of exercise, and you will need to shout and shout again and run with him or share in a sport that stretches him to the full. It may be a good idea to have him ready in his running clothes during the day so that when things get out of control you can simply grab him by the hand and go for a run to release the energy and calm him down.

DANCE AND MUSIC Music and movement are stimulating for everyone and an important aid in bringing your autistic child into the living, real world. Dance with the child, even if you feel like a puppet master moving unwilling arms and legs. Involve the whole family and friends—but only familiar faces as these children are frightened of people and the outside world.

Play music constantly, all day—classical, pop, anything at all to stimulate your child. If you don't have a piano, get a small keyboard and place your hands over your child's to make him play, or use an instrument he has to blow to elicit a sound, like a mouth organ.

PAINT Use large sheets of paper and bright colors in any way that will interest your child. Put paint on hands and feet, roll in it if that's the only way to bring him out of his indifference. This might be a therapy best suited to summers in the garden—and again, the whole family can join in. Given the opportunity, many autistic children show themselves to be exceptionally gifted at art and, indeed, music.

INCONTINENCE Self-sufficiency is important. Take your child's diapers away and make him wash his dirty clothes each time he soils them. You may have to hold his hands in the washing process, but in the long run this will be the easy way out as your child learns toilet training.

FEEDING Again, self-sufficiency is important. You may have to let your child get so hungry that the primeval instinct for survival takes over and he feeds himself.

All the advice given above involves you in a great deal of activity which forces the child to do something he hasn't the slightest inclination to do. The words "make your child" appear again and again and you will, again and again, have to force things. It is like trying to drag an enormously heavy weight from the bottom of a deep ocean, the ocean that lies between you. It will be difficult, to put it mildly, but it may be the only way to bring your child from his lonely recess into the world of communicating, human relationships.

ESSENTIAL OILS The essential oils are used to help an autistic child in two ways—as aids in both forming contact and releasing emotion.

Get the family to join you in a game, the object of which is to gain trust and exchange the unseen, unheard links that bind human being to human being on the subconscious level—which is the level on which the essential oils work. Play a game in which the child is blindfolded, given an essential oil to smell, and then asked to find the person in the room wearing that aroma. It is vital that all those involved in this game realize the necessity for absolute love and happiness during the proceedings. Whether the child guesses right or guesses at all is immaterial—still reward them with hugs and kisses (no material rewards). The child may be stiff as a board while all this is going on, but that doesn't matter either. Play the game often, every day for a month if only for ten minutes. Each person should always use the same essential oil—bergamot would be good—and choose something that they enjoy wearing.

You can make up your own games utilizing the subconscious effects of aroma on the sense of smell, but whatever you do, avoid using these aromas when there is any whiff of aggravation between other members of the household. The negative vibrations will be filtering through to the autistic child, even though he appears to be totally closed to them, and whatever aromas are around at the time will become associated with that negativity thus ruining their potential use in the future.

Massage: A body that is stiff and unyielding is no fun to massage, and if it recoils from the touch, even less so. Nevertheless, touch is what is needed. Make the whole exercise as stimulating as possible by playing music while you massage, and make sure that the half an hour or so that you need will be uninterrupted by telephone or visitors. Put aside a time when you know you will be able to give the massage your one hundred percent attention.

You can use a variety of essential oils and as the autistic child often has many other needs for which there are formulas throughout this book, choose whatever oils are applicable. The following two formulas are designed for autistic children and have been found useful:

TO ALLAY ANXIETY AND FEAR
MASSAGE OIL FORMULA

Bergamot	7 drops
Geranium	3 drops
Clary-sage	4 drops

Diluted in 2 tablespoons vegetable oil

TO STIMULATE
MASSAGE OIL FORMULA

Rosemary	5 drops
Basil	3 drops
Peppermint	2 drops
Lemon	5 drops

Diluted in 2 tablespoons vegetable oil

For the first six months massage the back of the child only. Use strokes that are firm and in control. Use the massage movement called effleurage, which is basically stroking, and to stimulate use the flat of the hand in circular, outward movements—clockwise with your right hand and counterclockwise with your left. After six months, the front of the body can be included in the massage. Use clockwise circular movements over the abdomen and solar plexus.

Head massage can be done at any time with the child sitting on the floor against your knees as you sit on a chair, or while he is sitting on your lap or whatever, but include it too in the back massage and back-and-front massage later on. Use gentle circular movements with your fingertips and put the oil on your fingers, rather than on the head itself, before massaging.

The work involved in caring positively for an autistic child is of saintly proportions, both in the minute-by-minute strains and the lengthy time required to bring your child out of his dark cage of fear and into the light of your love. But how much better to be actively involved in helping your child than leaving him in an institution which just babysits his terror or pumps him full of sedative drugs. The route will be enormously hard and I wish you all the patience and endurance you will need, but take heart in the knowledge that these children do respond to treatment and their first smiles and hugs will surely be your greatest lifetime accomplishment.

♦ CHAPTER 10 ♦
A WOMAN'S NATURAL CHOICE

WHETHER A WOMAN has children or not, her body is a complex machine for making babies which guarantees her spending 6.2 years of her life, as a well-known tampon advertisement points out, having periods. That's five days, thirteen times a year for thirty-five years. To this inconvenience, if not pain, some must add their days of premenstrual tension. The whole business continues until after the menopause.

The only break in this routine is pregnancy and, despite the myth that all women look and feel marvelous during pregnancy, this is when the body is going through dramatic hormonal changes and incurring great strains. Not only may there be morning sickness at the beginning of the term and extreme heaviness at the end, but sebum production increases and greasy or flaky areas may appear on the skin. Hair may become lank and fatty areas may develop over the body, besides the lump at the front. With all this going on it can be difficult to "bloom." However, if you take good care of yourself it is possible to go through a happy and healthy pregnancy.

It is important to bear in mind that your baby won't go without—you will. The baby gets the vital nutrients before its mother does and so the mother can very easily become depleted of nutrients. As a baby's absorption rate is so high, you have to take care of the water you drink as well as the food you eat. Any lead in the tap water will be absorbed by a fetus at a rate five times that of an adult, and in certain areas, pesticides have seeped into the water supply. It is therefore vital that pregnant women drink bottled water and use filtered water for cooking and the kettle—and don't forget to change the filters regularly. This is, of course, inconvenient and expensive, but it could prevent a lowering of your child's intelligence by lead and avoid known and unknown problems that may result from absorbing a wide variety of chemical pollutants. It is also wise at this time to avoid excessive exhaust fumes.

Your baby's care at this stage in its development is part and parcel of your own. From the moment you conceive, everything you eat or apply to yourself will be filtering through to your baby. If you develop an allergy, your baby could develop it too. If you have a reaction to a certain makeup, your baby could have a similar reaction. Even hair dye could travel into the system. Also, the baby will hear all the sounds you hear, so if you go to a rock concert you won't be going alone! It is especially important to take care of your psychological environment, because if you are tense your baby will be affected. This is the time to cut as much aggravation out of your life as possible, eat the best of everything, stock up with bottled water, and of course give up smoking. Indeed, this special care is ideally started even before you conceive.

Not all essential oils are safe to use during pregnancy, although many are. At this time the bias is towards the gentler oils—spearmint rather than peppermint, for example. These are the essential oils you can safely use during pregnancy:

PREGNANCY ESSENTIAL OILS

Tangerine	**Rose Bulgar**
Mandarin	**Rose Maroc**
Grapefruit	**Jasmine**
Geranium	**Ylang-ylang**
Chamomile Roman	**Lavender**

You can use the oils in a bath, shower, as a massage, or in one of the room methods. You shouldn't douche—with essential oils or with any other substance—unless advised by your doctor. Have a look at the chart on page 12 where you will find the minimum and maximum quantities of essential oils and the various methods of use. When you are pregnant you should always use the minimum quantities shown.

Problems in Pregnancy ◆◆◆◆◆◆◆◆◆◆◆◆

For many women pregnancy may entail a plethora of minor problems such as backache, swollen legs, heartburn, indigestion, and insomnia, or general aggravation in not being able to accomplish one's daily tasks with the usual efficiency. If this is so, you need spoiling! Here is a marvelous remedy which can be massaged into your back by a partner or friend on a regular basis and which will alleviate physical problems at the same time as uplifting your spirit. Use whichever rose essential oil you have handy or can afford; geranium would be a good substitute.

PREGNANCY PICK-UP BACK RUB

Rose	**Chamomile Roman***
Geranium	
Lavender	

Use some or all of these essential oils in equal proportions to a total of 30 drops per 2 tablespoons vegetable oil

*In some instances Chamomile German is more appropriate.

I remember well the heaviness of pregnancy. Perhaps only women who have experienced it can know how the tiredness seems to permeate every part of the body. Everything seems weighed down—the torso, of course, and the arms, legs, head and even, it seemed to me, the eyelashes.

If being pregnant is the ultimate "high," it is also the original "heavy" experience. But the uplifting qualities of the essential oils are a great help after a tiring day when the legs are swollen and the back aches. Pregnant women should use only 2–4 drops of essential oil in a bath. Choose your favorites or try the very relaxing combination of one drop each of chamomile Roman and lavender oils.

Morning Sickness

For morning sickness, a bowl of boiling water with 4–6 drops of spearmint oil added, placed on the floor by your bed overnight, will help keep the stomach calm. The aroma molecules will waft up and gently do their work as you sleep, and after using this method for three consecutive nights the morning sickness should be gone. Alternatively, put one drop on your pillow.

Stretch Marks

I have treated many women with essential oils during pregnancy and not one of them had stretch marks. And they all had wonderful babies. For the tummy-rub treatment the base oil is as important as the essential oils themselves, and here is a formula which has proved very successful:

MASSAGE BASE OIL

Almond oil	2 tablespoons
Wheatgerm oil	1 tablespoon
Borage seed oil	10 drops
Carrot oil	5 drops

Shake the oils together and use when needed

As this base oil comes to 3 tablespoons (plus the 15 drops), looking at the minimum-maximum chart again you will see that you need to add 12 drops of essential oil (for 2 tablespoons base) and 6 drops (for 1 tablespoon), giving a total minimum number of 18 drops of essential oil to 3 tablespoons base oil.

Massage wherever stretch marks may occur—the lower and upper abdomen, thighs, and buttocks. Use the oils regularly to prevent stretch marks. Here is an excellent synergistic blend you may like to try:

PREGNANCY TUMMY-RUB SYNERGISTIC BLEND

Rose Bulgar (or **Maroc**)	7 drops
Lavender	6 drops
Tangerine	5 drops

Mix into a concentrate using these proportions, then add 18 drops to the base oil quantity shown above; or add 2 drops per 2 teaspoons of base oil

Constipation

Every pregnant woman knows the importance of eating correctly during her nine months and while breast feeding. But doing so is by no means as straightforward as it used to be. In this age of chemical growing processes and irrigation an apple can no longer be guaranteed to be rich in vitamins C and B, and while liver was once recommended for its high iron content, animal livers now also contain high concentrations of the toxins fed to the animal during its lifetime. "Natural" foods may look natural but contain many unnatural products, so extra special care must be taken in choosing food at this time.

The unnaturalness of our food, together with hormonal changes, reduced exercise, and the sheer pressure on our digestive system during pregnancy, all conspire to make constipation a common complaint. It is important to avoid, however, because the toxins can seep back into the system. This is not the time to use chemical laxatives; instead stick to natural remedies which are, in any case, the basis of the chemical copies. Also, drink lots of mineral water and eat as many raw vegetables as you can. Good natural laxatives are dried fruits such as prunes and figs, and greens such as broccoli and cabbage. The bran content of your diet is essential now but avoid bran breakfast cereals because they are eaten with milk and sugar. Try instead the original muesli recipe devised by the Bircher Benner clinic in Zurich, Switzerland (see page 356). Eat this for a couple of mornings and you will find that your system has returned to normal. The oats clean the blood, take mucus from the bowel, and generally provide one of the most cleansing treatments you can take.

Another excellent way of clearing the bowel is to take a glass of water and add ¼ teaspoon of green clay, which is available in health food stores. As it passes through the intestinal tract the clay absorbs toxins and shows them the door! Yet another method involves psysillium husks, which are pure fiber and can be bought raw or in capsule form. Any of these methods will clean out all the rubbish lurking in the bowels.

Patchouli is an excellent intestinal cleansing oil and if you are prone to constipation it will be worth making yourself up a bottle of oil to use during pregnancy. Simply add 30 drops of patchouli oil to a bottle containing 2 tablespoons vegetable oil. To get everything going, rub the oil all over the abdomen in a clockwise direction. Start at the lower right-hand side, by the groin, and rub right up to beneath the breasts, across and down the other side, down to the hairline again. Cover the whole belly in slow, gentle, clockwise movements.

Hemorrhoids and Varicose Veins

The worst thing about constipation is that it makes you strain which in turn may cause hemorrhoids. Varicose veins and hemorrhoids are both dilated veins and their care and treatment are the same. Keep your legs up as often as possible, and for at least ten minutes a day lie with a pillow in the small of your back and another at the nape of your neck—not under the head. You may as well take advantage of this time of enforced inactivity to meditate on the well-being of your baby. Send loving, affirmative thoughts to the baby, for positive thinking makes positive things happen. Such thought projection is the oldest of treatments and one whose value is again being recognized.

To make an oil that will both prevent and alleviate varicose veins and hemorrhoids use the following:

Geranium	15 drops
Cypress	5 drops

Diluted in 2 tablespoons vegetable oil

Stroke the legs very gently, working upwards from ankle to thigh. The geranium will encourage the circulation of blood and cypress has an astringent effect upon the whole venous system. The oil will also help to balance the mind and alleviate doubts and anxieties. Remember that everything you inhale will reach your baby too—so breathe deeply now. (And by the same token, if a vehicle emitting particularly noxious fumes passes as you walk along the street, hold your breath until the worst of it has passed.)

The extra pressure on the legs caused by pregnancy makes varicose veins a common problem at this time. As well as keeping your legs up as often as possible try to exercise a little—even if only on the spot. Stroke your legs gently upwards while in a bath that contains 2 drops each of geranium and cypress. You'll obviously find this easier in month five than in month nine, but do the best you can. Lavender oil makes an excellent addition to this remedy, so add 2 drops if you have any handy. Foot baths also help, especially if you place a dozen or so small, round pebbles in the bottom of the bowl of water and rub your feet gently back and forth over them. Add 2 drops each of geranium and cypress essential oil to the bowl of water.

If you already have the problem of hemorrhoids, make yourself a cream by adding 15 drops of geranium and 5 drops of cypress essential oil to the contents of a small tube of KY jelly. Simply squeeze the jelly into a small jar, add the essential oils, mix very well and rub around the anal area when required. This treatment will not only alleviate the symptoms but prevent hemorrhoids occurring in the first place.

Flatulence

Flatulence is embarrassing at the best of times and is one of the conditions exacerbated by pregnancy. Wind in the stomach feels very uncomfortable—especially with so much pressure on all the internal organs—and can cause shortness of breath and palpitations. When the stomach expands this extra pressure can cause an angina type of pain which can be strong enough in some cases to be mistaken for a heart attack. When wind is expelled rather noisily this may be indigestion or may sometimes indicate something more serious, such as gallbladder problems, or even gallstones. But usually flatulence is functional—that is to say, unrelated to any disease of the organs—and in pregnancy the most common cause is swallowing air while eating too quickly or gulping large quantities of air during the day. If you are eating foods which have previously upset your digestive system, such upset will only be exacerbated by your present condition. Carbohydrate foods fermenting in the large colon often cause flatulence and it can be helpful to avoid foods which contain a large proportion of starch and cellulose—peas, potatoes, pulses, carrots, and onions. Try not to swallow air and breathe through the nose if you can. If you feel like belching, do, because you don't want the extra pressure at this time, but be careful not to take in another gulp of air just afterwards.

There are three essential oils which are helpful in combatting flatulence and which can be taken during pregnancy—dill, fennel, and spearmint. You can use any one of these individually to make an oil for the abdomen or mix two of the three. Dilute a total of 30 drops of your chosen oil or combination of oils in 2 tablespoons vegetable oil and rub over the abdomen several times a day. Alternatively, spearmint oil can be taken internally—but only in very small quantities once a day. Dissolve 3 drops in a tablespoon of honey and keep this mixture to use when needed. Once a day, take half a teaspoon of this honey and spearmint oil mixture in a small glass of boiled, warm water, being careful to sip slowly and avoid taking in yet more air.

Indigestion

Severe indigestion (or dyspepsia) is caused by various factors, from eating the wrong food to lack of muscular tone or an emotional problem. Depression, worry, overwork, or overstrain can all cause indigestion, as well as overeating. Basically, the cause is an increase in the acid of the stomach and most commonly it feels like a vague fullness or discomfort as soon as food is eaten. It is made much worse by worry and anxiety, and sometimes by excitement and pleasure. Sufferers experience backache, headache, insomnia, palpitations, loss of appetite, loss of strength, depression, and an obsessive attitude towards the bodily functions. There is usually not much pain as such, although the constipation, wind, and general disruption of the digestive system can add up to a pretty uncomfortable time.

If you suffer from dyspepsia you should consult your doctor, but there are still ways you can help yourself. First of all, start eating small meals every two hours or so—and eat slowly, chewing properly. Treat the constipation, and if there is flatulence as well it will usually clear up with that treatment. There are three essential oils which help in the treatment of indigestion—coriander, cardamom, and dill. Ideally, your treatment will be in a synergistic blend of all three because such a mixture has a symbiotic influence within the body. But any of the three can be used separately and dill is in any case a good oil to have in the house at this time because it will be useful for the baby.

INDIGESTION FORMULA

Coriander **Dill**
Cardamom

Make a synergistic blend using equal parts of these three essential oils
or
Use one oil only. Using a total of 3 drops, blend with 1 tablespoon honey. Put in an eggcup and store. Dissolve ½ teaspoon of the honey and oil mix in a little hot soya milk and sip after meals twice a day. *Do not exceed this dose.*

If you are experiencing pain with the indigestion, make an oil to rub over the abdomen and around the rib cage. Use a total of 30 drops essential oil to 2 tablespoons vegetable oil—again, the synergistic blend is best but any of the three oils may be used individually. Use a small amount, and only once a day. Also, avoid strong coffee, tea, spices, pepper, fizzy drinks, fatty foods, and smoking.

Nausea

Nausea usually clears up by the fourth month of pregnancy but some unfortunate women go to full term with that feeling of sickness morning, noon, and night, sometimes accompanied by vomiting. In part this is the result of a hormonal change or imbalance, for the increase in estrogen causes changes in the hypothalamus and then the gastrointestinal organs. Symptoms range from a simple loss of appetite to increased nausea and vomiting when smelling food. Not only is all this depressing at a time when one should be full of happiness but excessive vomiting is something that should be taken seriously in pregnancy.

ESSENTIAL OILS TO COMBAT NAUSEA

Coriander **Fennel** (at ⅓ the dosage of the others)
Cardamom
Lavender

As a rule, the dosage for nausea treatment should be low. For the following method use one drop each of coriander, cardamom, and lavender or three drops of either of those. Fennel is very strong and should be used at one-third the strength of the others—in the following treatment use one drop only. Blend the essential oil well into one tablespoon of honey. Dissolve ½ teaspoon of this mixture in half a cup of warm water to which you have also added the juice of a lemon or lime. Sip when needed.

The maximum dose for this treatment is four times per day for a period of six days. You can repeat the treatment if necessary after taking a break for ten days.

Another excellent treatment for nausea involves essential oil of ginger. Simply fill a bowl with boiling water, put in one drop of ginger per pint of water used, cover your head with a towel and inhale for five minutes with your eyes closed.

Bleeding

A small amount of blood loss sometimes occurs during the first three months of pregnancy and if this happens to you, call your doctor and go to bed. Bed rest usually takes care of the problem but if bleeding becomes heavy and persists this could result in a miscarriage so go to bed immediately and get somebody else to call the doctor *without fail* right away.

Cramps

Leg cramps in pregnancy are usually worse in the last months and can be caused by the position of the baby or by a calcium deficiency. They are often worse during the night or during an afternoon nap. French and Swiss women have been using the following foot bath with success for many years:

FOOT BATH FOR LEG CRAMPS

Geranium	5 drops
Lavender	10 drops
Cypress	2 drops

Place in a bowl of hot, but not boiling, water

You might also take a calcium supplement.

Cramps in the abdomen are a completely different subject and should always be checked with your doctor. Indeed, all your problems during pregnancy should be discussed with him or her, so make a habit of writing down everything that happens during your nine months—however minor—so that the doctor has a complete picture of your development and can treat any condition that warrants it. Make sure, too, that you attend all your prenatal appointments, no matter how inconvenient or unnecessary you may feel them to be, so that you receive regular urine and blood tests and can discuss everything that has been happening to you during this time.

Edema

One of the things you should remember to mention to your doctor or midwife is swelling, usually of the fingers or ankles. Edema, as it is known, is extremely common and is usually nothing to worry about, but if it occurs in conjunction with high blood pressure and protein in the urine it can indicate pre-eclampsia, or "toxemia," which should not be allowed to progress. If you experience swelling, spend at least ten minutes per day lying down with a pillow under your feet. The important thing is to have your feet higher than your heart, so merely sitting down will not do. One of the best treatments for edema is herbal tea—fennel and nettle are good, drunk twice a day. The following body rub formula also helps, rubbed over the ankles and legs (working upward, always massage toward the heart), the fingers and arms (in an upward direction), and especially on the back. Get your partner to rub the oil into your back for you; this allows the essential oils to get straight into the body via the central nervous system. Don't use the oil on the abdomen and only use once a day for ten days:

EDEMA BODY RUB

Ginger	3 drops
Cypress	2 drops
Lavender	2 drops

Diluted in 2 tablespoons vegetable oil

Exhaustion

Exhaustion can occur at any stage of pregnancy, especially if you already have one or two little ones to take care of. Here is a wonderfully reviving formula which you can treat as a synergistic blend and use for a body oil, bath, or foot bath. There's nothing to stop you using this remedy after the birth too—when you are just as likely to need it!

EXHAUSTION REMEDY

Lavender	10 drops
Grapefruit	10 drops
Coriander	10 drops

Use these amounts to 2 tablespoons vegetable oil for a body oil

or

Make a synergistic blend using equal proportions of each essential oil

If you have made the synergistic blend of oils use 6 drops for a bath; 5 drops in 2 teaspoons of vegetable oil for an individual body rub; or 4–5 drops in a bowl of hot but not scalding water for a foot bath.

Preparing for the Birth ◆◆◆◆◆◆◆◆◆

From about the seventh month you can help prepare the uterus for labor by drinking raspberry leaf tea. These leaves contain a substance called fragrine which relieves uterine pains by dilating the pelvic muscles. Use 1 teaspoon of raspberry leaf tea in a cup of boiling water.

A week before your due date start to soften the perineum by using an oil made of 5 drops rose Maroc to each 1 teaspoon almond oil. This tiny amount will last you the seven or so applications you will need but is very difficult to measure and store simply because of its size. I suggest therefore that you use a teaspoon of almond oil and add 5 drops rose Maroc to this and store it in an eggcup covered with plastic wrap. Once a day, rub a little oil along the perineum—the line of muscle and fibrous tissue which bridges the genital area and the anus. This will encourage elasticity in the area and help prevent tearing during childbirth.

The Delivery Room

Well, here you are . . . and there's no turning back! The baby has decided that it is time to arrive, or your body has decided it is time to let go, and one way or another, when you leave this room you will be a new mother. The baby has spent several weeks preparing for his entry into this new world and hormones released from the adrenal glands have been storing in the baby's body ready for the moment when he will have to rely on his own heart and lungs to sustain his life. The mother's uterus has been having trial runs of contractions during the pregnancy—sometimes hardly noticeable—and has been rehearsing for the big performance over and over again. Increased levels of progesterone have been softening up the pelvis, uterus, and cervix, as well as the surrounding muscles and ligaments.

"Labor," as it is so aptly known, is work. It is, indeed, probably the hardest work that a woman will do in her life. What we need to do is make the experience as easy as possible—for both the mother and the baby. Obstetric practices change from year to year and also vary from place to place, but these changes are determined to a large degree by the expectations and demands of the mothers themselves. We have a contribution to make and if our suggestions facilitate an easier delivery for both the mother and baby there's no reason to assume that midwives and doctors will object.

To ease the mother's task during delivery, massage is widely recommended these days, especially as the partner is often present to do the job. Using a special mix of essential oils, we can incorporate the benefits of massage with those of the oils and at the same time contribute towards the cleanliness of the air and ensure that the baby will have a pleasant aroma to greet him or her. During labor I recommend that you use Moroccan rose or geranium—either individually or blended together on a one-to-one basis, diluted in any base oil. If you still have some of the Massage Base Oil that would be ideal. As you can see from the chart below, rose and geranium both have excellent properties for use during delivery, and although a combination works very well, it really is important (and never more so) that the aroma of the oil you choose suits your taste. The massage oil can be used on the back through labor, but use it only once or twice on the abdomen during the first stage. The essential oil will help the uterus to do its job, but you don't want to overdo it because the baby will have to do his part of the job during the second stage.

OILS FOR THE DELIVERY ROOM

Rose

- Uterine relaxant
- Helps ligaments to soften, enabling the pelvic bones to expand; and to regain elasticity after the birth.
- Natural antiseptic
- Slight analgesic effect
- Good cardiac tonic

Neroli

- Works on the nervous system and facilitates easy breathing, especially during panting. Its calming effect increases the oxygen supply to the blood and brain and helps the woman to avoid hyperventilation.
- In low doses (1–2 drops per day on a diffuser) it has a sedative and calming effect; in higher doses, it is a stimulant.
- Antiseptic; disinfectant
- Confidence
- Antidepressant

Lavender

- Circulation stimulating
- Slight analgesic effect
- Calming
- Antibiotic; antiseptic, disinfectant; slight antiviral properties; antiinflammatory
- Promotes healing of open wounds—can be used instead of antiseptics.
- Accepted by everyone
- Good for headaches, fainting, and bringing around after shock.

Nutmeg

- Analgesic
- Calms the central nervous system; alleviates anxiety.
- Increases circulation—good for blood supply.

Clary-sage

This essential oil must not be confused with sage. Don't use sage for the baby's sake—it leaves too high toxic residues in the body. Clary-sage is a milder version, although still to be used with care.

Helps respiratory, muscular, and uterine systems.

Mild analgesic

Facilitates birth; uterine tonic

Euphoric

Helps breathing by calming the lower part of spinal cord.

Geranium

Circulation-stimulating. One of the best circulatory oils—and if the circulation is good, breathing will be easier.

Good for uterus and endometrium

Contractive effect—pulls together dilated tissues, so excellent for after the birth.

Good for the whole female reproductive system

Antidepressant, known for its uplifting effects

Babies are remarkably aware of the environment outside the womb. It is now thought that as well as being aware of the emotional state of the mother and the sounds she hears, the baby is also aware of the smells its mother inhales. If she is aware of this, the mother can prepare the environment so that it will be reassuring for the newborn baby. For a few days before the birth, at least, spend some time quietly relaxed listening to soft and gentle music, rubbing your tummy and letting your baby know that everything is all right. The same music can be played on a cassette player in the delivery room, thus reducing the contrast between the womb and the outside world. While you relax at home listening to the music and communicating with your baby, burn the essential oils you will be using in the delivery room in a diffuser so that all the senses become inextricably linked in baby's mind: relaxation, welcome, music, and aroma. When your baby is born it will be into an environment he or she recognizes as being related to the mother and, moreover, to the mother being relaxed.

Essential oils in the delivery room should be used in a diluted form—not so much to fragrance the room as to cleanse the air and provide a familiar, welcoming aroma for the baby. Mix your chosen essential oil or oils with a small amount of water and use on a diffuser or on a cotton-wool ball under the pillow or on a radiator. Don't overdo it; you don't need a great deal and you don't want the midwife to get spaced out! Lavender or neroli make excellent delivery room oils—used individually, not mixed.

Before the birth discuss with the midwife the possibility of having a cassette player and a diffuser in the delivery room, and ask for the lights to be turned down really low. If you are having a home birth none of these requests would be a problem, but hospital rules vary greatly and it is important that the staff know your wishes before the event. Some of the larger teaching hospitals have widely differing requirements from their patients, who come from all countries and all backgrounds, so they recognize the need to be informed of your particular wishes. If there are no complications at the birth, it is soothing for the baby to be placed close to the mother's heart as soon as possible after the birth. So let the staff know that this is important to you, rather than having the baby whisked away immediately. This should be one of the most precious moments of your life, so prepare thoughtfully for it—and it will be.

Postnatal Care ◆◆◆◆◆◆◆◆

Now it's time really to enjoy yourself and the baby. The essential oils are ideal to use after the birth, not only because of their excellent antibiotic, antiseptic, and disinfectant properties but because they are emotionally and spiritually uplifting. You can't use every essential oil at this time because you are still very delicate, but among those recommended here there is something for every mother to enjoy pampering herself with—in the knowledge that she's doing herself good at the same time! All those below can be used in a bath (4 drops) or incorporated into a body oil (a total of 30 drops per 2 tablespoons vegetable or nut base oil) or in any of the room methods. Don't use anything including essential oils, in a douche or sitz bath at this time. If you shower rather than bathe, simply put 4 drops of essential oil on your facecloth after you have finished washing yourself and wipe over your body.

POSTNATAL ESSENTIAL OILS

Rose	**Fennel**
Neroli	**Calendula**
Lavender	**Frankincense**
Nutmeg	**Myrrh**
Clary-sage	**Patchouli**
Geranium	**Bois de rose**
Grapefruit	

Infection

Infections after birth are fairly common for both mother and baby and, as usual, nature has provided help in that event. One can see this in action throughout the world and in the most primitive conditions as mothers apply a little colostrum—the food that comes from the breast for the first few days—to any infection the baby or she may have. Colostrum is packed with antibodies which give resistance to infections, which is why it proves to be such a remarkable remedy for all sorts of ailments from eye infections to cuts and wounds.

After the birth it is very important to keep the whole genital area clean and free from infection. Wash in saline solution and an excellent addition to the bowl or bidet in which you wash yourself would be one drop each of lavender and chamomile—Roman or German, either will do for this purpose. Swish the two drops of essential oil around in the water before lowering yourself in. This simple procedure ensures a chemical-free genital wash that is highly effective in both keeping infection away and facilitating healing.

If you do have an infection in the vagina or cervix following birth, use the synergistic blend formula given below. Put 3 drops in a bidet or bowl of water and bathe three times a day. Use warm water and ensure that you remain submerged for five minutes to allow the essential oils to do their job. This may not sound like long, but time can pass very slowly indeed in certain situations so have a watch handy and perhaps a magazine, and stay put!

The synergistic blend is well worth making up in some quantity because it will be very useful to treat all manner of possible minor infections in both the baby and the mother, especially during the first few months of susceptibility. Blend the essential oils in a clean, brown glass bottle that has a dropper for easy measurement:

SYNERGISTIC BLEND FOR INFECTIONS

Lavender	20 drops
Yarrow	10 drops
Chamomile Roman or Chamomile German	10 drops

Never use this synergistic blend neat and never use it, neat or diluted, in any bodily orifice—mouth, ears, rectum, or vagina (unless specifically directed, and then follow instructions carefully). For treating cuts, grazes, or open wounds, bathe the area with sterilized gauze which has been soaked in 1 pint of water to which you have added 2 drops of the synergistic blend above. Rashes on the baby's or mother's skin can be treated by mixing 1 drop synergistic blend per tablespoon of cream. Mix it in well with whatever lotion or cream you would usually choose for that purpose. If you have not been healing or recovering from the delivery as quickly as expected it indicates that your immune system is weak from the overwork to which it has just been subjected. The immune system can be boosted by massaging the whole body with a body oil made by adding 5 drops of the synergistic blend given above per 1 teaspoon vegetable or nut oil. If you have contracted an infection of the uterus, make a body oil using the same 5-to-1 proportions and massage over your stomach and lower back.

Care of the Breasts

Breast and nipple care becomes very important after a birth, for the comfort of the mother and well-being of the child. Cracked nipples are a fairly common problem and surprisingly painful. This reason alone would warrant taking good care of them, but the possibility of subsequent infection makes it vital. The formula below works very well, massaged thoroughly over the whole nipple and areola area. Also spend some time stimulating the nipples by rolling them between well-oiled thumb and forefingers.

CRACKED NIPPLE OIL

Almond oil	90%
Wheatgerm oil	10%
add	
Calendula essential oil	5 drops per 1 teaspoon base oil

You can also add calendula essential oil to vitamin E cream or petroleum jelly. These will have to be taken out of their tubes and placed in a small, clean jar. Mix the calendula essential oil in well, using 5 drops to each teaspoon of cream or jelly.

Whatever you put on the nipples to alleviate the pain of cracking, wash it off before you let your baby to the breast. I would suggest you do this as well with any preparation recommended by the hospital, even if you are told that it's all right to leave it there.

Breast abscesses can occasionally occur before birth but are more usual after a birth. The breast becomes hard and painful; often there is redness, a feeling of pulsation, and the breast feels very hot to the touch. You should always seek help from your doctor as this condition can lead to toxemia. Whatever treatment he or she decides to employ, use the following remedy in addition, because as well as relieving the redness and soreness, it decreases inflammation, is a natural antibiotic, and stimulates the autoimmune system:

SYNERGISTIC BLEND FORMULA
FOR BREAST ABSCESS

Chamomile German	15 drops
Lavender	10 drops
Eucalyptus	5 drops

Make up a concentrate using these proportions

Use 10 drops of the formula, placed in a saucer of warm chamomile tea. Soak a piece of muslin in the saucer and place over the breast, as you would a compress.

Repeat this treatment twice a day for five days only. If there is still discomfort after this time, prepare a massage oil using these quantities of essential oil (a total of 30 drops) in 2 tablespoons vegetable oil and rub over both breasts twice a day until the condition eases.

Breast Feeding

All agree that the best possible start in life for an infant is being breast fed, but sometimes this isn't as easy as the mother would wish. With the best will in the world, problems can still occur—from engorged breasts to a lack of flow; a weak mother or a baby that cannot suck strongly enough to stimulate the flow of milk. Whatever the problem, it can be equally distressing for both mother and baby and help should be sought, either from the midwife and health visitor or from one of the charities dedicated to helping mothers with nursing difficulties—such as the La Leche League which can be found in most areas. Essential oils cannot solve all breast feeding problems, but the following treatment will help if the supply of milk is insufficient for the baby's needs of if the mother is generally weak. The following three options are equally effective in increasing lactation, so choose which to use on the basis of which essential oil you already have or can easily obtain:

MASSAGE OILS TO INCREASE THE FLOW OF BREAST MILK

Fennel	15 drops
or	
Geranium	15 drops
or	
Clary-sage	10 drops

Diluted in 2 tablespoons good quality nut or vegetable oil

Use one essential oil only to make your massage oil—don't mix them for this treatment—and massage the breasts in a circular movement, starting under the arms, working inward and downward and then up between the cleavage. Do this once a day, remembering to wash the oil off before feeding your baby.

Postnatal Lift

Carrying a baby and giving birth is surely the ultimate example of human beings expending their energies to good purpose. But it does take a lot out of the mother. Here then is something for the woman who has been through a lot, given a lot, and would like to feel a lot better! This is an all-around oil which will bring you, physically and emotionally, back to normal:

POSTNATAL "LIFT" SPECIAL OIL

Nutmeg	7 drops
Bois de rose	6 drops
Frankincense	2 drops
Lemon	9 drops
Rose (any)	6 drops

Use these quantities to 2 tablespoons vegetable oil for a massage oil or body rub

or

Use these proportions to make a concentrate and use in a diffuser or room method, or as a perfume

This is a different formula from those found in the following section on postnatal depression, and one which every new mother will appreciate. If someone is looking for a treat to give you and you've already got more flowers than vases, suggest they get this synergistic blend together for you.

Postnatal Depression ◆◆

Pity the women who had postnatal depression before it was a recognized medical condition. They and their families could find no justification for the feelings of depression which overcame the new mother, often accompanied by rejection of her baby. It must have seemed the height of ingratitude for her to cry and bemoan what was, as we all logically know, the reason for gratitude and profound joy—the birth of a healthy baby. Now we know that when a woman loses the placenta at birth she loses with it a store of hormones which are essential to her emotional well-being. There are, indeed, women who today eat their own placenta after the birth and who report feelings of euphoria. What we now know is that the moment the placenta is delivered the front part of the pituitary gland swings into action and produces prolactin and oxytocin which are essential for the milk to "come in." We also know that progesterone injected immediately after birth seems to alleviate the symptoms of severe postnatal depression in susceptible women. Clearly, giving birth is a serious hormonal all-change and one that affects women differently.

There are degrees of postnatal depression, ranging from the "baby blues" which affects so many women around three days after the birth that it has come to be seen as an integral part of giving birth, to the frightening puerperal psychosis—a complete loss of sanity which affects about one woman in five hundred. And some women, of course, experience no depression at all.

Giving birth is not only the most profound chemical change a human body can go through in the space of a few hours, it's also the most profound social change for the mother and will affect every move she makes for the next decade, at least. There are many pressures after the birth of a child and many causes for concern. As well as the unrelenting demands of the baby itself, there is the unremitting round of washing and cleaning, relatives and friends all offering conflicting advice, a partner who may feel left out and jealous, single friends zooming off to exciting activities, and images of the perfect and happy mother in a thousand advertisements. And as if this weren't enough, there's the background fear that something will happen to the baby in its sleep. It is far better to be prepared for difficulties. We need to realize that profound changes have taken place in terms of hormones, the physical body, the psychological and social aspects, and try to nip in the bud any problems that could occur. As far as the essential oils are concerned, this is largely a matter of redressing the balance on the hormonal and emotional levels so that motivation, determination, and feelings of self-esteem aren't allowed to get out of balance. Socially, those around you need to recognize the complete change that has taken place in your timetable and give you a little time for yourself. With the essential oils and three hours a week from their partner, most new mothers will find they can not only cope but handle the situation with renewed confidence and energy.

Never forget that your baby's well-being depends on your own well-being and so anything you do to make your life easier and happier is all to the common good. Don't feel guilty about spoiling yourself. You have just spent nine months carrying the baby around and nourishing it, have been through labor, and committed yourself to a lifetime's hard work. Of course you deserve a little pampering—in fact, never have you deserved it more. Buy yourself a new outfit, have your hair done, and get yourself some lotions and potions to cheer yourself up. And there are no better potions for this time than the essential oils. Choose from the following list: these will make you feel special, calm you down, strengthen the nervous system, and in their own unique way lift depression.

"GOODBYE BABY BLUES" ESSENTIAL OILS

Bergamot	**Immortelle**
Neroli	**Mandarin**
Narcissus	**Geranium**
Clary-sage	**Rose**
Grapefruit	**Angelica**

You can use any of the above on their own or in any combination—up to a total of 30 drops in 2 tablespoons vegetable oil for a massage oil; up to 2–3 drops in a room diffuser; 4–6 drops in a bath; or simply dab on like a perfume.

You can start using the "Goodbye Baby Blues" oils as soon as you like after delivery. Take a bottle of massage oil into the hospital with you and rub it over your tummy and breasts, to restore tone to your skin and to make you feel great. If you're prepared for the baby blues you can nip them in the bud.

If you feel in need of a real lift, give yourself three hours a week for total indulgence. Ask your partner to babysit for that time, and if you are feeling guilty remember that he needs time to form a close bond with the baby, too . . . don't be possessive. Choose one of the single oils above or one of the following synergistic blends, pick up a good novel and retire to the bathroom. Run the bath and put in 6 drops of your chosen oil or synergistic blend of oils, swish it around and sink into the bath, breathing deeply to inhale the aroma. The combination of water, essential oils, and something to occupy your mind works wonders, so stay there as long as you want. Don't dash straight from the bath to care for your baby or make dinner; take your three hours totally for yourself. Retreat now to your bedroom and, taking your time, rub the body oil into your body, concentrating on the tummy, from breast to pubic line. Breathe deeply as you apply the oil and do some gentle stretching exercises. Putter about doing nothing in particular, painting your nails or whatever you want to do—even if it's just lying back on the bed thinking. Take your full three hours, ignoring all the sounds coming from the other room, and if you *still* feel guilty about leaving your baby in the hands of your partner, just remember that you have that responsibility for one hundred and sixty-five hours a week and he only has it for three! You are not asking for too much: you are trying to preserve your sanity for the benefit of the whole family, and it is surprising how just three hours of cushioned indulgence with the essential oils can strengthen and revitalize you.

BANISH THE BABY BLUES
SYNERGISTIC BLENDS

BLEND 1

Geranium	5 drops
Neroli	10 drops
Grapefruit	15 drops

BLEND 2

Bergamot	10 drops
Rose	2 drops
Clary-sage	5 drops

BLEND 3

Neroli	4 drops
Immortelle	8 drops
Mandarin	3 drops

BLEND 4

Angelica	5 drops
Geranium	8 drops
Bergamot	6 drops

BLEND 5

Grapefruit	10 drops
Geranium	10 drops
Mandarin	5 drops

Mix your synergistic blend of oils beforehand in a clean, brown glass bottle using the proportions shown. Then use 5 drops per 1 teaspoon vegetable oil when making the massage oil, following the directions on page 12. You can also form a synergistic blend for yourself by using the oils in the "Banish the Baby Blues" list and following the 5-to-1 formula.

Miscarriage ♦♦♦♦♦♦♦♦♦♦♦

Having a miscarriage is a highly emotional experience for a woman, as well as being a shocking and painful physical experience and a more subtle hormonal one. Even those women for whom the pregnancy was an "accident" can find themselves feeling deeply disappointed and empty. There may also be guilt and anger.

It doesn't ease the pain to learn that half of all pregnancies end in miscarriage, usually so early the woman doesn't notice. Nor to be told that one can always try again. A soul has been lost and there is grieving. For those who have repeatedly miscarried there are several areas of research which can offer hope. At the Harris Birthright Centre at St. Mary's Hospital, London, a treatment has been developed for a common problem, that of the woman's immune system rejecting the father's cells and baby and placenta tissue as "foreign." In successful pregnancies an immune response is made which prevents this happening; the new treatment stimulates antibodies by immunizing women with cells from the father's blood. Other research at the Middlesex Hospital, London, concentrates on adjusting the time at which the pituitary gland sends out its message so that hormones will mature the female egg, enabling conception to take place.

Women with rhesus negative blood, and those who do not know their blood group, should consult their doctor as soon as possible after a miscarriage that takes place after about eight weeks of pregnancy. This is because a woman with this blood type will have made antibodies against rhesus positive blood at the time of miscarriage if the baby was in the positive group, which one can't know. As a precaution, and to prevent these antibodies working against the next baby if that is in the positive group too, an injection called anti-D is routinely given within 72 hours to women who miscarry, or have a termination, and those who give birth to a baby in the positive blood groups. Without the injection, the next baby, if it has rhesus positive blood, will develop jaundice and may require a blood transfusion after birth.

The essential oils recommended for use after a miscarriage not only help to bring the body back into its pre-pregnancy state, they also heal on the emotional and spiritual levels. Choose a single oil or make yourself a blend using those given below, adding 5 drops of essential oil to each 1 teaspoon of base vegetable oil for a body oil and 6–8 drops in a bath:

ESSENTIAL OILS TO USE AFTER A MISCARRIAGE

Geranium	**Rose**
Chamomile Roman	**Narcissus**
Bois de rose	**Grapefruit**
Frankincense	**Palma rosa**

Or try this blend:

SYNERGISTIC BLEND TO USE AFTER A MISCARRIAGE

Frankincense	9 drops
Geranium	5 drops
Grapefruit	7 drops
Chamomile Roman	9 drops

Make a concentrate using these proportions.

Use 6 drops in a bath *or* 5 drops per 1 teaspoon base vegetable oil for a massage oil.

It is important to come to terms with the emotions you experience after a miscarriage so that anxiety doesn't affect your next pregnancy, because anxiety is in itself a cause of miscarriage. Exploring your feelings can be difficult to do because miscarriage is still a taboo subject and friends may tend to belittle the experience, all in good faith, with statements like "There was probably something wrong with the baby," "It happens all the time; you're lucky it didn't happen later," or "Well, it was an accident anyway, wasn't it?"—all of which attempt to close the door on the subject rather than opening it for discussion. If you find that you need someone to talk to who understands what an emotional upheaval you are going through, contact RESOLVE, Inc., a national self-help organization. See appendix for address.

Infertility ◆◆◆◆◆◆◆◆◆◆◆◆

According to an advertisement for one of the new ovulation-testing kits, "each year at least 250,000 women try to get pregnant and fail." Certainly being able to identify the period of peak fertility for a woman is a great help when trying for a baby, but unfortunately there are a plethora of reasons for infertility and for many couples success is dependent upon more than a trip to the pharmacist. Indeed, in both Britain and the United States one in six couples seeks help from the medical profession.

Reasons for infertility divide about equally between men and women at 40 percent each, with the remaining 20 percent of problems being attributable to subfertility, rather than infertility. When you add up the possible causes of the problems it seems a miracle that anyone makes a baby at all. First, you have to choose the right day to make love and there are only about 26 of those a year: as far as baby making goes, the other 339 days are a waste of time. Ten percent of infertile men ejaculate no sperm at all. Those with a low sperm count are producing less than the 60 millon per ejaculation needed so that just one has a chance of making it. A healthy sperm count is in the range of 60–125 million, which might seem an overabundance but which proves the degree of difficulty nature anticipates for the one sperm that will be successful. For some men, the problem is that the sperm they produce are deformed or diseased. For others, it's that the sperm don't have the mobility to wiggle to their destination. Another hazard is that the sperm may be coated in their own antibodies. Even provided that there are enough healthy and energetic sperm, they have to be able to speed along the system of tubes without getting stopped by a blockage. Once delivered into the vagina, the sperm face their major obstacle—the cervix. This is coated in mucus which some sperm cannot penetrate. Some women produce a mucus which repels or even kills off sperm. Now the sperm race to meet the egg. But has the woman's pituitary gland stimulated production of the hormone that will mature an egg that month—and at the right time? Polycystic ovarian disease may have interfered with the timely release of eggs. A frequent cause of infertility is a blockage in the fallopian tube which prevents the sperm and egg from meeting. There may be something wrong with the glycoprotein which lines the walls of the fallopian tubes and coats a fertilized egg as it travels down the tube to the uterus, or with the endometrium, the lining of the womb which must be prepared to accept it. These are just some of the known reasons for infertility.

Infertility is on the increase. This has been attributed to the fact that couples are postponing starting a family and in the interim contract an infection, sustain an injury, or take a drug which may cause the problem. The testes are the most sensitive organ in the male body to toxins and the increase in environmental and workplace pollution, including pesticides and heavy metals, is thought to be partly responsible for the fact that sperm counts appear to be going down. Radiation and alcohol also affect the production of sperm. Male fertility can be affected by an attack of mumps or by hormonal imbalances. Women are also at risk from hormonal factors, as from a wide range of conditions including endometriosis, salpingitis, pelvic inflammatory disease, gonorrhea, chlamydia, polycystic ovarian disease, and tuberculosis.

Because there are so many possible causes of infertility and because two people are involved, finding the problem can involve a couple in endless tests and medical examinations. This procedure puts enormous pressure on those who may already be demoralized and suffering a deep sadness from unfulfilled parental urges. Clearly, the essential oils can do nothing where the cause is structural but they can help with specific diseases: formulas for endometriosis, salpingitis, pelvic inflammatory disease, chlamydia, and polycystic ovarian disease can be found on pages 236–243. They can help too by adjusting the hormones and reducing stress.

There are at least eight hormones involved in conception and the essential oils I recommend have phytohormonal properties, that is plant hormones which imitate our own. Dr. Jean Valnet, a leader in the field of phytotherapy—a form of medicine widespread in Europe which utilizes essential oils—states that the oils work by giving the glands a new impetus. The significance of stress in conception is best illustrated by a well-known phenomenon: a couple try for years to conceive, decide to adopt a child, whereupon the woman becomes pregnant.

Here then are the essential oils for women:

ESSENTIAL OILS TO HELP
FEMALE INFERTILITY

Cypress	**Geranium**
Clary-sage	**Fennel**
Thyme	**Chamomile**
Nutmeg	**Roman**
Coriander	

UTERINE AND OVARIAN TONICS

Rose Maroc	**Melissa**
Rose Bulgar	**Geranium**

And for men:

ESSENTIAL OILS TO HELP
MALE INFERTILITY

Thyme	**Basil**
Cumin	**Cedarwood**
Sage	**Vetiver**
Clary-sage	**Angelica**

Treatment for men and women is the same except that women should start theirs on the last day of their period and men should continue treatment for at least three months. Choose a single oil or make a synergistic blend from your respective lists. Use 6–8 drops of your chosen essential oil in the bath; and make a massage oil using 5 drops of essential oil to 1 teaspoon of base vegetable oil. Rub the oil over the whole abdomen, the hips, across the lower back, and into the crease of the buttocks—but not as far as the anus. It is important not to forget the lower back area because this is where the nerves are that reach to the gonads or to the uterus and ovaries.

The permutations that are possible by utilizing the oils on the lists are endless but here are two good combinations for women:

MASSAGE FORMULAS FOR FEMALE INFERTILITY

FORMULA 1

Rose (any)	5 drops
Geranium	20 drops
Nutmeg	5 drops

Diluted in 2 tablespoons vegetable oil

FORMULA 2

Coriander	5 drops
Fennel	15 drops
Geranium	10 drops

Diluted in 2 tablespoons vegetable oil

With these formulas use 6 drops of geranium in your baths or, if you feel that stress is a strong factor in your situation, combine 3 drops of geranium with 3 drops of clary-sage essential oil.

There are various other factors involved in infertility that might be worth considering now. Zinc deficiency has been linked with both male and female infertility and it is possible nowadays to have your levels checked. In America the recommended daily intake for adults is 15mg and it is said that most British diets only provide 10mg; vegetarians may be taking in less than this. Good sources of zinc are fish, meat, green leafy vegetables, pulses, nuts, and wheatgerm; or put yourself on a course of zinc citrate. Organic vegetables contain more zinc than those grown with the help of fertilizers.

The fact that smoking hinders zinc absorption may account for the findings of a five-year survey of 4,000 women carried out by the Oxford Family Planning Association: women who smoked over 16 cigarettes a day failed to conceive twice as often as those who didn't smoke. The failure rate of lifetime nonsmokers was matched by ex-smokers and those who smoked fewer than five cigarettes a day. A high fiber diet and the birth control pill are also thought to hinder zinc absorption.

Further information about infertility and its treatments, as well as support groups, can be found through The National Association for the Childless (see page 227 for address). Various complementary medicine systems provide treatment for infertility, including homeopathy, acupuncture, and chiropractic; inquire from their respective professional associations.

Above all, keep hoping. Conception involves a fair amount of mystery and miracles are constantly taking place. I recently heard about a woman who conceived her second child normally after having to undergo in vitro fertilization treatment to conceive the first time because her cervical mucus made antibodies against her husband's sperm. Why her mucus should suddenly change is a mystery her doctors would love to solve, since identifying the reason could help many thousands of women. As it is, new solutions to the problem of infertility are being found almost yearly and many of the causes can be treated.

Menstrual Problems ◆◆◆

Menstruation affects women very differently. For some it is hardly noticeable. At the other end of the spectrum are the women who have three very distressing weeks per month. (Yes, that did read "weeks"!) During menstruation women may experience uterine cramps, water retention, bloating, constipation, backache, fatigue, headaches, migraine, nausea, vomiting, and even sinus problems and a runny nose. Premenstrual syndrome may bring additional emotional problems.

The fact that menstruation occurs remorselessly each month gives a good incentive to find a solution to any related problem. The essential oils have proved very successful in treating these problems, and they offer many women hope that "the curse" need not continue to live up to its name and impair the quality of their lives.

Premenstrual Syndrome

Premenstrual syndrome is a hormonal problem; it is thought that there are inadequate amounts of progesterone in the body in the days prior to menstruation. Because all the body's hormones work in an integrated, balancing way, other hormones which affect the salt and sugar levels are also involved in the way the syndrome expresses itself in any particular woman. Fluid retention is thought to be a crucial factor in the syndrome and as it affects all body cells, especially the brain cells, the symptoms can extend from weight gain to headaches and irritability. Indeed, the list of symptoms for PMS is extensive: swelling of the breasts, aches and pains, fatigue, loss of libido, changes in sleep and eating patterns, stress, tension, anxiety, irrational thinking, anger, frustration, depression, loss of concentration and memory. For some women PMS means that they find themselves weeping uncontrollably; others break out in spots. Any one of these symptoms is enough to make anyone pretty miserable, but add another one or two and you have a few days of sheer hell to contend with.

Unlike many other medical conditions, friends and family cannot see the cause of the trouble. Thankfully, the condition has at last been recognized as real and those women who find themselves behaving so irrationally that they end up in court for shoplifting or out of a job for throwing the typewriter at the boss may be freed and forgiven. But this doesn't alleviate the actual problem—which will return month after month unless treatment is given. Tranquilizers are often prescribed but these are merely calming and one can easily become dependent upon them, precisely because one needs them month after month. A course of vitamin B6 or evening primrose oil is more likely to prove beneficial.

However, aromatherapy and the use of essential oils have proved highly effective in treating this condition or, more accurately, conditions. As each woman experiences the syndrome in her own unique way it is impossible for me to provide one simple solution to everyone's problems. To a certain extent, you will have to find your own treatment from the information provided here. First comes a general list of oils that help; this information is then broken down into the oils most appropriate for PMS under the heads "violent/aggressive"; "weeping/depression"; "irritable/disagreeable"; and "apathetic/tired/listless." If you fall clearly into one of these categories, choose from the appropriate list of oils. If your symptoms cross two categories, mix and match your essential oils until you find a formula that exactly suits you. There is also great variation in the length of time any particular woman suffers from PMS. It can last anywhere from three days before the period to two weeks before and disappear between two hours after bleeding starts to three days after. In any event, start the treatment the day after the last day of your period and continue throughout two complete cycles (including the period) plus fourteen days. Then break for fourteen days so that you can see how your body is reacting and how you feel prior to the next period. If you find that the symptoms have gone, just have the occasional bath or massage using the successful essential oil or formula. The point is to use the oils in moderation; to find a formula that suits you so that you are essentially clear of the symptoms and only need use the oils as a crutch, when you feel the need. If the symptoms haven't gone after your two-and-a-half month treatment, try again with an adjusted formula. The essential oils are so delightful to use, this will not be in the slightest bit tiresome. In fact, you may find experimenting and having an excuse to use the essential oils a pleasure.

PREMENSTRUAL SYNDROME
ESSENTIAL OILS

Fennel	**Grapefruit**
Rose Bulgar	**Jasmine**
Rose Maroc	**Narcissus**
Geranium	**Jonquil**
Clary-sage	**Chamomile Roman**
Bergamot	
Nutmeg	

It is estimated that 40 percent of women suffer from PMS, and using combinations of the oils above it would be possible to make each one of them a unique blend. When making a blend, you can add the oils in equal proportions, or in innumerable ratios. You could also use the oils singly. In the specific categories below I have given the proportions that should be used in the given formula. For example, in the "weeping/depression" section the ingredients are in ratios of 9-12-9; add this number to 2 tablespoons base vegetable oil or make a synergistic blend in a separate bottle (which you will need for the bath anyway) and follow the proportions. In other words, the synergistic blend bottle would contain 90-120-90 drops of the ingredients if you put ten times the amounts given.

Use the synergistic blend in your bath and as a body oil. Rub over your abdomen, your hips, and your lower back to the coccyx—the lower end of the backbone, between the cleavage of the buttocks but not as far as the anus. Add 7–9 drops of your chosen essential oil or synergistic blend of oils to your bath, daily.

VIOLENT/AGGRESSIVE PMS

ESSENTIAL OILS

Narcissus	**Geranium**
Jonquil	**Parsley**
Nutmeg	**Palma rosa**
Bergamot	

FORMULA

Palma rosa	10 drops
Bergamot	10 drops
Geranium	10 drops

WEEPING/DEPRESSION PMS

ESSENTIAL OILS

Rose Bulgar	**Bergamot**
Rose Maroc	**Geranium**
Clary-sage	**Nutmeg**

FORMULA

Rose (any)	9 drops
Clary-sage	12 drops
Bergamot	9 drops

IRRITABLE/DISAGREEABLE PMS

ESSENTIAL OILS

Jonquil	**Clary-sage**
Nutmeg	**Chamomile Roman**
Bergamot	
Geranium	

FORMULA

Nutmeg	10 drops
Geranium	5 drops
Bergamot	15 drops

APATHETIC/TIRED/LISTLESS PMS

ESSENTIAL OILS

Parsley	**Grapefruit**
Clary-sage	**Fennel**
Bergamot	**Chamomile**
Geranium	**Roman**

FORMULA

Clary-sage	10 drops
Grapefruit	18 drops
Jonquil	2 drops

A friend of mine knew her period was imminent when she found herself rushing around the house cleaning everything in sight. No floor, wall, or surface would escape her frantic action. Every piece of clothing in the house found itself pristine clean and ironed, hanging in the wardrobe. It wasn't this that constituted her PMS but the profound listlessness that followed. Knowing that she was going to spend the next days totally motionless in a miserable heap in bed flung her into action just beforehand so that at least the house wasn't in as bad a state as she. To an outsider visiting for those few days, this must have seemed the house of a madwoman or of a woman of extremes, at least. It is to this propensity for imbalance and extremes that the essential oils address themselves when treating PMS. The exaggerated behavior so characteristic of PMS is brought into line so that the naturally quick-tempered woman won't become a violently aggressive one; the naturally weepy woman won't come to resemble Alice in her own pool of tears. Those who suffer violently from the syndrome might consider treating themselves to a couple of months with an aromatherapist—it would be well worth it to ensure that the essential oils bring you back to normal during the crucial premenstrual days.

Dysmenorrhea

A painful period can be anything from a dull ache to a violent cramp that causes you to double over. It is said that up to two-thirds of women suffer some sort of discomfort at some time or other. When emotional factors are involved and we feel particularly fragile, menstrual cramps are liable to be more severe than normal. Pains from other causes, a urinary infection for example, may be amplified during menstruation.

Painful periods fall into two groups: congestive dysmenorrhea, which starts a few days before the period and can cover the whole abdominal area; and spasmodic dysmenorrhea, which comes in a spasm of pain in the pelvis and/or lower back. In either case, avoiding constipation is a must at these times and anyone who has a history of period pains should consider undergoing colonic irrigation* if constipation is present as well.

* A water treatment that cleanses the intestinal tract.

ESSENTIAL OILS
THAT HELP DYSMENORRHEA

Chamomile	**Sage**
Roman	**Red thyme**
Cypress	**Nutmeg**
Geranium	**Peppermint**
Lavender	

Which oils are most effective will depend on what is causing the pain or cramps—and that can be many quite different factors. You will have to experiment with oils and formulas until you find what works for you. You might like first to try one of the following:

FOR STRESSFUL CONGESTIVE PAIN

Chamomile Roman	10 drops
Clary-sage	5 drops
Red thyme	15 drops

FOR SPASMODIC PAIN

Lavender	5 drops
Peppermint	10 drops
Nutmeg	10 drops
Cypress	5 drops

The above amounts should be added to 2 tablespoons base vegetable oil for a massage oil. Rub over the whole abdomen and lower back area, plus the shoulders. Do this daily, including throughout your period. In addition, choose one of the following essential oils or make a mixture to use in two baths during the menstruation. Leave a day's gap between the two baths—although you can, of course, bathe that day but without the oils.

Geranium	**Palma rosa**
Neroli	**Clary-sage**

Use 4 drops per bath

Menorrhagia

Heavy menstrual bleeding, or clotting in normal flow, or irregular bleeding at any time, all come under the heading of menorrhagia. These are not things that should be taken as part of "a woman's lot"; if you suffer from any of them you should be seen by your doctor so that the situation can be assessed. That's because uterine bleeding can also be a sign of uterine cancer or a fibrous growth and your condition must be diagnosed without delay. Often a "scrape" (or curettage) is done to remove the endometrium (lining of the uterus).

Once a proper diagnosis has been given for menorrhagia, use geranium and lemon essential oils in your daily bath. Get a small bottle and add equal amounts of these two essential oils not only so that they are conveniently ready but because in the bottle they will have the chance to get thoroughly synergized. You can also make a body oil using the formula below; this can be used daily at any time during the cycle:

MENORRHAGIA MASSAGE OIL FORMULA

Chamomile Roman	10 drops
Geranium	10 drops
Lemon	10 drops

Diluted in 2 tablespoons vegetable oil

Amenorrhea

Amenorrhea is the loss of periods. So-called "Bloody" Mary, Queen of Scots had amenorrhea for eighteen months and was sure she was pregnant, so the history books tell us. Which is not surprising, as stress is one of the causes of amenorrhea and Mary certainly had her worries. The menstrual cycle can also be stopped by disease of the ovaries, anorexia, physical or emotional shock, stress and emotional upsets, travel, or moving home or jobs. When the period stops during pregnancy and lactation it is known as "secondary amenorrhea" and is not a medical condition.

If amenorrhea is caused by an emotional problem, the menstrual cycle will usually return to normal once the problem has been sorted out. But the essential oils can hurry things along, as they work in both emotional and stressful situations as well as encouraging the cycle to start again through the reproductive system. All the following oils have a stress-combating component although the chamomiles are particularly good at this. You might like to refer to the "Stress" section on page 184 if you think these are very relevant to your amenorrhea, and put an additional 5 drops of an oil from that section into your 2 tablespoons massage oil. This is made by adding 30 drops of any single or combination of oils from the list:

ESSENTIAL OILS THAT HELP AMENORRHEA

Chamomile German	**Geranium**
Chamomile Roman	**Cypress**
Yarrow	**Fennel**
	Clary-sage

Or use the formula:

Yarrow	4 drops
Chamomile Roman	15 drops
Geranium	11 drops

Diluted in 2 tablespoons vegetable oil

Massage this over your abdomen and lower back every day for at least two weeks. You can, in addition, do the bath treatment using oils from the list above or the formula. I particularly recommend clary-sage, geranium, and fennel. This is a two-part treatment involving a bath of hot water and a bowl of cold water. Add 6–8 drops of one of the essential oils into both bath and bowl; lower yourself alternately three times into the bath of hot water, where you stay for ten minutes, then the bowl of cold water where you stay for five minutes. The total treatment takes forty-five minutes.

Menopause ◆◆◆◆◆◆◆◆◆◆◆◆

Menopause is often approached with dread. Over the years I have heard all manner of worries expressed by my patients: will I get hairy and grow a moustache; will my face collapse and lines appear all over it like a railway junction; will I lose my libido—or, worse, will my man lose interest in me?

What many people do not realize is that menopause can start quite early—in a woman's thirties—and so many of the attractive women in their thirties and forties that one might see and envy for their glamour and femininity are actually going through or have gone through menopause. On the other hand, some women continue to menstruate well into their fifties.

What I try to point out to those who are worrying themselves unnecessarily is that menopause actually brings many advantages. First, you don't have the bleeding and pain of menstruation every month. Contraception ceases to be a problem. If you have suffered from PMS or migraines induced by monthly hormonal changes, this will all go. One's love life doesn't change except that now that the fear of pregnancy has gone, and the "time of the month" inconveniences, it is possible to enjoy sex more and—perhaps—more often.

Certainly, we shall all get old. But menopause need not be the beginning of some inevitable decline. In the first place, menopause is a gradual process which takes place over several years. Secondly, it is often men, not women, who sink into old age and while the woman still wants to enjoy sex, he finds getting an erection more and more difficult (although that is not a physiological inevitability, but a reflection of his attitude). It is crucial that a woman doesn't allow the attitudes of her culture to affect her self-confidence at this time, and in some southern European countries where women traditionally start wearing black to signify their lack of fertility at the onset of menopause this is obviously easier said than done. But cultural attitudes throughout Western society are pretty negative towards those in the older age brackets too and it is easy for a woman—and her man—to pick up the subtle messages put out by the media and advertising industry. However, if your man is giving you a hard time because you are going through "the change of life" remind him about Liz Taylor and all the other fabulous older beauties—and remind yourself that you can always change your man if he doesn't change himself!

Yes, we've all heard about hot flashes and have come to expect them, unfortunately. But the majority of women experience no symptoms at all. *Reader's Digest* carried out a survey and found that only 25 percent of women had any symptoms. Of these, 70 percent experienced hot flashes; 40 percent depression; 30 percent sweating; 25 percent fatigue; and 15 percent had skin and hair changes. Experience in my practice over the years confirms these figures. Other problems may be bloating and water retention, constipation, vaginal dryness, circulatory problems, varicose veins, and osteoporosis.

The new hormone replacement therapy (HRT) is thought to be the wonder cure for all these problems, and although the idea of taking something extracted from mares' urine doesn't much appeal to me, it does seem to halt the progression of bone mass characteristic of osteoporosis and for some women it has certainly been a great help. At present, however, there is some controversy over the question of whether HRT increases your chances of developing other physiological problems.

But there are other safe ways to help yourself. Good nutrition, using cold-pressed cooking oils, taking vitamins and evening primrose oil, are all beneficial. Also very helpful are the essential oils:

ESSENTIAL OILS FOR MENOPAUSE

Clary-sage	**Sage**
Geranium	**Rose Maroc**
Jasmine	**Bergamot**
Bois de rose	**Coriander**
Nutmeg	**Red thyme**

You can use any of the above singly, or make yourself a blend from the list. Alternatively, use one of the formulas below for specific symptoms.

Sweats and flashes are caused by the irregular function of the blood vessels when they constrict and dilate. This increases the blood flow, raises the temperature, and slightly increases the heart rate. Probably the main discomfort is embarrassment when you suddenly turn red or break into a sweat while in the company of other people. Avoiding stimulants like tea, coffee, and alcohol is a good idea, and evening primrose oil is reported to work well with some women, especially those who have hot flashes.

Use the following formulas while the symptoms occur and additionally if you so wish:

HOT FLASHES FORMULA

Clary-sage	10 drops
Geranium	11 drops
Lemon	7 drops
Sage	2 drops

Dilute in 2 tablespoons vegetable oil

or

Make a synergistic blend and use on a 5-to-1 basis (5 drops-1 teaspoon) as a massage oil

Massage all over the body and use 5 drops of the synergistic blend in a bath whenever you wish.

DAY AND NIGHT SWEATS FORMULA

Grapefruit	10 drops
Lime	10 drops
Sage	5 drops
Thyme	5 drops

Dilute in 2 tablespoons vegetable oil
or
Make a synergistic blend and use on a 5-to-1 basis as a massage oil

Massage all over the body and use 5 drops of the synergistic blend in a daily bath.

WATER RETENTION AND BLOATING FORMULA

Fennel	5 drops
Juniper	5 drops
Lemon	15 drops
Peppermint	5 drops

Dilute in 2 tablespoons vegetable oil
or
Make a synergistic blend and use on a 5-to-1 basis as a massage oil

Use every day. Massage in the abdominal area and lower back. Use 5 drops of the synergistic blend in the bath daily.

CIRCULATORY PROBLEMS FORMULA

Geranium	10 drops
Peppermint	5 drops
Rose Maroc	10 drops
Patchouli	5 drops

Dilute in 2 tablespoons vegetable oil
or
Make a synergistic blend and use on a 5-to-1 basis as a massage oil

Massage daily. Always massage in the direction of the heart. If it's the legs that are affected, massage from feet to thigh; if the hands, massage from fingers, up the arm; and if the whole body is affected, massage front and back of the torso. And use 5 drops in the bath daily.

You only need to use a small amount of the massage oil because even as little as a teaspoon should be enough for the whole body if you apply it lightly. The oil should disappear into the skin, rather than leave an oily residue on the surface. The base vegetable oil is merely the medium through which one can deliver the essential oils to the body surface so they can penetrate the skin; this isn't meant to be a skin moisturizing treatment.

Many of the symptoms of menopause mentioned earlier have treatments which can be found elsewhere in this book.

Pelvic Pain ◆◆◆◆◆◆◆◆◆◆◆

The medical profession has come in for a great deal of criticism from women for their diagnosis and treatment of pelvic pain. Probably some of this has been fair and some unfair. Pelvic pain has many causes and it is not as easy as it may seem to make a correct diagnosis. In this section we shall be looking at just some of the conditions that cause pain and, as you can see, there are many. Read the whole section before deciding which, if any, applies to you. And then discuss all the possibilities with her doctor.

The greatest criticism women have is that doctors don't take their pain seriously. Often, after a very cursory examination, the woman will be put on a course of antibiotics, and when these do nothing to alleviate the problem another antibiotic is prescribed, and then another until the woman realizes she's been on antibiotics for years and still has the pain. At this point the doctor may prescribe tranquilizers—that is if tranquilizers weren't prescribed in the first instance, as they often are.

Sometimes it is not the doctor's fault that the problem cannot be identified. It was only in 1986 that doctors at St. Mary's Hospital Medical School, London, identified enlarged veins in the pelvis as a cause of pelvic pain. It was not until the researchers had examined the pelvic veins with X-rays after they had injected the wall of the womb with opaque dye and watched it draining away that the problem could be identified, because in a normal examination the woman lies down and in that position the veins empty.

Conversely, doctors can sometimes be blamed for taking a woman's pain too seriously. According to Dr. Patrick Hogston of the Princess Anne Hospital in Southampton, England, many women who have received extensive gynecological investigations and perhaps surgery are actually suffering from irritable bowel syndrome—which certainly need not be treated so that one loses one's ability to conceive. Indeed, many women have the experience of doctors' overenthusiasm for surgery. One woman I know who had had years of unexplained pelvic pain collapsed one day and awoke to find herself in a hospital bed with a doctor there holding a clipboard and form he wanted signing. They were going to open her up and he wanted permission to remove anything he felt was the cause of the problem. She immediately got up and dressed and went to the safety of her home. She decided to test for food allergy and found eggs to be the cause of the problem. She cut out eggs and any product with eggs and the pain went. Now, some years later, her body seems to have adjusted chemically and she can once again enjoy a boiled egg—with her two-year-old son.

Endometriosis

Endometriosis is estimated to affect well over one million women in Britain—a staggering figure. And stagger is the word: the pain can be unbearable. This is a very mysterious and previously unrecognized condition for which the cause has not yet been found. It involves a type of endometrial cells, which normally line the uterus, traveling to other parts of the pelvis and, indeed, elsewhere in the body. How the cells grow outside of the uterus is a great mystery for which at present there are three main theories: they pass through the fallopian tubes into the pelvic cavity; the cells travel in the blood and lymph channels; or that these are remnants of embryonic tissue that weren't placed properly, as it were, and which become active when puberty activates the hormones.

The condition is sometimes diagnosed when the woman complains of severe pain with menstruation or sex but can only be confirmed when a laparoscopy is performed. This involves the insertion of a fiber-optic tube through the skin to examine the abdominal cavity. Often, the diagnosis is made when the woman undergoes examinations to find the cause of her infertility. The rogue endometrial cells can gather into very large clumps and attach themselves to any comfortable niche—around the ovaries, fallopian tubes, intestines, and lungs. I have seen cases where the tissue has found its way to the arms and even the cheeks.

Early diagnosis is important to avoid repeated surgery or partial or full hysterectomy as the cells cause increasing havoc to the reproductive organs. An estimated 40 percent of sufferers may become infertile. Signs to watch out for are pain during sex, menstruation, or ovulation; heavy and irregular bleeding; and pain when clearing the bowels or urinating. Sometimes there are no symptoms and the problem is only identified during infertility examinations.

Present medical treatment is usually Danazol, a testosterone-like drug. Its side effects can be disastrous. These are recognized by the manufacturers although the patient is seldom informed of the trouble she might be letting herself in for, probably because the doctor knows there is little choice in the available treatment. Side effects of Danazol include hot flashes, sweating, vaginitis, itching, weight gain, decrease of breast size, hairiness, loss of libido, ceasing of menstruation, lowered voice, acne, nervousness, and instability. Which might be worthwhile if the drug works for you.

Obviously, endometriosis is a very serious problem which encompasses every aspect of womanhood from fertility to beauty. But there is hope. Aromatherapy is one of the most effective ways to rid yourself of—or at least put into remission—endometriosis. Exercise, swimming, good food, and vitamin supplements all help, as does "de-stressing"—taking a good look at your lifestyle, identifying the stressful areas and trying to cut them out. This is a condition that must be handled with care and that means using a properly qualified therapist, who has accurate information and uses absolutely pure essential oils.

But this is a book about do-it-yourself and there are some things you can do without professional help. Try to get a friend to give you massages—they are tremendous for de-stressing. In addition, use the following two-part treatment.

The bath treatment involves taking alternate hot baths and cold sitz baths. Run hot but not uncomfortably hot water into the bath and prepare a bowl of cold water for the sitz. A baby bath or dishwashing bowl will do as you need to lower your rear end into it, and "sitz." (Ideally, you need to sit in waist-deep water and in clinics there is equipment to facilitate this. But with ingenuity you might be able to find a piece of suitable equipment—try a garden center for large plant pots!) Now put 9 drops of the synergistic blend formula into the hot bath only.

ENDOMETRIOSIS BATH
SYNERGISTIC BLEND

Geranium	10 drops
Rose Maroc	5 drops
Cypress	2 drops
Nutmeg	10 drops
Clary-sage	8 drops

Blend these 35 drops or more in these proportions

Stay in the bath for at least fifteen minutes and then move to the cold sitz bath. Stay there for five minutes and then get back into the hot bath. You may need to add a little hot water to the bath so that it is still comfortably warm second time around. The number of times you go in and out of both baths—a complete cycle—depends upon the severity of your case, but aim for between two and four cycles. The object of the exercise is to get the blood vessels to contract and dilate, and it should be carried out daily.

If you find it impossible to "sitz" you can use an ice pack instead. Or, come to that, a packet of frozen peas! Place whatever you are using on your sacrum area—the big bony point on your lower spine, just above the coccyx. Hold it there for five minutes and then get back into the hot bath, as above. Make sure you place the ice pack or pea packet in a towel so that you don't get ice burns.

The second part of the treatment involves massaging twice a day with the following formula. Massage over the whole of your abdomen and over the hips.

ENDOMETRIOSIS MASSAGE OIL
SYNERGISTIC BLEND

Clary-sage	5 drops
Rose Maroc	5 drops
Geranium	10 drops
Nutmeg	10 drops

Dilute in 2 tablespoons vegetable oil
or
Make a synergistic blend using these proportions and 5 drops per 1 teaspoon base vegetable oil

If the pain is particularly bad during menstruation make up a separate bottle of massage oil using double the quantities —60 drops of essential oil to 2 tablespoons vegetable oil—and use this during the week before each period is due. This double-strength oil should be used three times a day on the same areas as above. So even if you are at work take the bottle in with you and do it at lunchtime. No excuses—this is your uterus you are trying to save! For the abdominal/hip massage you will need only a little oil—about the size of a quarter as it sits in the cupped palm of your hand.

Salpingitis

Salpingitis is an inflammatory condition of the fallopian tubes caused by the streptococci and staphylococci bacteria. It sometimes follows acute appendicitis or an abortion, and can cause a great deal of pain in the lower abdomen. Other symptoms are fever, vomiting, and vaginal discharge. If left, it can become a chronic condition producing heavy periods, pain on intercourse, and inflamed ovaries. The danger is that scarring will obstruct the fallopian tubes and lead to an ectopic pregnancy or infertility. Surgery is sometimes necessary.

Unfortunately it is difficult to diagnose and symptoms can go on for a few months. If salpingitis is diagnosed it must be treated immediately. You will probably be prescribed antibiotics, but use the two-part essential oil treatment given below as well. The essential oils make the body more receptive and gear it towards healing, and are themselves antibiotic.

You should rest in bed for as long as possible. Eat fresh food, especially fruits and vegetables, and drink plenty of mineral water. In addition, take vitamin C to tolerance levels—that is, as high as possible without it causing diarrhea. Massage one of the following formulas over the whole of your abdomen three times a day:

SALPINGITIS MASSAGE OIL FORMULAS

FORMULA 1

Lavender	10 drops
Thyme	5 drops
Tea tree	10 drops
Chamomile Roman	5 drops

Diluted in 2 tablespoons vegetable oil

FORMULA 2

Cinnamon	9 drops
Red thyme	9 drops
Lavender	5 drops
Chamomile German	7 drops

Diluted in 2 tablespoons vegetable oil

You should also use a cotton tampon soaked in essential oils. This should be inserted into the vagina during the day; make sure to remove it before going to bed at night. There is a choice of two treatments: make your choice dependent upon which ingredients are most speedily arranged.

Simply soak the cotton tampon in one of the following mixtures:

SALPINGITIS TREATMENT:
COTTON MIXTURE A

Lavender	3 drops
Niaouli	3 drops
Chamomile Roman	3 drops
add to	
Honey	3 teaspoons
Clay*	1 teaspoon

Blend together well

* The clay could be any clay; green is best.

From this blend take half a teaspoon and mix it into 5 ounces warm water in a bowl. Soak the tampon and insert into the vagina three times a day.

SALPINGITIS TREATMENT:
COTTON MIXTURE B

Chamomile German	3 drops
Lavender	2 drops
dissolved in	
Glycerine	1 teaspoon

Add to 1 cup warm water

Soak the tampon and insert into the vagina twice a day.

Chlamydia

Pelvic pain is just one of the symptoms of chlamydia. Other symptoms include flu-like effects, fever, conjunctivitis, painful bowel movements; and profuse vaginal discharge in women and discharge and/or bleeding from the penis in men. If the infection spreads to the uterus, urination may become frequent and painful and periods may become heavier and more painful. It can also affect the liver and cause conjunctivitis and pneumonia in unborn babies. Untreated, chlamydia attacks the fallopian tubes, causing infertility. One of the main problems with the condition is that it can be symptomless until it becomes severe. Another is that the symptoms come and go and are dismissed as just routine, inexplicable "women's problems."

Chlamydia is one of the most common sexually transmitted diseases in the world. It is often associated, rightly or wrongly, with gonorrhea. It is estimated that there are 170,000 new cases of chlamydia each year in Britain and the effect on those who have it—and those who don't know they have it—is very saddening indeed. One survey found chlamydial infection present in 100 of 200 women who were seeking in vitro fertilization because they had fallopian tube damage. Of 39 who had previously had an ectopic pregnancy, 27 were found to have had chlamydia. All sexually active people with more than one partner should occasionally have a checkup at a special clinic, and women who have had an ectopic pregnancy should take particular care to visit a clinic where the chlamydia test is available.

Before 1970 it was thought that chlamydia trachomatis, the organism responsible, was a virus because it thrives in live cells. Now it is known to be a bacterium. It seems to prefer attacking young women, and particularly those on the birth control pill or with an IUD, although this may simply be because young women have more partners and neither method provides the safety of barrier methods of contraception such as the condom.

Chlamydia trachomatis is a hardy little organism and it needs attacking on all possible fronts. As well as the antibiotics the doctor will prescribe, use the following treatment because the essential oils put the body into good condition as well as themselves being antibacterial and antifungal.

ESSENTIAL OILS TO FIGHT CHLAMYDIA

Tea tree	**Niaouli**
Eucalyptus radiata	**Red thyme**

Here is a very effective synergistic blend which can be used by women for the cotton tampon method of treatment and by men and women in the alternate bath treatment:

CHLAMYDIA SYNERGISTIC BLEND

Tea tree	15 drops
Niaouli	5 drops
Lavender	5 drops

Blend using these proportions

Put 4 drops of the above into half a pint of warm water and soak the tampon. Insert twice a day, morning and evening. Remove before going to bed and use a new tampon each time.

The two-part treatment should be followed by both men and women. The first part consists of alternate baths. Use the bath and a bowl or pan—a dishpan or a baby bath will be fine—and put warm water into the big bath and cold into the dishpan . . . less torturous than the other way around! Add 5 drops of the synergistic blend to both baths and lower yourself into them alternately four times over a twenty minute period. Do this three times per week.

In addition, massage daily over your lower abdomen using the following formula:

CHLAMYDIA MASSAGE OIL FORMULA

Red thyme	10 drops
Tea tree	15 drops
Niaouli	5 drops

Diluted in 2 tablespoons vegetable oil

AV1 (Dermatect)* can be substituted for both the alternate bath and massage oil treatments. Use 30 drops of Dermatect to 2 tablespoons vegetable oil.

*See list of suppliers.

Pelvic Inflammatory Disease

Pelvic inflammatory disease (PID) is an umbrella term which covers several inflammatory conditions. Pelvic pain and abdominal tenderness are classic symptoms. Too often, PID is a term used to describe specific conditions, chlamydia and salpingitis among them, and far too often it is given as a diagnosis when no other more specific diagnosis is made. Use of antibiotics is the usual catchall treatment that all too often misses.

As more research is carried out on women with recurrent PID it is becoming clear that their partners are re-infecting them over and over again with a condition that is more often than not symptomless in the male partner. One survey at St. Thomas' Hospital, London, found nongonococcal urethritis present in 46 partners of 58 women being treated. Over 75 percent of these men had no symptoms. Clearly, a woman looking for an accurate diagnosis of her pelvic pain should consider asking her partner to go to a special genito-urinary clinic for testing.

Any inflammatory condition can be helped by the chamomile family of essential oils, and their effectiveness is increased by the synergy with lavender. The following treatment will not conflict with any antibiotics being prescribed:

PELVIC INFLAMMATORY DISEASE SYNERGISTIC BLEND

Peppermint	10 drops
Chamomile German	10 drops
Lavender	5 drops
Bergamot	5 drops

Make up a bottle of synergistic blend using the above proportions and add 6 drops to each bath. In addition, make a bottle of massage oil using 5 drops synergistic blend to each 1 teaspoon of vegetable oil and rub over the whole of the abdominal and pelvic area (but not near the genital region), including the lower back, twice a day.

Pelvic Pain Syndrome

The veins which serve the female reproductive organs are unique in human physiology because they have no valves and can dilate during pregnancy to three times their normal state. It is presumed this is so that they can better serve the growing placenta and the baby. In some women, however, these veins dilate in the nonpregnant state and cause pain. Typically, the pain is dull with occasional sharp pangs. Sometimes the pain can be so bad that the woman is admitted to the hospital, where appendicitis or an ectopic pregnancy are suspected and the woman undergoes unnecessary surgery. Although most women experience the pain on one side most of the time it usually also occurs on the other side on some occasions. It is exacerbated by walking or lifting heavy objects and is worse during or after sex when blood is directed to the reproductive area. Other symptoms of pelvic pain syndrome (PPS) are backache, vaginal discharge, and headaches.

Women with PPS are often labeled neurotic by their doctors because the condition is difficult to diagnose. When the woman's pain is taken seriously and exploratory surgery is carried out, the blood drains out of the veins in the lying down position and so nothing wrong can be seen. If, however, a follicular cyst is discovered during the examination this may be thought to be the cause of the problem and may be removed, leading to tubo-ovarian scar tissue which can impair fertility. Another danger for women presenting pelvic pain for diagnosis is that they will be given antibiotics to treat so-called pelvic inflammatory disease when this is not actually the problem and the antibiotics will do nothing to alleviate the condition. When the next bout of PPS comes along it is taken as a recurrence of the inflammation and more antibiotics are given, and so the cycle continues—possibly for years.

For PPS the following essential oils are recommended:

PELVIC PAIN SYNDROME
ESSENTIAL OILS

Nutmeg	**Black pepper**
Clove	**Ginger**
Bergamot	**Geranium**
Coriander	**Thyme**
Rose	

Treatment involves twice daily massage and three times weekly sitz baths. Ten days before your period is due begin to massage twice, in the morning and evening, and continue for at least eight weeks. You can make your own formula using the list above, to a total of 30 drops per 2 tablespoons base vegetable oil, or use the formula below. Massage front and back from waist to knees:

PELVIC PAIN MASSAGE OIL FORMULA

Nutmeg	5 drops
Geranium	15 drops
Black pepper	5 drops
Ginger	5 drops

Diluted in 2 tablespoons vegetable oil

The second part of the treatment involves alternate warm and cold sitz baths. This is not meant to be either pleasurable or sadistic, merely to cause alternate dilation and contraction of the veins to disperse the engorgement or constriction of blood in the pelvic veins. Follow the bath treatment three times a week, and do at least two cycles each time.

PELVIC PAIN SYNERGISTIC BLEND
FOR WARM BATH

Ginger	5 drops
Rose	2 drops
Bergamot	8 drops

Make a concentrate using these proportions.

Use 3 drops of this in a warm bath run to hip level; sit for ten minutes.

COLD SITZ BATH

Coriander	1 drop

Stay in for five minutes

If you cannot obtain the essential oils to make up this treatment, use 5–6 drops of a single oil or combination of oils from the main list above in your regular baths. And if you have all the oils for the sitz treatments, use the PPS essential oils in your usual baths as well.

Gynecological Problems ◆◆◆◆◆◆◆◆◆◆◆◆◆◆

Thrush (Candida)

This is one of the most common, annoying, and irritating infections that women have to deal with. Thrush is on the increase due to the use of antibiotics, the birth control pill, to stress and tension, and various other ingredients of modern life. The constant irritation can cause depression and, one way and another, thrush can be a plague on sexuality. Indeed for some couples it puts a stop to all sexual activity. The fungus Candida Albicans is responsible for all the trouble and can be transmitted from partner to partner. Some researchers think that men are the carriers, although they don't always carry the symptoms. If you have a partner it is as important for him to get treatment, whether he has symptoms or not.

The real problem with thrush is that it can lead to more dangerous conditions such as nonspecific urethritis (NSU) which may make urination very painful and can, in turn, lead to Reiter's disease, which is a form of crippling arthritis, and inflammation of the cervix. Thrush is no minor aggravation; it needs to be taken seriously and treated.

Thrush thrives on sugar so the first thing to do is change to a wholefood, sugar-free diet. Bicarbonate of soda also helps to clear the condition, as do garlic, yogurt, and of course, nature's essential oils.

Thrush can completely exhaust people —and their relationships. Judith was nineteen when she came to see me for thrush. She had had only one lover, her current boyfriend Peter, and yet she had already come to the conclusion that sex was more trouble than it was worth! Thrush had so worn her down that she was depressed, irritable, and tired; sex was impossible because her vagina had become raw and her work was suffering because her ability to concentrate was being impaired. As a result of her troubles Judith couldn't sleep and had begun to eat all the wrong foods —purely for comfort.

It was very sad to see such an attractive young woman on the downward slope just because of a horrible little fungus. She and Peter had already been to the doctor together and tried the usual treatment: pessaries, creams, and antibiotics, which had only made the condition worse. She was desperate.

First, I changed her diet to a wholefood one—the only sugar allowed was the natural sugar of fruits and fruit juices. She was advised to cut out all coffee and tea and to take three tablets of Acidophilus daily. These are freeze-dried bacteria which enter the system and wage war on Candida Albicans (the only form of biological warfare we should be talking about!). Whether you have thrush or not, these Acidophilus tablets are well worth knowing about because they encourage the growth of "friendly" bacteria which means that the body can do a better job of elimination. Keeping the intestines clean, eliminating bad breath and flatulence, improving the complexion, and reversing the damage caused by antibiotic treatment are just some of their benefits.

The mucous membrane of Judith's vaginal tract was completely raw and she could hardly bear to urinate, so my first concern was to make an essential oil cream for her to apply to the delicate area to relieve the soreness and awful itch. You can do this yourself by adding 2 drops of any of the essential oils that appear on the list that follows to 1 teaspoon of either vitamin E ointment or KY jelly. Judith's discharge was very thick and heavy and I treated this with yogurt and essential oil, first in a douche and then in a thicker solution inserted into the vagina every day for two weeks.

When I saw Judith again after two weeks she looked a different person. The scowl she had worn on her last visit had gone and she was no longer nervous. The symptoms, she told me, had gone. Peter had played his part too. Here is the treatment I had advised for him.

THRUSH TREATMENT FOR MEN

Change of diet, as above
Three tablets of Acidophilus daily

Tea tree	5 drops
Patchouli	5 drops

Combine and add 1 drop to a bowl of warm water and wash under the foreskin twice a day

and

Dilute in 2 tablespoons vegetable oil and apply under the foreskin once a day. See page 266 for further treatment.

Now that you know you are not going to be reinfected by your possibly symptomless partner, take a look at the essential oils which will help to clear up your case of thrush:

ESSENTIAL OILS FOR CLEARING THRUSH

Chamomile German	**Geranium**
Yarrow	**Rosemary**
Marjoram	**Tea tree**
Cajeput	**Myrrh**
Eucalyptus	**Thyme**
Lavender	**Patchouli**

There are several ways to treat thrush, so find the one most effective for you. First, the yogurt way. The yogurt used here must be whole-milk, natural, white, unpasteurized, and with the live acidophilus culture—obviously, no additives or preservatives. If you can't find a "live" yogurt that fits the bill, forget this method for now.

Using yogurt with essential oils provides a dual action—the lactic acid and "friendly" bacteria of the yogurt plus the antibiotic and antifungal properties of the essential oil. You can prepare a carton of yogurt for this purpose and keep it in the fridge. This method is very effective if you have a lot of soreness and itching:

Chamomile German	5 drops
Lavender	5 drops
Tea tree	5 drops

Add to a 4 ounce carton of yogurt (as above) and stir well

Now we get to the fun part—trying to get the yogurt mixture into the vagina! Use either an applicator for inserting pessaries or a tampon applicator. If the latter, remove the tampon and scoop as much yogurt into the applicator as you can (in the end which normally holds the tampon). You will need to close off the end of the applicator that normally pushes the tampon into the vagina; either use a piece of adhesive tape or plug it tightly with cotton wool. Insert the applicator now as you would with a tampon. This will enable you to get as much yogurt mixture into the vagina as is necessary. Use once a day until the condition has cleared up.

Another way of using yogurt is to dilute it in warm spring water until a thick fluid has been obtained. Then add the following essential oils:

Geranium	3 drops
Marjoram	2 drops
Patchouli	1 drop

Add to 4 ounces yogurt and spring water and stir well

Place this mixture into a douche and wash out the vaginal tract twice a day. If you don't have a douche, here is another method but it is not as effective and therefore takes longer to clear the thrush away. Put the yogurt and essential oils into a bowl of warm water and lower yourself into it, submerging the whole genital area. Open the vagina with your fingers and push as much water as you can with the palm of your other hand into the vagina. If you find this too difficult, just open the vagina as wide as possible and allow the solution to enter. Alternatively again, soak a tampon in the yogurt mixture and insert into the vagina once a day in the morning, making sure to remove the tampon at night.

Thrush can also be treated by using the vinegar and water methods. The vinegar should, of course, be an entirely natural product with no additives or preservatives—apple vinegar is excellent. It is important that the vinegar should be sugarless as the thrush fungus thrives on sugar. Vinegar can help to restore the acid balance of the vagina.

THE VINEGAR TREATMENT
FOR THRUSH

To 2 tablespoons of vinegar add

Lavender	2 drops
Rosemary	2 drops
Tea tree	2 drops

Mix together well, then add to 2½ cups warm water

When you have the completed solution, soak a tampon in it and insert into the vagina. Do this daily, in the morning, remembering to take it out at night. Alternatively, use the entire solution in a douche, daily for three days. If you would prefer to use a bath method, add the solution made up as above to a bath that has been run until it is at hip level and add 1 tablespoon of rock salt, as salt also helps to heal the mucous membrane. (The salt addition, however, can only be used in the bath method, not the douche or tampon method.)

When the mucous membrane of the vagina is inflamed and very sore it is sometimes better to use yet another method—bicarbonate of soda. This works in the opposite way to the yogurt or vinegar method as it increases the alkaline content of the vagina instead of the acid content, making the vagina too alkaline for the fungus Candida to grow.

THE BICARBONATE OF SODA
TREATMENT FOR THRUSH

Dilute ½ tablespoon bicarbonate of soda in 2½ cups warm water

and

Dilute

Lavender	2 drops
Yarrow	2 drops

In 1 tablespoon vegetable oil

Mix together as well as possible

Although water and oil don't mix, do as best you can and don't worry about it as this is an effective way to use the soda with the essential oils of nature. You can soak a tampon in the solution and put it in the vagina, daily, remembering to take it out at night. Alternatively, use the entire solution in a douche, daily for three days. And if you prefer the bath method, pour the entire solution into a bath that has been run up to the level of your hips. One way or another, you're going to banish the nasty little thrush fungus from your life!

Vaginal Infections and Inflammation

When treating the vaginal tract you must remember that undiluted essential oils can burn the delicate mucous membrane tissues and so they must be used in a diluted form. There are various methods to treat these conditions—just find the method included here that you are most happy with using.

If you have an infection where there is a large amount of discharge it is important that you should see a medical practitioner before attempting self-treatment as this could be a sign that there is something more seriously wrong. Also, your sexual partners should be seen by a practitioner and all sexual activity should stop until the infection has cleared up. If you absolutely can't say "no" to sex, use a condom as this reduces the risk of passing the infection back and forth between you.

Trichomonas

Here is a synergistic blend formula for trichomonas. As you know by now, you make up the synergistic blend and then add the recommended number of drops taken from this concentrate, depending upon the method you intend to use. It is important that whatever method you choose you should keep up the attack—use the essential oil remedy regularly and do not be tempted to double the dose, thinking you will be doubling your chance of recovery—instead use for twice as long. Follow the method preparations as described in the section on thrush.

TRICHOMONAS SYNERGISTIC BLEND

Tea tree	5 drops
Cypress	4 drops
Lavender	8 drops
Red thyme	3 drops

CHOOSE YOUR METHOD FROM THESE:

- 8 drops in a Sitz Bath, daily
- 4 drops in yogurt
- 4 drops in yogurt and 2½ cups water
- 4 drops in bicarbonate of soda and 2½ cups water
- 4 drops in vinegar and 2½ cups water
- 2 drops in 2½ cups water on a tampon
- 5 drops per teaspoon vegetable Massage Oil—use twice a day, morning and night (keep the unused ½ teaspoon in an eggcup for the evening massage).

Now let us look at the essential oils that can help to clear up some of the other debilitating infections and inflammations that women are prone to:

ESSENTIAL OILS TO HELP CLEAR VAGINAL INFECTIONS

Cinnamon	**Red thyme**
Juniper	**Origanum**
Hyssop	**Tea tree**
Lavender	**Eucalyptus**
Rosemary	**Cypress**
Sage	**Niaouli**
Clary-sage	

ESSENTIAL OILS TO HELP
CLEAR INFLAMED VAGINAL TISSUES

Chamomile German	**Tea tree**
Lavender	**Eucalyptus**
Yarrow	**Angelica**

Many conditions can be helped by the use of essential oils—you may like to experiment yourself, taking care to follow the golden rules for the use of douches, or choosing one of the other methods outlined here.

SUMMARY OF METHODS OF USE

DOUCHES
If specified, you can douche once a day for three days each week. Always add the oils to spring water that has been warmed.

SITZ BATH
Drop formula into bath of water run to hip level. Sit there for at least 15 minutes.

TAMPON METHOD
Soak tampon in mixture of essential oil and other ingredients, as directed. Place in vagina in morning and take out at night.

CREAMS
Add formula to 4 ounces vitamin E ointment or KY jelly.

MASSAGE OILS
Add formula in proportion to a total of 30 drops per 2 tablespoons any vegetable oil including soya, almond, sunflower, borage seed, evening primrose, jojoba.

GLYCERINE
Available from any pharmacy, glycerine makes essential oils less harmful to vaginal mucous membrane and lessens irritation. Add essential oils to glycerine before adding this mix to water.

Some Other Conditions

Here now are some formulas you may like to try for those common and persistent problems. The methods are options—you can use up to two methods at any one time.

LEUKORRHEA is a noninfectious, catarrhal-type discharge from the vagina, usually caused by an overproduction of dead cell, usually in a thick, white substance:

FORMULA

Clary-sage	2 drops
Juniper	2 drops
Red thyme	1 drop

Dilute in 2 teaspoons glycerine

METHOD OPTIONS
Sitz bath, daily
Massage, daily
then
In 2½ cups water
Douche, daily for 3 days a week only

NONSPECIFIC VAGINITIS gives a heavy discharge, usually white or yellow and sometimes streaked with blood. The vagina is very sore and itchy and there may be a burning sensation on urination:

FORMULA

Lavender	2 drops
Cypress	1 drop
Hyssop	1 drop

Dilute in 2 teaspoons glycerine

METHOD OPTIONS
Sitz bath, daily
Massage, daily
then
In 2½ cups water
Tampon, daily
Douche, daily for 3 days a week only

VAGINALIS GARDNERELLA (Hemophilus bacteria) is an infection of the vaginal secretion. It is normally present in the healthy vagina but gets troublesome when the vagina becomes too alkaline, making the vagina very itchy and giving a white or gray discharge:

FORMULA

Lavender	1 drop
Tea tree	1 drop

Dilute in 1 teaspoon vinegar plus ½ teaspoon lemon juice

then

In 2½ cups water

METHOD OPTIONS

Tampon, daily
Douche, daily for 3 days a week only

ATROPHIC VAGINITIS isn't really an infection but an inflammation of the genital walls caused by a decrease in the female hormone estrogen. This can leave the vagina exposed to infection.

OIL METHOD

Chamomile German	5 drops
Lavender	5 drops
Clary-sage	5 drops

Dilute in 2 tablespoons hazelnut, safflower or almond oil and use at least 2 teaspoons a day, tampon or massage

CREAM METHOD

Yarrow	5 drops
Lavender	5 drops
Clary-sage	5 drops

Add to 4 ounce jar of cream and insert into vagina using either fingers or applicator

Clearly, there are a great variety of possible infections and if you have a discharge you must certainly get it diagnosed accurately. If you intend to try self-treatment with the essential oils it is important that you use the absolutely pure product so please see the section "Blending and Mixing" which gives advice on how to identify the pure product and find suppliers. Also, if you intend to use the douche method, read that section too before starting your treatment with essential oils. I can assure you, however, that providing you follow all the directions carefully, you may find a solution here that has hitherto eluded you.

Polycystic Ovarian Disease

Ovarian cysts are abnormal growths, usually filled with fluid, that are liable to bleed or to become twisted in places, causing pain. It is estimated that 100,000 women in Britain have POD. As well as the pain, other effects are weight gain, hairiness, and various hormonal upsets. And for 28 percent of those who fail to ovulate, it is the reason for their infertility. For POD I recommend the following formula gently rubbed over the abdomen once a day:

POLYCYSTIC OVARIAN DISEASE SYNERGISTIC BLEND

Clary-sage	10 drops
Fennel	10 drops
Geranium	7 drops
Rose	3 drops

Add these amounts to 2 tablespoons vegetable oil

or

Make a synergistic blend using these proportions and use 6 drops to a bath, and make an oil using 5 drops synergistic blend to 1 teaspoon vegetable oil

Uterine Prolapse

Difficult or repeated childbirth can stretch the ligaments that hold the uterus in place, causing the uterus to displace and drop. In severe cases the uterus may protrude out of the vagina; in mild cases, no more than an unpleasant dragging sensation is experienced. There are not usually any side effects except that pressure on the bladder sometimes causes slight incontinence. Surgery is often performed; or a ring-pessary is fitted around the cervix to hold the uterus in place.

There are no magical oils to repair the elasticity the ligaments have lost but there are a few oils that can help relieve the feeling of pressure. Exercise is of the highest importance. Stand with your legs about two and a half feet apart (or six inches more than is comfortable) and pull the muscles up from the vagina as if trying to stop yourself while urinating. Do this as many times as you can manage during the day, while washing dishes or cooking, for example; it need not take time out of your day.

Also use the following oil, rubbed over the lower abdomen and back twice a day:

UTERINE PROLAPSE LIGAMENTS AND MUSCLE TONER

Nutmeg	10 drops
Rosemary	10 drops
Lemon	10 drops

Diluted in 2 tablespoons vegetable oil

Baths with nutmeg and lemon essential oil also help—2 drops of each every time you bathe.

Uterine Cancer

Uterine cancer is a malignant growth situated in the womb. This type of cancer is most usually found in postmenopausal women. High risk groups include the childless and women who have a later menopause. If you have any bleeding from the vagina or an offensive discharge after the menopause, go to the doctor right away. Don't leave it, as time is always of crucial import in cancer treatment, which consists of chemotherapy, irradiation, and surgery.

Home treatment with essential oils involves alleviating the stress and anxiety that is an inevitable consequence of this condition and treating the skin before and after irradiation to prevent radiation burns. To begin with here is a choice of oils from which you can make a tummy rub; these have been found very useful by many aromatherapists treating patients with uterine cancer:

UTERINE CANCER OILS

Geranium	Always make sure you include 50 percent to any mixture

Use a total of 4–6 drops in baths

or

Cedarwood	**Rose**
Niaouli	**Myrrh**
Lemon	

Use 5 drops essential oil to 1 teaspoon vegetable oil when making the tummy rub oil

In my practice I have seen many burns that could have been avoided if essential oils had been used beforehand. This formula is for the treatment of all irradiation burns:

IRRADIATION FORMULA

Lavender	10 drops
Chamomile German	5 drops
Chamomile Roman	5 drops
Tagetes	5 drops
Yarrow	5 drops

Diluted in 2 tablespoons vinca-infused oil
or
2 tablespoons marigold-infused oil

The base oil that you use for this treatment is very important. Vegetable oils will do, but much better options are vinca and marigold. The periwinkle, from which vinca is made, is known to contain certain alkaloids which in some cases can suppress the cancerous cells when taken in the form of drugs. If you have the plant in your garden make an infused oil, following the instruction on page 326. If you don't have the raw material, dried vinca, which should be available at any good herbalist, can be used instead. Use this as your base oil. A second option is marigold-infused oil. This shouldn't be tagetes—the African marigold—but just the humble old garden marigold.

Apply the oil once a day to skin that is absolutely clean and dry. Cover the whole torso, including the lower back and abdomen, and pay particular attention to the trauma area. In the case of the uterus, rub well into the tummy; in the case of breast cancer, into the breasts; and so on.

Try to start using the oils at least two or three weeks before the irradiation treatment is to begin. Sometimes one isn't given an exact date, so start as soon as you are told you are having treatment so that you are prepared even if you are called to the hospital without warning. Don't use it on the days of treatments but use it in between and for at least a month after your last irradiation treatment.

If you are having chemotherapy, use the irradiation formula as well—but again, not during the actual days of treatment.

For any loss of hair due to cancer treatment, help can be given by daily massage of the scalp with jojoba oil. When the hair grows again it will be lush and thick.

Treatment with essential oils will not conflict with the treatment given by your doctors. You should not neglect to visit your doctor for referral to specialists in the field relevant to your condition. Complementary treatments should be that—complementary. However, there are many things you can do to help yourself. The Bristol Cancer Center (address in appendix) has information on ways to fight cancer with dietary changes and relaxation methods. I cannot stress enough that to prevent the spread of cancer we must make the body as nonhospitable as possible to rogue cells. This means eating properly and alleviating stress wherever possible. Increase your dose of vitamin C, avoid using commercial chemical body and food preparations, and assume as natural a lifestyle as you can manage.

Cervical Cancer

The thought of cancer is terrifying for all women, and as cervical cancer is virtually 100 percent curable in its pre-malignant state, getting a Pap smear regularly should be obligatory for all.

It is thought that a virus is at least partially responsible for cervical cancer and that it is sexually transmitted. This doesn't mean that a woman has been promiscuous, simply that she has slept with one man or more. The increasing incidence of cervical cancer—especially among the younger age group—is attributed to the reduced use of barrier methods of birth control since the advent of the pill.

Cells in the precancerous state could stay that way for up to ten years and it is the cells that are detected by the Pap smear. Nowadays the use of the laser has made treatment fairly straightforward and noninvasive. Symptoms range from irregular bleeding or "spotting" between periods to bladder problems and pain on intercourse. Some women just report "feeling uncomfortable" inside. There should be no need to say this again—but anything unusual should always merit a visit to your GP. A survey by the Jessop Hospital for Women in Sheffield, England, confirmed that laser treatment doesn't impair in any way a woman's ability to bear children. Another study by researchers at the Middlesex Hospital in London found that almost half the women there because of genital wart infection developed precancerous signs within a year. They recommend women treated for genital warts have a regular colposcope examination. An Australian survey confirms the Middlesex Hospital findings and points out that women who were under twenty-five when the virus was first diagnosed are at particular risk. Clearly, if you fall into this category you must take yourself off to be examined on a more than regular basis.

We cannot say that essential oils prevent or cure cancer because no studies have been carried out. However, natural products certainly play a part. One of the oils used is carrot and the Imperial Cancer Research Fund found that beta-carotene—the vegetable form of vitamin A which carrots provide—is important to prevent the growth of precancerous cells. In a survey of 300 women, it was found that beta-carotene levels were a quarter lower in women with the precancerous cell changes. The researchers recommend an increased intake of beta-carotene as a protective and it can be found as a pill in health food stores, most plentifully among the vegetable group in carrots, followed by green leafy vegetables, apricots, prunes, and peaches. Apart from its vitamin qualities, essential oil of carrot is a powerful cleansing agent which stimulates the liver and gall bladder. I recommend it added to grated, raw, or cooked carrots. Make a carrot soup and add 4 drops to each bowl—and eat several a week. If you prefer, add 2 drops of carrot oil to a teaspoon of honey, and take once a day for two weeks after laser treatment.

Cervical cancer has been associated with stress and, of course, having the disease can add more distress. To alleviate any stress and fear in women with cervical cancer I recommend the following essential oils:

CERVICAL CANCER ESSENTIAL OILS

Geranium	**Rose**
Carrot	**Niaouli**
Benzoin	**Lavender**
Lemon	**Clove**
Frankincense	**Cypress**
Myrrh	

Make yourself a blend using the list above and add 6–8 drops to your bath. For a body rub add 5 drops of essential oil to 1 teaspoon base vegetable oil. There are some delightful oils on the list, and with a little experimentation you will be able to mix yourself a treatment that smells so appealing you will forget that this is a medicinal treatment and experience it simply as a body and mind pampering delight. You may use the oils singly if you prefer.

Alternatively, follow my formulas:

FOR BATHS

Geranium	10 drops
Lavender	5 drops
Frankincense	5 drops
Benzoin	7 drops
Lemon	10 drops

Make a synergistic blend and add 6–7 drops to each bath

FOR BODY OIL

Benzoin	10 drops
Cypress	10 drops
Geranium	10 drops
Carrot	5 drops

Blend all together and add to 2 tablespoons vegetable oil

Massage the oil well into your lower abdomen, hips, and lower back, at least twice a day.

Try to adopt as positive an attitude as you can in the circumstances and do what you can to help yourself. According to a five-city American study a few years ago, women who have smoked regularly at some time in their lives are twice as likely to develop cervical cancer as those who have not. The more recent the smoking, the greater the risk. Clearly, it would seem sensible to put as far a distance as possible between tomorrow and the end of smoking. So give up today if you can. Diet is an important aspect of cancer care, and I suggest you write to the Bristol Cancer Center for further information on this, or refer to the many books on the subject. Relaxation is important, so take up yoga or some other relaxation method.

Other Common Problems ◆◆◆◆◆◆◆◆◆◆◆◆◆

Cystitis

Cystitis is the inflammation of the bladder and, sometimes, its outlet to the urethra. It is extremely painful and troublesome and is suffered by many women—some estimates say 50 percent of the adult female population. They feel a frequent need to pass urine, often necessitating getting up many times during the night, only to find that there is little urine to pass but even passing that small amount is very painful. Cystitis is usually caused by bacterial infection and sometimes by minor bruising of the urethral tube and bladder during sexual intercourse (often called "honeymoon" cystitis for obvious reasons). Treatment of the bacterial form should be prompt to ensure that infection doesn't spread to the kidneys.

The bacteria that cause cystitis can become resistant to antibiotics, elevating an acute case into a chronic one. It is very important to drink a lot of fluid—at least two pints of water a day, but avoid tea and coffee. Treatment with nature's essential oils is particularly effective.

OILS TO TREAT CYSTITIS

Rosemary	**Clove**
Thyme	**Cajeput**
Sage	**Cinnamon**
Savory	**Lavender**
Pine	**Fennel**
Niaouli	**Cumin**
Marjoram	**Coriander**
Oregano	**Cypress**
Hyssop	**Eucalyptus**
Basil*	

* See following reservations regarding the use of basil.

You can make up your own formula for a massage oil from the list above, although do not use basil on its own. All the others can be used singly but basil should not exceed one-third of the component parts of a formula, or less. You can use one of my massage oil formulas below, designed for addition to 2 tablespoons vegetable oil, or one of your own. Massage daily, rubbing the oil over your lower abdomen, hips, and lower back. Do this until relief is obtained —in some women that is just two days and in others, two weeks. I have no doubt that you will know when relief comes and when to stop your treatment.

MASSAGE OIL FORMULAS FOR CYSTITIS

FORMULA 1

Basil	10 drops
Lavender	10 drops
Pine	10 drops

Diluted in 2 tablespoons vegetable oil

FORMULA 2

Sage	5 drops
Oregano	5 drops
Niaouli	20 drops

Diluted in 2 tablespoons vegetable oil

An essential oil sitz bath is also very effective in treating cystitis. But, again, do not use basil in sitz baths. Run a bath to the level of your hips . . . and sitz! You can also use a bidet or a bowl. Any of the methods mentioned can be used on their own or in conjunction with a daily massage—it really depends on the time available to you and the degree of your complaint. Here are my sitz bath formulas:

SITZ BATH FORMULAS FOR CYSTITIS

FORMULA 1

Eucalyptus	5 drops
Cinnamon	2 drops
Niaouli	5 drops

FORMULA 2

Rosemary	5 drops
Hyssop	5 drops
Savory	5 drops

FORMULA 3

Cumin	5 drops
Pine	5 drops
Cajeput	5 drops

FORMULA 4

Lavender	5 drops
Marjoram	5 drops
Coriander	5 drops

Varicose Veins

This is one of the conditions where prevention is all important. No one wants to have to wear trousers whatever the fashion to conceal unsightly protruding veins. Nor do we want the aches and fatigue that go with them and can be more difficult to hide. Camouflage makeup is mucky and inconvenient, and anyway cannot hide the protrusions. Support stockings and tights are fortunately nowadays more glamorous than they used to be, and they do have a part to play in prevention.

People who stand all day are at greater risk of developing varicose veins because the blood cannot circulate. Aim to take a walk at lunchtime if your job is a threat to your good looking legs; and everyone confined to a chair all day at the cash register or office should get up from the desk and stroll around from time to time. If the boss asks what you are doing, tell him you are preventing your legs becoming the subject of a workers' compensation case!

If you already have varicose veins, support stockings and tights may help a little to relieve the tiredness caused by the veins, although they do nothing to alleviate the condition itself. That's because 20 denier support can't put enough pressure on a dilated vein to send the blood back around the body and up to the heart. An awareness of the potential problem should encourage us all to take care of our feet and legs. As well as using the essential oils in foot baths, sitz baths, and massage oils, try to put your feet up for a while in the evening after work. Eat good, healthy food and avoid constipation. Take plenty of exercise, and find time to relax—and there's no better time to do that than after a foot and leg massage with the following:

VARICOSE VEIN PREVENTATIVE MASSAGE OIL

Peppermint	5 drops
Cypress	10 drops
Lemon	5 drops
Geranium	10 drops

Diluted in 2 tablespoons vegetable oil (a nut oil is effective here)

Always massage in the direction of the heart, from the foot and up the leg. If your feet and legs feel tired after heavy work, carrying the shopping, or just spending a day out, massage the oil well into the legs, when you get home and again before bedtime.

Foot baths are very good at preventing varicose veins. For the following treatment you need two bowls to put your feet into—one filled with hot water and the other with cold water to which you have added a few ice cubes. Add 2 drops of lavender to the cold water and 2 drops of geranium to the hot. Now put both feet in the cold water and leave them there for five minutes; then put them in the hot water for five minutes. The cold constricts the blood vessels and the hot dilates, sending the blood back around the body. This treatment is also good for tired and swollen legs.

If you stand all day make the effort at least three times a week to have a half-hour foot bath, followed by a leg massage. Use 2 drops of geranium in a bowl of warm water for the foot bath and the massage oil formula above. Then put your feet up and relax. It could be done while watching TV, catching up on paperwork, or peeling the vegetables for dinner. But a more effective treatment is just to sit back and relax completely—what a hard life!

Heart Disease

Men and women over sixty-five are more likely to die of heart disease than any other cause. Lower down the age scale, women figure less than men—two men to one woman in the over fifties age group and five men to one woman in the under fifties. Because men figure so prominently in the statistics, most research has been carried out on them—to the extent that there prevails a myth that women don't suffer heart trouble. Also, there is a shortage of information about women's symptoms. This is important because their symptoms are different from those of men. According to Dr. Millicent Higgins of the Framingham Heart Disease Epidemiology Study, women's symptoms may be missed or misdiagnosed. This can be catastrophic because although men are more susceptible to heart attacks, women are twice as likely to die as a result of them.

Women should beware of pressure or pain in the chest. This may be intermittent over a period of time. Diabetics, who have trouble with their circulation anyway, are particularly at risk. Smokers aren't doing themselves any good, and if you smother your potatoes in butter, I'll say goodbye now. So, cut out all fatty foods and eat fewer dairy products. Use olive oil, which studies show to be beneficial to the heart. Eat more fresh fruit and vegetables—they will save your heart and keep you slim. Ensure periods of complete relaxation and aim for de-stressing—by taking a daily soak in the bath or a monthly trip to the masseur, whatever suits you so long as you get off the merry-go-round *some* time. According to Professor Morris, chairman of the Fitness and Health Advisory Group to the Sports and Health Education Board, England, a brisk walk for half an hour daily could reduce by half the risk of heart disease. Perhaps you should walk to work. Plus, do ten minutes' general exercise in the privacy of your home—there's no need to go into mega-routines and you will be more likely to persevere if you don't get too ambitious.

All circulation-stimulating essential oils are good for the heart. Alternatively, try my special heart formula. Rub over the entire front of your torso in a clockwise direction:

PREVENTATIVE HEART CARE FORMULA

Geranium	14 drops
Hyssop	4 drops
Rosemary	8 drops
Peppermint	4 drops

For the massage oil
If to be used weekly these amounts to 2 tablespoons vegetable oil
or
If to be used daily these amounts to 3½ ounces vegetable oil

Make a synergistic blend using the above proportions and add 30 drops to your chosen bottle of base oil. Also, add 4 drops of the synergistic blend to your bath: and as you lie back, inhaling the delicious aroma, you'll agree that prevention is better than cure.

Osteoporosis

The dowager got her hump from osteoporosis. Her bones got thin and porous and she got a spinal fracture. Forty thousand women in Britain this year will break a hip. You and I may notice nothing until we break a leg. We may think of bone as solid mass and unchanging, but it is a living substance, constantly "remodeling," slowly replacing itself. A child renews its skeleton every one to two years; an adult takes just over a decade. But after about forty we're on a losing curve, and what we are losing is calcium and bone strength. Women are five to six times more likely than men to suffer osteoporosis, and the vast majority of these are in the postmenopausal group. Their susceptibility is attributed to estrogen loss at this time. It used to be thought that once lost, bone mass could not be replaced, but recent studies have shown that mild exercise can increase lumbar spine bone mineral content while lack of exercise allows levels to drop. This is an important discovery because the usual alternative for postmenopausal women is just to watch their bone mass fade away inexorably at the rate of about 2 percent a year. Compared to the menstruating women's 0.2 percent, the acceleration is frightening.

Estrogen replacement therapy is sometimes given at or soon after menopause but cannot replace lost bone mass and carries its own risks. So prevention is by far the best approach to osteoporosis. It is conjectured but not yet proven that an active life gives the higher bone density we need to see us through the later years. A similar "in the bank" factor takes place with calcium —enough before we are thirty-five to forty increases our chances of being able to hold up our backs later. But calcium intake is not such a straightforward procedure. Some women are trying to avoid the dairy products—milk and cheese—that provide most calcium. Others are allergic to them. And calcium can be drawn out of the bones by coffee. Foods we may consider A1 in dietary terms—certain raw vegetables and fruits among them—can hinder calcium absorption. Finding the perfect regime to give the optimum calcium absorption level in any particular person would require a computer: taking into consideration whether or not we smoke, drink alcohol or coffee, and what we eat. Even tap water would have to be in the calculation, as it can provide up to 200mg per day—if you live in a hard water area. Most bottled brands of water give the calcium content on the label. Calcium supplements may be an option but if you lack a particular enzyme, you could get kidney stones.

But while becoming an expert on the complexities of calcium, phosphates, oxalic acid, vitamin D, and all the rest, why not jump into a nice relaxing bath with one, two, or three of the following:

ESSENTIAL OILS

Ginger	**Chamomile German**
Rosemary	**Lemon**
Hyssop	**Thyme**
Fennel	**Benzoin**
Cumin	

Sage	**Cajeput**
Chamomile Roman	**Geranium**
Yarrow	**Nutmeg**
Carrot	**Mace**
Oregano	**Clove**
Black pepper	**Niaouli**
Peppermint	**Bay**

Any of the oils can be used singly in the bath, or make a combination to suit your taste—a total of 4 drops to a bath. In addition, make a body oil and put a generous amount on the most susceptible joints—hips, knees, elbows, wrists, and ankles—before you get into the bath and then massage these areas well once you are actually in the bath. The massage oil can be made by combining any of the oils on the main list or by following my formulas:

MASSAGE OIL FORMULAS

FORMULA 1

Ginger	10 drops
Nutmeg	7 drops
Carrot	5 drops
Chamomile Roman	8 drops

FORMULA 2

Benzoin	7 drops
Thyme	4 drops
Black pepper	8 drops
Fennel	11 drops

FORMULA 3

Lemon	10 drops
Hyssop	5 drops
Rosemary	10 drops
Niaouli	5 drops

FORMULA 4

Cumin	5 drops
Peppermint	15 drops
Bay	10 drops

If you are fit and healthy, without a creak or groan emanating from your bones, use the above formulas—or 30 drops chosen from the main list—in 3½ ounces vegetable oil for long-term use. But if you feel susceptible to osteoporosis use the above formulas, or 30 drops chosen from the main list in 2 tablespoons vegetable oil, daily. Postmenopausal women are clearly in the risk group, along with diabetics, thin white women, women who have had anorexia nervosa or arthritis, or anyone whose mother had osteoporosis. You should also consider the more concentrated treatment if your knees make a grinding noise when you bend, if you are losing height, or your posture seems to be collapsing in on itself, and if you are experiencing creaking joints. Some women just feel there is something "wrong" with their bones. Living in a soft water area can also make you more susceptible as soft water contains less calcium.

As well as being applied to the joints in the bath, the oils may be used as a body massage, and a full massage on a regular basis would be an excellent preventative measure. A good mineral and vitamin supplement should also help.

Raynaud's Disease

Imagine what it would be like to feel the cold so much that you have to wear iceworkers' gloves to take a packet of fish sticks out of the freezer. I have known women who suffer so badly with this condition that even if they put five pairs of socks on before they go out, their feet will soon be purple and their legs a veritable paint palette with patches of red, orange, royal blue, mauve, and white showing through the color of their skin. Arriving at a party looking glamorous is a bit difficult when you peel off three pairs of gloves and put away your portable pocket heater only to reveal blue hands.

Raynaud's Disease isn't catching and is not really a disease, more a physiological phenomenon relating to the arteries and the sympathetic nerves supplying them. Normally, blood heat is conserved in the cold by the muscular walls of the arteries constricting a certain amount. Conversely, when it is warm outside, the arteries relax and allow blood to the surface of the skin where it can cool down. In Raynaud's sufferers, the arteries go into spasm when it is cold, starving the skin of blood. This then turns the skin numb and white and then, as the tissues lose oxygen, blue. As the spasm ends, oxygenated blood flows again, turning the skin red and sometimes causing throbbing pain.

An attack can last for minutes, days, or weeks, and the sufferer may not know whether a particular attack will last ten minutes or two weeks. The oddest thing can set off an attack—using a power drill, or smoking a cigarette, or holding a bag too tightly. Nine out of ten sufferers are women. Raynaud's Disease isn't usually dangerous but in extreme cases it can lead to frostbite and gangrene. You should have the symptoms diagnosed to make sure the cause is not due to an obstruction in the body pressing on the arteries or a connective tissue disorder, for example. Also, certain drugs can cause the Raynaud's symptoms.

Luckily for Raynaud's sufferers, the essential oils provide an extremely effective remedy to their problem, as many of my patients' case histories show. I shall always remember the young mother who after treatment was able, for the first time she could remember, to go out during the month of January in just her stockings and shoes. Winter was no longer approached with dread.

See how simply and vigorously the essential oils help you. Choose from these oils to make your own formula, or follow that given below:

RAYNAUD'S DISEASE ESSENTIAL OILS

Nutmeg	**Rose Maroc**
Mace	**Palma rosa**
Clove	**Lavender**
Black pepper	**Fennel**
Geranium	**Rosemary**

The treatment is a two-part regime of baths and massage, using two formulas on alternate weeks. Here is the formula for the first week:

RAYNAUD'S DISEASE
SYNERGISTIC BLEND FORMULA 1

Nutmeg	15 drops
Lavender	5 drops
Geranium	10 drops

Make a synergistic blend using these proportions
or
Use these amounts to 2 tablespoons vegetable oil for a massage oil

Bathe twice a day—in the morning and before going to bed—using 6–8 drops of the synergistic blend. The water should be hot but not uncomfortable and while you are sitting there, massage your fingers and toes. Add 5 drops of synergistic blend to each teaspoon of vegetable oil to make the massage oil and apply it all over your body except your face. Get your partner or a friend to massage your back for you. Pay special attention to your toes and fingers but do the whole lot—arms, legs, bottom, tummy, chest, and shoulders. Do this daily. If an attack is on, use the massage oil as often as you like and double up on the fingers and toes.

If your toes and fingers are always extremely painful and your skin is perhaps fragile, add 50 drops of tagetes essential oil to 2 tablespoons of made-up massage oil as given in the formula above. This may seem rather a lot to add, but you are reading it right. Use this formula massage oil during the first two weeks.

Now to the second formula, which is used alternately with Formula 1 until the condition eases off and relief is obtained. Use exactly as directed above—in the bath and as a massage oil, for a week.

RAYNAUD'S DISEASE
SYNERGISTIC BLEND FORMULA 2

Black pepper	10 drops
Geranium	10 drops
Nutmeg	10 drops

Make a synergistic blend using these proportions

Eat lots of onions and fresh garlic and also take garlic capsules. Cut out coffee and tea and drink herbal teas instead. Try rosehip with a drop of cinnamon, orange, or nutmeg essential oil. Although essential oils cannot cure the condition, they can help in easing the symptoms. And if you can drag yourself away from your delicious tea, I'll see you at the ice rink!

Breast Care ◆◆◆◆◆◆◆◆◆◆

We decorate our breasts with pretty lace bras, show them off in revealing clothes, feed our babies from them, and allow our menfolk to fondle them. And yet, even though it could save our lives, how many of us examine our breasts for lumps? Not enough of us, that's for sure. We probably spend more than the five minutes a month needed for examination worrying that our breasts aren't big enough, or small enough, or. . . .

On the subject of breast cancer I would say just one thing. Consider giving up commercial deodorants because these contain aluminum salts which stop perspiration and yet aluminum is a poison which could be absorbed into the skin. Stopping this natural method of excreting toxic substances—which is what perspiration does—is as silly as putting a stop on the other natural methods of excretion. It is bound to lead to trouble. (Those who know about the dangers of aluminum have for many years stopped cooking in aluminum pots.) The pores under your arms need to breathe and so try to avoid deodorants as much as possible, and use a natural product available from health food stores when you really feel the need—when going to a social gathering or whatever.

If you already have breast cancer and radical surgery is proposed, use the soothing massage oil before surgery and the toner massage oil after—both formulas follow. Those having irradiation treatment should refer to the irradiation formula on page 249.

If surgery is proposed for another reason—the removal of a nonmalignant cyst or for a silicone implant, for example—use the toning massage oil before surgery to prepare the breasts and the soothing massage oil afterwards.

If you do find a lump in your breast, do not jump to conclusions. Over two hundred thousand women in Britain each year go to their doctors worried out of their minds and nine in ten will be worrying unnecessarily. The majority of women who go to their doctors about a pain in the breast have a cyclical-related problem to do with the hormone prolactin. Obviously, you must see a doctor if you have a lump or pain. However, essential oils do help all manner of breast problems. They also prevent stretch marks—a common problem due to the fluctuation of breast fatty tissue with dieting.

So, you've done your monthly check and you're fine. Right, now we can firm and tone. Exercise is a must—grip your hands or wrists and exercise the pectoral muscles by pushing the arms together so they come up against the invisible force created by your arm pushing in the opposite direction. Then massage over the whole of the breast area in circular movements, once a day:

BREAST TONING MASSAGE OIL

Geranium	5 drops
Lemongrass	10 drops
Parsley seed	5 drops
Carrot	5 drops
Clary-sage	5 drops

Combine and add to 2 tablespoons vegetable oil

If your breasts are sore, use this soothing formula twice a day:

SORE BREAST SOOTHING MASSAGE OIL

Chamomile Roman	10 drops
Geranium	5 drops
Lavender	10 drops
Carrot	5 drops

Combine and add to 2 tablespoons vegetable oil

Breast Abscess

This is a collection of pus created by bacterial infection, which occurs if an inflammation has been allowed to progress. Women who are lactating should refer to the treatment given on page 223. The treatment here involves three parts. First, apply 2 drops of neat lavender essential oil over the abscess area. Then make a compress by taking a bowl of warm water, adding 5 drops each of tea tree and lavender essential oil, soaking a small piece of material in this, and applying to the area. Also, use the following massage oil formula, applied over both breasts. These three things should be done daily.

BREAST ABSCESS FORMULA

Tea tree	10 drops
Lavender	10 drops
Chamomile Roman	10 drops

Diluted in 2 tablespoons vegetable oil

Cystic Breast Disease

A change of diet seems to help this condition tremendously, as do the essential oils. Try cutting out tea, coffee, and pop drinks and opting for fruit drinks, bottled water, and herb teas. A rapid improvement and even remission of the condition has been found with evening primrose oil in two double-bind, placebo-controlled trials at the Hospital of Wales, Cardiff, and the University of Dundee in Scotland. Have an aromatherapy treatment once every six weeks or get your partner or a friend to massage your back as often as they can with the following formula. You, meanwhile, massage the breasts daily:

CYSTIC BREAST DISEASE FORMULA

Lavender	10 drops
Cypress	5 drops
Chamomile Roman	15 drops

Diluted in 2 tablespoons vegetable oil

♦ CHAPTER 11 ♦

THE NATURAL CHOICE FOR MEN

LIFE IS A STRAIN for most of us, and for men the pressure is very often taken by the heart. The figures are shocking. Forty percent of men who die in the forty-five to sixty-four age group do so as a result of a coronary. Sudden heart attack strikes down men from the age of twenty-two onwards with alarming regularity, and it's thought that there are more than a million men in the forty to fifty-nine age group whose blood pressure is so high that it puts them at three times the risk of developing serious heart disease as those with low blood pressure. But when was the last time you had yours checked?

While some of the 160,000 people who die of heart disease in Britain each year could blame their tragic early demise on hereditary factors, the rest could probably have done a great deal to prevent their poor hearts packing up so early. According to recent government figures, fewer than half the medical records kept by general practitioners show recent blood pressure measurements. By comparison, 75 percent of Americans have their blood pressure checked every six months. But if you know that your blood pressure is taking you into a high risk category, you might heed the well-advertised warnings and stop smoking, eat more healthy food, and exercise more.

Slowing down is essential for those who already have a cardiac problem, and probably good advice for everyone, but who can afford to let up when the pressure to succeed is so great and the competition so formidable? Often it's the man who appears to have everything under control who develops a problem with his heart and it comes as a great surprise to everyone. "He looked so healthy," they say.

Heart Care ♦♦♦♦♦♦♦♦♦♦♦

As prevention is better than cure, we start with a formula that reduces stress, improves the circulation and nervous system, and also lowers high blood pressure:

HEART CARE FORMULA

Rosemary	1 drop
Hyssop	1 drop
Bergamot	1 drop

Use in a bath
or
In 1 teaspoon vegetable oil for self-massage

In recent research carried out by Edinburgh University it was found that men who have had heart attacks or suffer from angina have less essential fatty acids in their body than men with no heart trouble. This implies that it is the lack of vegetable oils, fish, and fresh green vegetables, rather than the over-consumption of saturated animal fats that causes the problems. The two factors are of course related in that someone who uses butter regularly is unlikely to use polyunsaturated fats simply because he is already using one form of fat and none of us spreads our toast twice! Also, if you have meat, which includes animal fat, for a meal, that precludes you having fish. It's a question of choice, and in preventative heart care it seems to make more sense to go for fish and vegetables rather than steak and buttered baked potato. This research is, however, merely a refinement on the old advice: lower your cholesterol intake.

Those who already have a heart problem should, in addition to the above and following dietary advice, try to have an aromatherapy treatment once a month. If this isn't possible, adapt the self-massage techniques outlined on pages 409–411 once a week, and use the essential oils in your bath at least twice a week. You might also like to look into chelation therapy which claims, by giving massive doses of vitamins E, C, A, B-complex, plus other vitamins, minerals and trace elements, to stimulate production of the antibodies which break down the dangerous plaque coating of the arteries. In China, ginger has been known as a heart strengthener for thousands of years, and oil of ginger happens to be one of the essential oils recommended for use in heart care.

Choosing from the two lists below, use the oils singly or in combinations—to a total of 5 drops in a bath, or a total of 30 drops per 2 tablespoons vegetable oil for the massage. You can create marvelously sensual aromas for yourself that will also be doing you a great deal of good:

HEART CARE ESSENTIAL OILS

TO STIMULATE CIRCULATION

Geranium	**Hyssop**
Rosemary	**Black pepper**
Rose Bulgar	**Cardamom**
Rose Maroc	**Ginger**
Egyptian rose	

TO ALLEVIATE STRESS AND STRAIN

Bergamot	**Cypress**
Clary-sage	**Basil**

Many of these oils smell spicy and masculine and are used in the most exclusive men's aftershaves and toiletries, and finding an oil or combination that suits your aroma preference won't be too difficult. Here is a formula you can try—either in a bath or as a massage oil. It is precisely because of heart care considerations that massage is always done working towards the heart, and in this case concentrate on your shoulders, the back of your neck, and both sides of your arms. This formula stimulates blood circulation and strengthens the nervous system while dispelling anxieties and helping you to relax:

MORE HEART CARE FORMULA

Cardamom	2 drops
Geranium	1 drop
Clary-sage	2 drops
Bergamot	1 drop

Use in a bath

or

In 2 teaspoons vegetable oil for a full body massage

or

In 1 teaspoon vegetable oil for self-massage

Body Awareness ◆◆◆◆◆◆

The human male is socially conditioned to ignore biological signs that protect him from stress and illness. All too often the fatigue that warns him against going on any further and protects him from exhaustion is pushed aside heroically, or it may be that a sense of duty or the circumstances of his responsibilities prevent him from taking heed of the warnings. Whatever the reason, pushing yourself beyond the limits of healthy fatigue over a period of time leads to the gradual breakdown of body systems.

Having body awareness is being able to chart the difference between extending and overextending ourselves. The problem with this whole subject is that once we have become exhausted it is difficult to recognize that things have gone too far. We blame the escalated problems, frayed tempers, and fractured relationships on other things.

You can be pretty sure you are heading for trouble when you find you have no reserves for unexpected situations. Even something as simple as the phone ringing—again—can seem like a huge aggravation. Your goodwill seems to be wearing very thin indeed, but you may experience it as a feeling that the world is full of idiots and incompetents. Some men get into the state of being unable to distinguish between what is good for them and what is bad for them, and this sensation of turning in circles and getting giddy brings an unnerving sense of lack of control. A common sign that things are not as they should be comes when your wife asks you to mow the lawn and you think she's just asked you to climb Mount Everest. Every little molehill has become a mountain. By asking you to do these insurmountable tasks, your wife is seen to be picking at your self-esteem. "She's a nag," you tell yourself on the way to the bar and escape. Naturally, this causes more friction in the family unit, arguments become commonplace, sleep becomes impossible, sexual relations dwindle, and divorce seems inevitable. "You're impossible to live with," says the wife. "My wife doesn't understand me," says the husband.

A crucial factor in this grim scenario is the pressure imposed by society on men always to be able to handle life's problems. Employment brings enormous pressures but not as great as those that result from being unemployed. Mental ill-health is greatest among the unemployed, and those who drink heavily are fifteen times more likely to find themselves on the psychiatrist's couch as those who do not.

Denying that problems exist is a common practice among men, and it is a well-known fact that men find sharing their emotional problems difficult. This is a complex subject to do with the way our society is structured, and not really within the scope of this book. But what results from all this is a commonly felt, deep sense of isolation among men, and that shows up in the horrifying statistics of male suicide. According to the Dean of the Royal College of Psychiatrists, Dr. Jim Birley, "Suicide is the second most common cause of death in young men after accidents." Five men under thirty-five kill themselves compared to one woman in the same age group. Over all ages, the ratio is two to one, with 3,000 male deaths a year to 1,500 female deaths. In the last ten years the incidence of suicide in men between thirty-five and forty-four has risen by 46 percent compared to a decline in the figures for women of 6 percent. Clearly, men are finding it hard to cope with life, even if they present a tough exterior to the world—or perhaps it is precisely because of that.

So why not admit it? You sometimes feel anxiety, rage, and despair. You are tired: tired of trying to succeed, tired of feeling responsible for feeding the family, tired of younger men being promoted over you, tired of watching other people accumulate consumer goods, tired of feeling like a loser, tired of trying to maintain success, tired of the job, tired of looking for a job—just tired, tired, tired!

Mental and physical exhaustion manifests itself in a myriad different ways. Common manifestations are angina pectoris, high blood pressure, low blood pressure, fluid retention, ulcers, bowel disorders, breathing problems, hyperventilation, and inexplicable pains. And the problem is that the lifestyle can become addictive. Betablockers which are so often prescribed in these situations do not provide an answer to the fundamental exhaustion, and of far more use is the awareness to recognize the symptoms for what they are. Looking at how family and friends react to you is also helpful. If they jump out of the window every time you enter the room, you know that it may be time to slow down. Pushing yourself beyond the limit to get the house painted over the weekends, or keep the lawn looking like the center court at Wimbledon is all very commendable, but is it worth it if it makes you so grumpy that nobody dares talk to you? And think about that pain you have in the leg or back—it may have more to do with sheer exhaustion than rheumatic problems.

Relaxation is the key word, but without help it is easier said than done. For someone in an exhausted state massage provides a particularly good way of relaxing, although it may take six or more sessions for relaxation to be complete. Using the essential oils not only helps the body to cope but enables an exhausted person to sleep so that reserves of energy may be put back. A rested person is also better able to deal with emotional situations and can avoid the dramatic emotional swings characteristic of the exhausted state.

FIRST STEP ESSENTIAL OILS TO HELP EXHAUSTION

Vetiver	**Marjoram**
Frankincense	**Lavender**
Bergamot	**Melissa**
Chamomile Roman	**Benzoin**
	Clary-sage

FIRST STEP EXHAUSTION MASSAGE FORMULA

Vetiver	2 drops
Frankincense	5 drops
Bergamot	5 drops
Marjoram	8 drops
Clary-sage	5 drops
Chamomile Roman	5 drops

Diluted in 2 tablespoons vegetable oil

Exhaustion is not overcome by stimulating the body further. The key to regaining a normal state of affairs lies in using oils that work through the nervous system to calm and relax. This is the first step, and it is a process of deprogramming so it will take time—don't expect miracles overnight. Use the formula above or make your own from the selection of oils and massage into your whole body every night. If you have a partner who can do this for you, all the better. When you are sleeping well and find that you can forget about the list of things you have to do, move on to step two.

SECOND STEP ESSENTIAL OILS TO HELP EXHAUSTION

Lavender	**Black pepper**
Rosemary	**Neroli**
Basil	**Lemon**
Ginger	**Lime**
Sandalwood	**Grapefruit**

SECOND STEP EXHAUSTION MASSAGE FORMULA

Lemon	10 drops
Rosemary	10 drops
Basil	8 drops
Lavender	2 drops

Diluted in 2 tablespoons vegetable oil

Use the second step formula, or one of your own made from the second step list of essential oils, in the mornings. Continue to use the first step massage oil in the evenings, leaving it on overnight. Alternate in this fashion until you feel that your body and mind have regained their former strength and balance.

Exhaustion can lead directly to either hypertension or hypotension—high or low blood pressure. Both can be dangerous. If this is the case with you, choose from the lists below to make a massage oil—use 30 drops of essential oil to 2 tablespoons vegetable oil.

TO LOWER BLOOD PRESSURE

Lavender	**Marjoram**
Melissa	**Clary-sage**
Nutmeg	**Lemon**
Hyssop	**Rosemary**

TO RAISE BLOOD PRESSURE

Thyme	**Cinnamon**
Clove	

The Reproductive System ♦♦♦♦♦♦♦♦♦♦♦♦♦♦♦

The male genital system is a complex production and delivery network which consists of many parts. As well as the penis and scrotum, there are the testes, prostate gland, seminal vesicles, vas deferens, and urethra, all connected by a system of tubes. The interrelationship between the whole means that a breakdown in any one department can cause problems with output and relationship difficulties between management and the client!

But, joking apart, an awareness of potential trouble spots within the network is important to ensure a smooth running operation and the continuation of delivery. One such spot is the testicles, because testicular cancer is the most common cancer in young men and it's on the increase. This is a cancer that has a 90 percent cure rate and the men who don't make it into that figure are usually those who didn't go to their doctor until months or even years after they noticed changes in that department. The two testicles are often slightly different in size, but when one begins to change in relation to the other, or its consistency changes, or you feel a hard lump or nodule, it is time to visit your doctor. Swelling can be painless and quite generalized and the testicle may feel numb or slightly numb. Other symptoms are back pain, dull aches in the lower abdomen or groin, tenderness, a wart type growth on the foreskin or glans, a pus discharge, blood passed in urine, pain on urinating, or the need to pass urine frequently. Men who have a testicle that didn't drop into the scrotal pouch must make a special note of the above because statistics show that they are ten times more likely to develop this cancer. However, all men should make a point of checking for any changes in their testicles once a month. Do this in the bath, while the supporting muscles are relaxed, by rolling each testicle in turn between the thumbs and fingers of both hands. Make this a habit, and you could save your own life.

Many of the symptoms listed above could relate to all sorts of other conditions and it goes without saying that anything unusual should be checked by your doctor. Passing blood in urine, for example, may have nothing to do with cancer and may be related to conditions as diverse as tuberculosis and overenthusiastic sexual activity. Sores in the genital area could indicate all sorts of things, including diabetes and sexually transmitted diseases. And talking of these, infections are often passed back and forth between a couple because in one partner the symptoms are absent. If your partner has a sexually transmitted infection, whether you have symptoms or not you must get an examination. You could be the innocent cause of her trouble and untreated infections can cause infertility—in the male as well as the female.

Thrush

Thrush is often thought of as a woman's problem, but it affects men too. It is caused by the fungi Candidiasis or Moniliasis which live in the bowel or stomach and infect not only the genitals, but the skin, mouth, and even the fingernails. Essential oils used in baths or in the sponging method, can help clear this condition, as can massage. Thrush is treated with antifungal oils, of which savory and patchouli are particularly effective. Use your chosen method daily until the condition goes:

ANTITHRUSH BATHS

Patchouli	6 drops
Bergamot	2 drops
Italian everlasting	2 drops

Savory	6 drops
Bergamot	2 drops

Savory	1 drop
Patchouli	2 drops
Lavender	2 drops

Use these quantities in a bath *or* half these quantities in a sitz bath *or* on a sponge or facecloth for sponging

The following synergistic blend can be used in a bath or massage oil. The massage oil should be applied all over the body and used once a day until the condition has cleared.

ANTITHRUSH SYNERGISTIC BLEND

Niaouli	5 drops
Patchouli	10 drops
Tea tree	5 drops
Balsam de Peru	5 drops
Lemon	5 drops

Use 4 drops in a bath
or
5 drops in 1 teaspoon vegetable oil for massage

Trichomonas

Trichomonas is another infection that is easily passed between a couple and which can be difficult to eradicate for that reason. It causes inflammation of the urethra in men. Make up your massage oil using the formula below and massage the vertebrae from your waist down, pass your hands over your hips and then massage your upper and lower abdomen. Massage and bathe daily until the condition goes:

TRICHOMONAS MASSAGE FORMULA

Patchouli	8 drops
Palma rosa	8 drops
Italian everlasting	8 drops

Diluted in 2 tablespoons vegetable oil

TRICHOMONAS SITZ BATH FORMULA

Oregano	4 drops
Bergamot	4 drops

Dilute in a bowl of water, lower yourself in, stay there for two minutes

Pains and Sores

Any pain or sores on the penis must be seen by a medical practitioner. Do not ignore them. Pain can mean kidney, bladder, or prostate disorders. Sores can be caused by sexually transmitted diseases, gout, diabetes, and lack of hygiene. Cleaning with salt and essential oil every day will help to relieve soreness and heal sores:

SOOTHING BATHING SOLUTION

Lavender	2 drops
Natural rock salt	1 teaspoon

In 1 pint of water

Washing around the genitals is important for health and relationship happiness alike. Washing well under the foreskin can be helpful in combating genital smell, and the antibacterial and antiviral qualities of essential oils go some way towards providing the protective, preventative aspect of "safe sex." For the genital wash, pour 2½ cups of warm water into a bowl, dilute your essential oils in the water and wash the penis and scrotum, taking care to use the water and not just neat essential oil —which you'll be able to see streaked through the water because oil and water don't mix. If you prefer, mix the two drops of essential oil first in half a teaspoon of pure alcohol or vodka as this dissolves the essential oil and makes dilution in the water easier. Use only the essential oils listed below which, although broken into their most useful therapeutic roles, are all excellent additions to the wash.

All too often the diagnosis of male genital conditions is vague and you are told that you have "a bacterial infection," "a viral infection," or "inflammation." If you cannot find in this section the condition that specifically relates to you, use the essential oils which come under the headings that are most relevant to your symptoms:

ESSENTIAL OILS
FOR THE MALE GENITAL AREA

INFLAMMATION

Chamomile German	**Yarrow**
Chamomile Roman	**Lavender**
	Hyssop

INFECTION

Tea tree	**Niaouli**
Lavender	**Patchouli**
Eucalyptus radiata	**Oregano**

SWELLING

Cypress	**Lavender**
Hyssop	**Calendula**
Eucalyptus peppermint	**Chamomile German**
Eucalyptus	**Juniper**
Rosemary	

Abrasions

The delicate mucous membrane of the penis can suffer minor abrasions during intercourse, or the foreskin can split, either of which may lead to infections. Treatment with essential oils is very effective—the antibacterial properties of lavender help to avoid infection in the splits while encouraging healing:

FOR MINOR ABRASIONS
OF THE PENIS

Lavender 3 drops

In a bowl of water; wash twice daily until healed

Inflammation

Never be tempted to use neat essential oil to speed up the process of reducing swelling—the essential oils must be diluted as directed. Here are two methods of treating an inflamed, swollen testicle:

ANTIINFLAMMATORY 1
FOR SWOLLEN TESTICLE

Hyssop 6 drops

In a sitz bath
or
In 1 pint of cold water for sponging

ANTIINFLAMMATORY 2
FOR SWOLLEN TESTICLE

Chamomile Roman
Chamomile German
Yarrow

Add 15 drops of any one oil to

Lavender 15 drops
Jojoba or almond oil 2 tablespoons

There are many antiinflammatory essential oils and they are best applied by sponge or washcloth. This method can be used for the penis as well:

COOLING FORMULA
FOR PENIS AND TESTICLES

Chamomile Roman
Chamomile German
Yarrow

Any one or combination to a total of 4 drops to 1 cup water
or
2 drops of any, mixed with 2 drops lavender to 1 cup water

Balanitis

This is an inflammation between the penile glans and the foreskin. It can be caused by lack of hygiene, by dirt trapped in clothing, or even by fibers of cloth which have become caught there. Balanitis causes the foreskin to swell and a pus to be discharged from underneath. It can cause a burning sensation when urine is passed. As in any conditions with symptoms of this sort, a diagnosis must be sought from your doctor to rule out venereal disease. Bathe the area twice a day with the following:

Lavender 5 drops
Chamomile German 5 drops

In a bowl of warm water to which 1 teaspoon salt has been added

Also apply a small amount of the following oil around the inflamed and infected area:

Thyme linalol 3 drops

Diluted in 2 teaspoons jojoba oil

Hydrocele

Fluid which gathers in the layers of tissue around a testicle is often harmless and painless but it can cause swelling and discomfort. The testicle will usually need to be supported by a jockstrap and the fluid will need to be drawn off. The problem with this condition, however, is that it may recur.

Massage is the best way of reducing the fluid—and that means massage of the whole body as well as the swollen testicle. Water massage, as outlined in the cellulite section (page 146), is very helpful.

Massage once a day for fifteen days using the following:

HYDROCELE MASSAGE OIL

Juniper	10 drops
Fennel	5 drops
Lemon	10 drops
Hyssop	5 drops

Diluted in 2 tablespoons almond oil

If your problem is a swollen scrotum, use the following formula massaged around the scrotum and groin twice a day:

SWOLLEN SCROTUM MASSAGE OIL

Juniper	5 drops
Hyssop	5 drops
Cypress	10 drops
Lavender	10 drops

Diluted in 2 tablespoons almond oil

Orchitis

Orchitis is an inflammation of the testes. It is usually a complication of mumps although gonorrhea is sometimes the cause. It can occur at any age. Symptoms are painful swelling of the testes, fever, and pain when passing urine, and these can take two weeks or more to subside. In the case of mumps, bed rest is essential, as in any type of viral invasion. Treatment is in two parts, body massage and testicle massage, using two different oils twice a day:

ORCHITIS BODY MASSAGE OIL

Oregano	5 drops
Tea tree	10 drops
Lemon	10 drops
Hyssop	5 drops

Dilute in 2 tablespoons vegetable oil and massage over the whole body

ORCHITIS TESTICLE MASSAGE OIL

Lavender	10 drops
Chamomile German	10 drops
Cypress	5 drops
Palma rosa	5 drops

Diluted in 2 tablespoons vegetable oil

Prostatitis

There are many causes of an inflamed prostate gland and prostatitis can be chronic or acute. Symptoms are pain, a burning sensation when passing urine, lower abdominal pain, heaviness, the inability to retain urine, frequent urination, fever, and a general feeling of tiredness and lethargy. It can occur at any time and is most uncomfortable.

Massage around the lower abdominal area, over the lower back, and around the sacrum with the following formula as needed, to a maximum of three times a day:

INFLAMED PROSTATE MASSAGE OIL

Lavender	5 drops
Cypress	10 drops
Eucalyptus radiata	10 drops
Thyme linalol	5 drops

Diluted in 2 tablespoons vegetable oil

Intertrigo

Soreness and inflammation can affect skin that is in contact with another skin surface, especially in a damp, sweaty area such as around the groin. Bacteria cause much of the trouble and the skin can take on a disagreeable odor. The problem can be caused by obesity, and incontinence in babies and the elderly.

Bathe the affected areas with the following wash twice a day for one week:

Lavender	5 drops
Eucalyptus peppermint	10 drops

Diluted in 2½ cups water

Make up the following talc using pure, pharmaceutical grade talc which is available from many pharmacists. Mix the ingredients thoroughly, in a blender if available, and dust over the area after washing:

Pure talc	4 ounces
Lavender	10 drops
Rosemary	10 drops
Chamomile German	10 drops

Varicocele

A varicocele is a varicose swelling of a vein leading from the testicle, usually on the left side for anatomical reasons. The soft swelling is usually harmless and often painless but it can ache, especially after you have been standing for long periods. Treatment is in two parts.

Massage around the lower abdomen and sacrum daily with:

Geranium	15 drops
Cypress	10 drops
Chamomile Roman	5 drops

Diluted in 2 tablespoons vegetable oil

Also, apply an ice-cup (see page 96) to the swelling once a day and afterwards massage it with:

Hyssop	2 drops
Cypress	5 drops

Diluted in 1 teaspoon evening primrose oil

This quantity is enough for two applications.

Other Problems ◆◆◆◆◆◆◆

Foot Odor

Having feet that smell less than sweet is by no means an entirely male problem, but men do seem more prone to it. This embarrassing and inhibiting problem can be caused by a number of fungal disorders as well as by bad dietary habits such as overindulgence in bottles of beer and fast food over a period of time. If a fungal infection is your problem, add 2 drops of tea tree essential oil to the foot powder formula below:

FOOT ODOR POWDER

Baking powder	1 tablespoon
Sage	2 drops

Put the baking powder in a plastic bag, add the sage oil, shake the bag well. Allow to dry, and separate mixture by running a rolling pin over the bag.

Add a zinc supplement to your daily diet, as this can help enormously. Bathing the feet in a bowl of water with 2 drops of essential oil of sage, every day for a week, will help too. Dust the feet regularly with the foot powder above and also leave half a teaspoon in your shoes overnight—this will provide good bacterial protection. Tap the powder out in the morning. Change your shoes regularly too.

Jock Itch

"Jock itch" is a familiar problem to men, especially sportsmen, and is often caused by wearing tight underpants or jeans. The symptoms are a scaly type of itchy rash, and it can become painful. The fungus germ that causes this infection of the skin, Tinea cruris, thrives in a moist area so you need to ensure that you keep the groin area as clean and dry as possible. Boxer shorts help to keep the air circulating. An oily area is also better for keeping the fungus at bay which is why it features in the two-part treatment below:

"JOCK ITCH" TREATMENT

Lavender	**Tea tree**
Cypress	**Patchouli**

Dilute 2 drops of any one essential oil in a bowl of water. Wash area, dry well.

Using 2 drops of any one essential oil diluted in 1 teaspoon vegetable oil, apply to area morning and night.

Pruritus Ani

This is a rather unglamorous problem better known as itching of the anus. It has a multitude of causes, from soap, clothing, or the chemicals in toilet tissue to antibiotics and laxatives. Because the anal area is moist and warm it is an ideal breeding ground for fungi and bacteria. Hairs around the anus can catch bacteria from food residue passing through the rectum. Eating especially hot food can cause a burning soreness in the area which leads to itching and irritation; and some people in a highly emotional state tend to perspire in this area more than normal and this can lead to an itchy anus. Try not to use soap when washing and instead bathe the area twice a day, preferably after passing stools, using the synergistic blend treatment below:

PRURITUS ANI
SYNERGISTIC BLEND TREATMENT

Geranium	5 drops
Lavender	4 drops
Bergamot	3 drops

Make a concentrate using these proportions and add 2 drops of the concentrate to a bowl of water and bathe the anus

Hemorrhoids

While we are in the general area, let's discuss hemorrhoids. This is a problem that seems to affect men quite considerably, and is best treated early on. Start to drink plenty of water and take vitamin E supplements. Many people have reported complete relief of the symptoms after following the treatment below for seven to ten days:

HEMORRHOIDS TREATMENT

Cypress	2 drops
Geranium	2 drops
Peppermint	2 drops

Dilute in 2 tablespoons wheatgerm oil or 1 ounce KY jelly and apply several times a day

Hernias

The human body is a miracle, and we have all no doubt at some stage asked ourselves, "How does it all manage to hang together so efficiently?" Well, sometimes it doesn't, and bits protrude from their designated compartment and push into another area where they don't belong. These protrusions are called hernias and they occur where there are weaknesses in the supporting structures. Hernias are often associated with men because they are affected by one of the most common types, an inguinal hernia. The weak point in this instance is the gap in the abdominal muscles through which the testes descended into the scrotum and through which the vessels must pass, so it can never be sealed off. It is through this gap that a loop of intestine or some other abdominal structure can slip. There are several weak spots in the human anatomy and hernias can affect women and babies as well.

All hernias should be seen by a doctor and some types are worrying because they can become "strangulated"—that is, a loop of intestine at the entrance to the hernia becomes pinched and obstructed, when gangrene can set in. Generally the main problem is discomfort and soreness, with perhaps pain on coughing or when making bowel movements. By gently persuading the hernia back into place manually and using certain essential oils to help heal the fibrous tissues at the split, it is not uncommon for hernias to be completely healed.

The following treatment applies to inguinal hernias, hiatus (or diaphragmatic) hernias, and incisional hernias—use the oils that apply to your condition. In all cases massage the area with your respective massage oil in the following way.

HERNIA EXERCISE Lie on the bed or floor and spend a few minutes breathing deeply. Yoga breathing is excellent. With gentle circular movements, using the palm of your hand, massage over the area with the massage oil. While you are doing this, relax and breathe deeply. If you have a large hernia, gently use the heel of your hand, and if you have a small hernia, use your fingertips, and slowly and gently persuade the protuberance back into place. Note that the word used is "persuade," not "push"; pushing will only cause more damage. Now relax for a moment before again repeating the circular movement and gentle persuasion. Alternate in this way at least ten times. Finally, relax in this same position for ten to fifteen minutes. Try to repeat this whole procedure as often as you can each day—twice a day at least.

INGUINAL HERNIA As we have already discussed, this rupture is in the abdominal muscles above the scrotum. The bulge can be quite large. It appears just above the groin and can extend into the scrotum itself. Make your massage oil by using a total of 30 drops of essential oils from the list, or by following the formula:

ESSENTIAL OILS

Rosemary	**Basil**
Geranium	**Lavender**
Cypress	**Ginger**
Hyssop	

FORMULA

Ginger	10 drops
Basil	5 drops
Lavender	8 drops
Rosemary	7 drops

Diluted in 2 tablespoons vegetable oil

HIATUS HERNIA This is both a male and female problem and is so common after middle age that it is almost considered a normal result of getting on in years. The rupture here is through the diaphragm, the layer of muscle and fibrous tissue that separates the chest and belly cavities, and is most commonly found where the esophagus passes through to the stomach—the stomach pressing up into the gap being the usual problem. It is important to avoid overeating as this exacerbates the condition.

ESSENTIAL OILS

Coriander	**Rosemary**
Cardamom	**Ginger**
Fennel	**Basil**
Lavender	

FORMULA

Coriander	10 drops
Rosemary	7 drops
Ginger	8 drops
Fennel	5 drops

Diluted in 2 tablespoons vegetable oil

INCISIONAL HERNIA This is caused by scar tissue failing to heal, usually after an abdominal wound or operation incision has become infected.

ESSENTIAL OILS

Lavender	**Palma rosa**
Neroli	**Lemon**
Tea tree	**Ginger**
Geranium	

FORMULA

Palma rosa	10 drops
Lavender	10 drops
Ginger	5 drops
Neroli	5 drops

Diluted in 2 tablespoons vegetable oil

The Liver ◆◆◆◆◆◆◆◆◆◆◆◆◆

The liver is one of the most crucial organs in the human body, quietly helping with digestion, synthesizing proteins, and neutralizing poisons—whatever abuses we subject to it. Not until three-quarters of its cells have been damaged does it cease working. Its silence is one of the things that makes a liver problem difficult to know about until things have been allowed to progress too far. Even when the damage is already quite extensive we may simply feel generally unwell or have indigestion or we may lose weight.

Alcohol is by far the biggest problem a liver has to deal with, and while it is neutralizing this poison so that the rest of the body is protected, it can itself become poisoned. So next time you have a double whisky and ruminate on how the world puts its troubles on your shoulders, just remember that you are leaning on your liver and that it, ultimately, gets the brunt of the world's problems. This is literally true, for the liver also has to process all the toxins we take in from the environment, and the chemicals we inhale at work, and many drugs designed to help other parts of the body cause poisoning to the liver in the process. Needless to say, all the toxins in the junk food we throw into our supermarket cart end up in the liver, and while "convenience" foods may be convenient to us, they are extremely inconvenient to our poor poisoned livers.

Cirrhosis of the Liver

This is a chronic, progressive disease caused mainly by alcohol and is more common in men. Healthy liver cells are replaced by fibrous tissue which hardens the liver and compresses the blood vessels. The drinking may simply be compounding a problem of toxicity, leading to cirrhosis. Or cirrhosis may be the result of poisoning by chemicals such as cleaning fluids, by certain drugs, or even anesthetics. The hepatitis B virus can also lead to cirrhosis, as can an accumulation of bacteria in the liver.

Although a normal liver has a tremendous capacity to regenerate its damaged cells, tissues damaged by cirrhosis only regenerate their damaged selves. It is therefore vital to stop further damage, and that means giving up alcohol—whether it was the cause or not. In all cases, the concern is to prevent further deterioration of the tissues by subjecting them to fewer toxins. Red meat, fish, chicken, wheat, and dairy products should all be stopped because these contain traces of chemicals and pollutants used in their growth. Also, cut out tea, coffee, and citrus fruit juices.

Instead, eat raw or steamed vegetables—organic, as far as is possible—grains (not wheat), pulses, nuts, and all fruits except citrus. Pineapple is a good fruit for the liver because it contains bromine, a substance which is extremely helpful in the treatment of all liver conditions. It should be eaten every single day, in whatever form—fresh, as juice, and even in tins (the only tinned product allowed). Spinach is another goodie that should be eaten every day. Get a book on the Hay diet, a system of food combining, which could be useful too. Bottled or boiled, cooled water is the only drink allowed, apart from vegetable and fruit juices—except, of course, citrus fruits. Take 1000mg of vitamin C a day, and vitamin A in the form of beta-carotene and a multi-vitamin B are essential.

To help elimination of the toxins, do skin brushing as outlined in the cellulite section (page 147), take daily showers, saunas whenever possible, and ask a qualified therapist to do lymphatic drainage for you. Daily massage is a great help, and you can do this yourself. If you do take all these steps you will have a fast and complete recovery and the previous signs of tingling, numbness, loss of libido, weakness, and a gray and dirty-looking complexion will go—and you'll feel and look great!

During this liver cleansing period, use only the essential oils listed below—and that is for any purpose whatsoever, including skin care. This limitation is necessary because essential oils have to be excreted through the system just like any other substance and the recommended oils contain biochemical substances which are beneficial at this time.

CIRRHOSIS OF THE LIVER
ESSENTIAL OILS

Chamomile Roman	**Myrrh**
Chamomile German	**Calendula**
Lavender	**Frankincense**
Geranium	**Neroli**
	Rose

FORMULA

Chamomile German	5 drops
Lavender	5 drops
Frankincense	2 drops
Calendula	2 drops
Rose	5 drops

Dilute in 3 ounces almond oil to which you have added 1 teaspoon borage seed oil

Hepatitis

Hepatitis is an inflammation of the liver which is caused by three viruses.

HEPATITIS A is found in children and young adults who acquire it through food contaminated by flies, and feces.

HEPATITIS B affects people differently: in some cases the viral infection passes after a few months, in others it remains present in the system forever. People carrying hepatitis B present the same problems of possible infection to doctors and dentists as do those with the AIDS virus. Like AIDS, it is passed by infected injection needles, blood transfusion, and sexual intercourse.

NONSPECIFIC HEPATITIS is a fairly new strain of the virus and has not been completely identified as of this writing, yet it is very common.

In all cases of hepatitis bed rest is advised because the patient may experience drowsiness, nausea, rashes, vomiting, confusion, and even unconsciousness. All the body fluids are contagious and precautions must be taken. Care must even be taken when handling clothes. Follow the dietary advice given for cirrhosis of the liver, and carry out the toxin elimination methods too. In all cases of hepatitis, use only the essential oils in the following list:

ESSENTIAL OILS FOR TREATING HEPATITIS A, B, AND NONSPECIFIC

Chamomile German	**Cinnamon**
Chamomile Roman	**Tea tree**
Yarrow	**Eucalyptus lemon**
Calendula	**Eucalyptus radiata**
AV1 (Dermatect)	**Thyme**
Oregano	**Patchouli**
Cypress	**Immortelle**

Use the essential oils in baths or massage oils. Use the following formula for the first two weeks:

HEPATITIS:
FIRST TWO WEEKS MASSAGE OIL

Chamomile German	10 drops
Thyme	5 drops
Cinnamon	2 drops
Tea tree	10 drops
Patchouli	3 drops

Diluted in 2 tablespoons vegetable oil

HEPATITIS:
FOLLOWING WEEKS MASSAGE OIL

Eucalyptus radiata	10 drops
Chamomile German	5 drops
Tea tree	5 drops
Eucalyptus lemon	10 drops

Diluted in 2 tablespoons vegetable oil

Also seek the advice of an aromatherapist for antiviral essential oil formulations tailored to your particular needs.

Balding ◆◆◆◆◆◆◆◆◆◆◆◆◆◆

Male self-image can be greatly reduced by baldness and this despite the fact that a correlation has been shown between baldness and high levels of testosterone and thus, virility. Nevertheless the dream of many balding men is that a magic drug or substance will be found to restore the hair of their youth.

Several new drugs have recently been identified that will in some cases stimulate hair growth. The idea is that these locally applied substances stimulate atrophied hair follicles into producing hair growth, and what has excited and fascinated the researchers is that these are drugs which are used in the treatment of hypertension: they dilate blood vessels, stimulate cell division and, in the process, encourage hair growth. These developments do not come as a surprise to aromatherapists, who regularly use any number of essential oils which have the same function. Not only that, but essential oils, unlike chemical drugs, are harmless to the body if used correctly. So while the pharmacists continue with their testing, aromatherapists and the trichologists who have studied essential oils will continue stimulating hair growth in atrophied hair follicles.

Hereditary factors do, of course, come into the balding problem. But reducing the aging factor in the whole body by keeping the cell functions healthy and vigorous also delays the hereditary factor in balding.

While you are doing the balding treatment that follows, do also employ the essential oils to work on the whole of your system—especially the circulatory and lymphatic systems. Look through the book and find something that would help you in other areas, or simply make up a massage oil with some of the essential oils below and use that as a body rub for the period of your balding treatment. You could make some excellent masculine-smelling oils to suit your own taste. Also, use the oils singly or in combination—4–6 drops—in baths.

ESSENTIAL OILS TO STIMULATE HAIR GROWTH

Rosemary	**Sage**
Neroli	**Hyssop**
Lavender	**Thyme**
Geranium	**Lemon**
Basil	**Grapefruit**
Ginger	**Cypress**
Cedarwood	

As a simple measure to strengthen hair, add 1 drop of rosemary oil to a cold water rinse when you have finished washing your hair. There's no need to rinse the rosemary out—it will give your hair a nice shine—and the cold water stimulates the blood capillaries, causing them to contract and thus stimulating the movement of nutrients from the blood and into the bulb of the hair, or follicle, which feeds the hair.

The Treatment

This treatment will prevent hair from falling out, strengthen and make thicker the hair you still have and, in some cases if the hair follicle is still productive, bring back a fluffy, downy hair. Premature balding can be lessened by the oils but don't be impatient—treatment must be continuous and don't expect to see results for about four months. However, patience is rewarded with a bonus—while you are following the treatment you may find that you won't catch colds, coughs, or flu, and any sinus problems will be helped too. First make your synergistic blend of oils:

PREMATURE BALDING SYNERGISTIC BLEND

Rosemary	3 drops
Geranium	4 drops
Lavender	5 drops
Cypress	4 drops
Cinnamon	2 drops
Juniper	2 drops

Blend together in these proportions

Each day take one drop from the bottle of synergistic blend and mix it with ¼ teaspoon of water and rub it into the head. Rub the bald area first and then rub well into the rest of the scalp. Don't rub too hard. Night is the best time to do the treatment because that's when the body is working hard to regenerate itself. In the mornings use a hypo-allergenic shampoo, which is to say one that doesn't contain detergent. The important thing is to stick to the treatment, but discipline is made easy by the fact that it smells so good.

To really wake the scalp up, special efforts have to be made during the first two weeks of treatment. On alternate days put the formula on your head as usual and then wrap the head in a hot towel, Turkish turban style. Leave it in place for two or three minutes and then rub the head all over with an ice-cup (see page 96). When your scalp is icy cold, apply another hot towel. Repeat this alternate hot and cold procedure at least five times, then apply the formula for a second time and leave it on the scalp overnight.

On the fifteenth day, take 2 teaspoons of oil of jojoba and massage it well into the whole scalp. This is rather a lot of oil, but slick your hair back and keep the oil on for as long as possible—one hour is the minimum. If you use hair gel to get the wet look or to make different styling effects, start using jojoba oil instead. It's a liquid wax and will be feeding your hair with nutrients.

The Skin Fitness Regime ◆◆◆◆◆◆◆◆◆◆◆◆◆◆

I have yet to meet a woman who would agree with Ovid's statement made some three thousand years ago that "men should not care too much for good looks; neglect is becoming." After all, who wants to kiss a flaking, dehydrated skin with shaving rash and spots? A rough skin might not turn the boss off—unless she is a woman—but this is a very competitive society and if the stress and fatigue show, the boss might decide you are looking a bit rough and give the promotion to someone else—someone with a bright and clean image. This need not be someone younger because the older man can be very attractive and sexy if he takes care of himself, and facial lines add character. Neglect, on the other hand, shows a careless, perhaps lazy character—and that attitude could have as bad an effect on the job as it does on the image.

Certainly someone thinks so, because the male cosmetics business is booming. Of course, it's not called "cosmetics" but "bioengineering," "moisturizers" have become "balm," and instead of "gently smoothing out wrinkles," male products "combat the rigors of stress and fatigue."

The rigors of the male lifestyle, however, do mean that men's skin suffers different abuses from that of women. Fishermen out on the raging seas are beaten by howling winds and the drying effect of working in a foundry can only be imagined by most of us. After each sweaty shift of cutting coal deep beneath our feet, miners emerge covered in grime, and certainly one of the most grueling experiences my skin has endured was a day of mixing cement—it was weeks before the dryness and soreness went.

Men are thicker skinned—literally—than women, and although this means that they age more slowly it also means they will spend hours digging in the garden without due respect for the elements. Some men's image will prevent them from covering themselves with factor eight suntan lotion when the sun emerges. And many businessmen spend a fair amount of their time locked up in the drying environment of airplane air-conditioning and do nothing to combat its effects, and then wonder why they look terrible when they arrive for the meeting.

In certain respects male and female skin is the same. In each square centimeter there are two hundred nerve endings, twenty-five pressure sensors, twelve sensors for heat, and two for cold. There are approximately seven hundred pores, one hundred sweat glands, and fifteen sebaceous glands. We all have about a dozen hairs and hair follicles per centimeter, but hormones ensure that male hairs are thicker and therefore more visible. Men also produce more sebum which, combined with the additional thickness of their skin, ensures that wrinkles do not come so early. However, the thickness of male skin means that when middle age comes the wrinkles can be deeper. The thickness of male hair leads to several problems. It can trap sebum and dirt when unwashed and soap particles when cleaned, and the generally protected skin underneath gets sensitive during winter and can suffer badly when exposed to bright sunshine. Hairy chests, backs, and shoulders suffer especially from all these problems, and when the hairiness is excessive it may be worth having it removed by electrolysis.

Facial hair is of course a major distinguishing feature between male and female skin, and the average man will spend nineteen weeks of his life standing in front of the mirror with a shaver of some sort in his hand. The sheer inevitability of having to shave every morning has driven most men, at some time in their lives, into the decision to grow a beard or at least a moustache, but whatever the length or nonlength of your facial hair, special care must be taken of this portion of your face. It is these aspects of facial fitness that we discuss here; turn to the general beauty section for preparations to use elsewhere.

Shaving

Shaving every day is rather like scraping sandpaper over your face, robbing it of its protective layer of skin cells and sebum, each time revealing new sensitive skin. As you know, problems can occur as a result. A good pre-shaving product should cause the hairs to swell up and allow them to be cut more easily, but even simple water can reduce the hair's strength by 40 to 60 percent. If you have a particularly tender, dry, or flaky skin, apply a moisturizing oil to the skin before your shaving cream, at least for a while until the skin's condition improves. Try to use a new blade as often as possible and shave downward, in the direction of the hair growth, twice. Your shaving cream should be as natural and gentle as possible and avoid anything that is drying or aggravating to your skin. Use plenty of water to rinse the skin afterwards.

AFTERSHAVE SPLASH Here is a formula for a refreshing, antiseptic, and spot-clearing aftershave. You can vary the essential oil content and make your very own designer preparation:

Witch hazel	4 teaspoons
Rosewater	2 ounces
Cider vinegar	2 teaspoons
Tincture of benzoin	2 teaspoons
Bay	6 drops
Lemon	6 drops
Lavender	2 drops
Rosemary	10 drops
Lime	3 drops

Add the essential oils to the benzoin and shake well for at least a minute. Then add the witch hazel and shake again; then the rosewater and vinegar and shake again.

Some kind of moisturizing medium should always be used by men to protect them from the pollutants in the environment, so apply a face oil (see pages 124–127) and wipe off the excess with a tissue.

No matter how careful you are, shaving brings many problems:

SHAVING CUTS Make up this shaving cut mixture to keep in the bathroom cabinet for when it's needed. Put all the ingredients in a bottle and shake it well each time before using. Dab a little onto cuts to stem bleeding and as an antiseptic.

Witch hazel	2 teaspoons
Lavender	10 drops
Yarrow	10 drops

SHAVING RASH This can be brought on for no apparent reason, but here is a remedy that usually has very quick results. Spread a small amount over the rash after shaving, leave it on for a few moments and then wipe off the excess with a tissue:

Lavender	10 drops
Chamomile German	10 drops
Calendula	5 drops

Diluted in 4 teaspoons evening primrose oil

SHAVING ITCH The above formula works equally well for the itch that often accompanies a dry skin left after shaving. Make it up as above but dilute it further by adding the total ingredients shown above to 2 tablespoons of soya bean oil.

SHAVING INFLAMMATION AND SENSITIVITY This formula should be splashed on the face after shaving if your skin is inflamed and sensitive after you shave:

Tincture of myrrh	2 teaspoons
Rosewater	2 tablespoons
Chamomile German	10 drops
Lavender	5 drops
Peppermint	2 drops
Lemon	1 drop

Dilute the essential oils in the tincture of myrrh first and then add to the rosewater. If you have a still and can make chamomile water, or if you make an infusion of chamomile, that can be substituted for the rosewater. Shake the bottle well after preparing, and shake again before each use.

MASKS When the beard area gets shaved each morning, with all the attendant dangers of drying on that part of the skin, there can be a noticeable imbalance between this and other areas of the face, especially if those other areas are greasy—spotty nose or forehead, for example. Exfoliating masks are ideal for men who have an oily complexion. Use one of the masks in the beauty chapter, pages 119–122, to get rid of the excess oiliness and dead skin cells around the upper facial area.

Beards

During the six weeks or so that it takes for a beard to grow to a reasonable length, problems may be caused by ingrowing hairs. Products used on beards need to be good for the skin too because beards can trap sebum and debris, which may cause an odor as well as spots. Beards also need to be shaped. In times past all these aspects of beard care would have been carried out by a barber, but today most men have to take care of their own beards.

A beard in good condition, shiny, healthy, and well groomed, looks great; but a dull-looking, bristly, patchy one perhaps with spots underneath, looks scruffy and feels horrible to you and your lady-friend alike. Essential oils diluted in a conditioning medium are extremely useful during the growth period, and also make a good conditioning treatment for the beard that is already grown:

ESSENTIAL OILS FOR THE BEARD

Rosemary	**Lemon**
Lavender	**Cypress**
Thyme linalol	

CONDITIONING MEDIUMS

Avocado oil **Jojoba oil**

BEARD CONDITIONING FORMULA

Rosemary	10 drops
Lavender	5 drops
Thyme linalol	5 drops
Lemon	10 drops

Diluted in 4 teaspoons almond oil plus 2 teaspoons jojoba oil

During the growth period apply some of the conditioning oil around the beard area once a day, massaging in well and wiping off the excess.

If your beard has already grown, use the oil as a conditioning treatment by massaging it into the beard and skin before taking a bath. Wash it off afterwards using boiled, cooled water.

◆ CHAPTER 12 ◆

ESSENTIAL HELP IN THE MATURING YEARS

THERE IS GREAT variation in the attitudes of different societies towards their citizens of maturing years. In China, age rules, with the younger members deferring to the wisdom of experience. In many Western societies, however, older people are made to feel obsolete and given no role to play. Is it any wonder that many feel worn out before they really are?

Most old people *feel* themselves to be the same as they were in their youth. Experience might have made them think differently about a few things, but that's about it. Reconciling the inner feeling with the outer reflection can be difficult for many older people, especially in a society which venerates accumulation in everything but years. But getting to know the essential oils can help us mature gracefully by bringing the body more into line with the young person we feel inside. Remember, you are never too old for an activity unless you are physically incapable of doing it. Where's the law that says you can't go disco dancing at eighty?

Whatever you do, make this time of your life one of enjoyment. Once you are retired there is more time to enjoy the simple pleasures of life, like music, having lunch on the lawn, and visiting interesting places—not to mention starting up magazines and other businesses! So it's time to wake up to the challenge. Of course, we all need a little help sometimes, so if you wake up feeling listless and tired, here is the regime for you: when you get up, have a fruit juice and take a bath or shower using the essential oils below. If you take the bath, lie back and breathe deeply, inhaling the delicate revitalizing aroma molecules:

"WAKE UP" FORMULA
FOR THE MATURING YEARS

Bergamot	*Bath:* 3 drops *Shower:* 1 drop
Basil	*Bath:* 1 drop *Shower:* 1 drop
Peppermint	*Bath:* 1 drop *Shower:* 1 drop

Now do a few exercises—not a Jane Fonda workout, more like a cat stretching in the morning. Just stretch each muscle as best you can, paying attention to each part of the body in turn. If you find that as far as exercise is concerned, the mind may be willing but the body is not, things will seem much easier after the wake up bath or shower because the oils stimulate circulation as well as the respiratory, nervous, muscular, and skeletal systems.

By this time you'll be ready for a balanced, wholefood breakfast. It is very important at this time of life to take care that the toxins that have built up in your body over the years don't lead to aches, pains, or even rheumatism or arthritis. Do try to eat regularly and well—you need your nutrients as much as ever, if not more.

Whatever you do, enjoy.

Circulation ♦♦♦♦♦♦♦♦♦♦♦

For many older people bad circulation can be a problem, particularly in the hands and feet. To treat this, add 30 drops of geranium oil to 2 tablespoons of vegetable oil and rub it on yourself, from the hand to the elbow and from the foot to the knee. Indeed the more of your body you can get the oil on, the better. You can also put it on your face, and as geranium is one of the best revitalizing oils it will improve the texture of your skin and make it firmer and smoother. As well as making you look good, geranium cheers you up because it is a highly effective antidepressant.

For a more comprehensive discussion of this subject see Raynaud's Disease, page 256.

Swollen Ankles and Feet ♦♦♦♦♦♦♦♦♦♦♦♦♦

Ankles can swell for many reasons, including arthritis, rheumatism, varicose veins, high blood pressure, fluid retention, and even constipation. Resting with the feet up is always an effective measure, as is a pebble foot bath. Place a dozen or so smooth, round pebbles in a bowl of warm water and then add:

Cypress	1 drop
Lavender	1 drop

Roll the soles of your feet slowly over the pebbles for a few minutes, then dry your feet. Massage from the feet, as low as you can manage, then the ankles and upwards towards the knees, including behind the knees, with the following oil:

Fennel	15 drops
Cypress	15 drops

Diluted in 2 tablespoons vegetable oil; also, drink plenty of water

If the swelling happens in hot weather, before massaging the feet and ankles get a piece of ice and put it in a plastic bag and rub it around the back of the knees until they feel quite cold, then rub it in the center of the soles of your feet.

Leg Cramps ♦♦♦♦♦♦♦♦♦♦

Night cramps can cause a great deal of anguish, not only from the pain which can last up to ten minutes while the muscle is in spasm and make even the bravest of us scream, but from the interrupted sleep pattern which results. A cramp is a painful contraction of a muscle which cannot be relaxed, and in this instance it most often occurs in the calf muscle.

The Swiss have a way with cramps that must have been adopted from the Chinese, and it does work. You just hold your big toe, pressing on the nail and applying very firm pressure on both the front and back.

But prevention is the best option. Calcium and zinc supplements are recommended, as are garlic capsules and quinine. Warmth and massage are also important. This is the massage oil to use:

LEG CRAMPS MASSAGE OIL

Rosemary	10 drops
Hyssop	5 drops
Lavender	5 drops
Marjoram	10 drops

Diluted in 2 tablespoons vegetable oil

Before going to bed, massage the whole leg in an upwards direction and lastly, massage the feet. Then put on a warm pair of socks (forget about glamour—jumping around holding your foot isn't glamorous either). This should be done every night for at least two weeks. Treating recumbency cramps is also a deprogramming process—you have to prevent the message that says there'll be a cramp every night.

Incidentally, one of the most effective ways to combat cold feet during the night is to place a soft pillow between the sheets at the end of the bed and use it as a sort of hot water bottle. The difference is that while a hot water bottle starts warm and gets progressively colder during the night, the pillow starts cold and gets progressively warmer as it absorbs your body heat. If you can heat the pillow on a radiator before putting it in the bed, you have the best of both worlds.

Varicose Veins ◆◆◆◆◆◆◆◆

There are two interconnected systems of veins in the legs—the deep and the so-called "superficial," which are near the surface. It is the latter which are prone to the unsightly and painful condition known as varicose veins, in which they become swollen because the valves aren't working properly or the muscular tissue lining the walls of the veins relaxes, sometimes as a result of a hormonal imbalance. Although they are not dangerous, varicose veins do cause a great deal of discomfort when you stand, swelling in the feet and general fatigue, and in bad cases the veins rise from the surface of the skin giving it an uneven texture, sometimes with darkened, knotted areas. Inflammation can occur, and varicose veins are prone to bruising and varicose ulceration.

General massage may cause damage to the fragile capillary wall, but as essential oils can be highly beneficial by lessening the pressure on the defective valves you can apply them, but only when using a particular massage technique. Please note that you should not use other massage techniques with this condition. Grip your ankle gently and using the whole of the hand, sweep upwards in one gentle movement, using one hand only.

DAYTIME VARICOSE VEIN MASSAGE OIL

Geranium	10 drops
Cypress	15 drops
Hyssop	5 drops

Diluted in 2 tablespoons vegetable oil

NIGHTTIME VARICOSE VEIN MASSAGE OIL

Parsley	30 drops

Diluted in 2 tablespoons vegetable oil

If you can't get hold of hyssop for any reason, make the daytime massage oil using 15 drops each of geranium and cypress. And if you have a very bad family history with this condition add 10 drops of peppermint oil to the formula.

If you use the essential oils neat to make a synergistic blend, in the proportions given for the massage oil formula, this can be added—10 drops at a time—to foot baths. Why not have a foot bath, massage with the formula, and then put your feet up for an hour? To round the treatment off completely, sip a cup of peppermint tea while you are sitting there. Alternatively, make up a mixture of 2 tablespoons of honey and 4 drops of peppermint and take 1 teaspoon of this mixture in a cup of hot water. You should try to have two of these honey and peppermint drinks each day.

It is important to avoid constipation as this increases the pressure on the veins. Use plenty of onions and garlic in your cooking and eat raw parsley whenever you can. Garlic capsules and vitamin E supplements are a helpful aid in the treatment of varicose veins. Walking is the best form of exercise for anyone with this condition, but any gentle exercise is better than none. After long periods of standing, sit with your feet at the same height as your head.

Varicose Ulcers ◆◆◆◆◆◆◆

According to one survey 400,000 people in Britain at any one time suffer from leg ulcers and of these a quarter have the more serious condition of open sores. If these become infected they may become serious, and if healing cannot be accomplished a skin graft may be the final option. All this starts with an innocent-looking discoloration of the skin or a papery look, which results from an inadequate supply of oxygen to the skin, often from having varicose veins. The size of varicose ulcers can vary tremendously and although they are generally painless, a knock to the area can change that happy state in a flash.

Nutritional supplements must be taken, including zinc, vitamins E, C, and D and beta-carotene (vitamin A). Eat only fresh foods and drink herbal teas. Avoid dairy products, alcohol, tea, and coffee. Bed rest is often recommended but spend as much time as possible with the affected leg up. If you have varicose veins, follow the treatment recommended in the previous section. Treatment of the ulcer itself is simple: the following oils and synergistic blend are to be used to bathe the area and on dressings.

VARICOSE ULCERS ESSENTIAL OILS

Lavender	**Chamomile German**
Tea tree	**Thyme linalol**
Eucalyptus peppermint	**Geranium**

SYNERGISTIC BLEND

Lavender	10 drops
Geranium	5 drops
Thyme linalol	5 drops
Eucalyptus peppermint	10 drops

Use 2 drops of essential oil to a cup of water—this gives you plenty, not only to bathe the area of the ulcer itself but the whole of the leg. Do the unaffected area first, and then the ulcerated area. Now apply a dressing to the ulcer itself. Make this by placing 4 neat drops of one of the essential oils above onto a sterile piece of gauze. Change the dressing every day.

Insomnia ◆◆◆◆◆◆◆◆◆◆◆◆◆

As we grow older we need less sleep, and this can become a problem if we hold on to the idea that everyone needs a good eight hours' sleep each night. The fact is that many people function very well throughout their lives on five or six hours. A vicious circle may begin after retirement when catnapping becomes possible during the day, and this leads to waking during the night because the body just doesn't need so much sleep.

Generally people sleep a lot longer than they think they do, with the loss of sleep being exaggerated. "I haven't slept all night" can, on examination, really mean that someone woke a couple of times for two or three minutes. The time involved becomes amplified by the aggravation it caused.

There's nothing wrong in waking with the dawn chorus, but if you are starting to worry about it, feel tired all day, or are mentally unalert then you possibly have true insomnia. There are several possible causes if this is the case, including pain, cramps, fatigue, diet, stimulants, and even insufficient food. Removal of the cause, if possible, is the first and most important step. If the problem is diuretic and you frequently need to pass urine during the night, cut down on fluids, especially before going to bed. Flatulence can cause pain and discomfort and is often caused by eating too late—so eat earlier. Fatigue is caused by working late into the night, and even reading can cause overstimulation and the tired-but-can't-sleep syndrome. Look at your habits in the hours prior to going to bed. Stimulants—and tea is one—should not be taken after four o'clock if you go to bed at ten. Remove all external disturbances such as a ticking clock or a humming electrical machine.

Emotional problems and anxiety are more difficult to control, but even these can be helped by using the essential oils and listening to relaxing music before you settle down. You might also try changing the lightbulb in your bedside table lamp to a low voltage, soothing, colored one. A light shade of pink is an excellent color, as are certain tones of light green; but red and blue should be avoided. Make sure you have good ventilation in your bedroom because stuffiness is often the cause of waking in the night. A little brandy with the last meal of the day often helps to send you off and is much better for you than sleeping pills. Most importantly, stop worrying about not sleeping!

The essential oils below can be used in a warm, sensuous bath—as opposed to a stimulating hot or cold one—before bedtime. You may prefer to use them in a foot bath. Also, they can be used in an oil which can just be gently rubbed onto any convenient-to-reach parts of the body. A diffuser in the bedroom works well too, used overnight. The oils starred below are only relaxing when used in low doses—too much and they become a stimulant—so do bear that in mind when using them. Don't use more than 3 drops in a bath, for example.

ESSENTIAL OILS FOR INSOMNIA

Lavender*	**Benzoin**
Marjoram*	**Clary-sage**
Chamomile Roman*	**Vetiver**
Nutmeg*	**Hops**
	Valerian

*In low doses.

GENERAL SYNERGISTIC BLEND FOR INSOMNIA

Clary-sage	3 drops
Vetiver	2 drops
Valerian	1 drop
Lavender	2 drops

Use 3 drops per bath

or

2 drops in 1 teaspoon vegetable oil for a body rub

WARMING SYNERGISTIC BLEND
FOR INSOMNIA

Benzoin	4 drops
Nutmeg	3 drops
Chamomile Roman	2 drops

Use 3 drops per bath

or

2 drops per 1 teaspoon vegetable oil for a body rub

FOOT BATH SYNERGISTIC BLEND
FOR INSOMNIA

Lavender	1 drop
Marjoram	3 drops
Chamomile Roman	3 drops
Valerian	1 drop

Use 2 drops in a foot bath

Breathing Difficulties ◆◆◆◆◆◆◆◆◆◆◆

The three most common types of breathing problem are painful breathing, having a panting, shortness of breath type of breathing, or noisy, wheezing breathing. These are dealt with separately in this short section.

PAINFUL BREATHING (Pleuritic respiration) is often an indication of a serious disorder of the lungs, muscles, or bones. It can be accompanied by a cough, which is also painful, and inflammation. The most likely cause of painful breathing is fibrositis, although chest injury or pneumonia should be ruled out before following this treatment. Use the following essential oils to make your own massage oil, or use the formula, and rub all around the chest area and the back too, if possible (this also applies to myositis):

ESSENTIAL OILS FOR
THE TREATMENT OF FIBROSITIS
CAUSING PAINFUL BREATHING

Eucalyptus peppermint	**Rosemary**
	Ginger
Eucalyptus blue mallee	**Chamomile Roman**
Hyssop	**Nutmeg**
Frankincense	**Cinnamon**

FORMULA

Nutmeg	5 drops
Cinnamon	2 drops
Eucalyptus peppermint	10 drops
Ginger	10 drops
Rosemary	3 drops

Diluted in 2 tablespoons vegetable oil

SHORTNESS OF BREATH can become a problem when old age brings lack of mobility. You will be forced to alter your lifestyle no matter how much the rest of you says "go" if you find yourself breathless when climbing the stairs or walking to the end of the garden, not to mention going to the store. The causes of this type of breathlessness are many and it must be taken seriously because it can be the forerunner of other respiratory diseases.

Another type of shortness of breath is brought on by mental or physical anxiety—taking a driving test or riding in an elevator, for example, although almost anything can spark it off. You may find that it stops spontaneously when you sigh or laugh.

With all kinds of breathing difficulties it helps enormously if you learn to control your breathing. Practice taking deep breaths, like sighs, and holding them for a few seconds before releasing. Also, as you breathe in, raise your arms above your head and lower them as you breathe out—this will exercise the muscles. Increasing the circulatory flow will help you too, and keeping your feet warm will improve things. Use the following essential oils to make your own massage oil, or use the formula, and massage daily all over your torso. Also, use the oils in hot baths, breathing in the steam.

ESSENTIAL OILS TO HELP OVERCOME INCREASING BREATHLESSNESS

Eucalyptus lemon	**Geranium**
	Hyssop
Rosemary	**Benzoin**
Cardamom	**Marjoram**
Juniper	**Thyme**

FORMULA

Benzoin	15 drops
Geranium	5 drops
Hyssop	10 drops

Diluted in 2 tablespoons vegetable oil

NOISY BREATHING can be wheezy or hoarse and it can come suddenly (acute) or be a chronic wheeze that increases in intensity. Often the simple common cold is to blame, but the cause may be more serious, such as an obstruction, asthma, bronchitis, or certain viral infections.

For acute conditions, rest and steam inhalations are often all that are needed. Float 4 drops of eucalyptus or hyssop on a bowl of hot water and breathe as deeply as you can for at least five minutes. Your head needs to be covered with a towel to keep the steam in and you will need to come out for a second or two every now and again. Keep your eyes closed when under the towel.

Steam in the bedroom helps at night. Boiling a kettle repeatedly helps to clear the room of dry dust particles. Sitting in a steamy bathroom will help too. Chronic conditions need massage and steam every day. Massage with the following formula over the chest first, then the neck and the back if at all possible:

NOISY BREATHING MASSAGE OIL

Eucalyptus	15 drops
Rosemary	10 drops
Hyssop	5 drops

Diluted in 2 tablespoons vegetable oil

Bronchitis ♦♦♦♦♦♦♦♦♦♦♦♦

Bronchitis is inflammation of the bronchi, the air passages in the lungs. It can be acute or chronic. During the acute stage there is often wheezing, expectoration of phlegm, and a persistent cough, and there may also be a headache or fever. The condition usually clears up within three weeks but is nevertheless extremely distressing. You should keep warm and stay in bed and avoid all smoke, whether from cigarettes or fires. When the cough is painful and dry, gentle inhalation of essential oils during the night will help tremendously. These can be used in a diffuser, or any of the heat room methods, or in a bowl of hot water —6 drops, whichever method you choose.

As a virus is often the root cause of the problem, with secondary infection being caused by bacteria, refer to the lists of essential oils to deal with these on pages 396–397. The oils can be used in whatever inhalation method you decide to use. Also make a massage oil and rub it on to the chest, all around the ribcage and along the entire length of your front torso, from the throat and neck to your abdomen. If you can, get someone to rub the oil on your back as well. A lump of sugar with 1 drop of eucalyptus on it, taken three times a day, will help to fight the infection.

All types of eucalyptus essential oil are useful in the treatment of bronchitis and there are four types on the list below. Of these, I prefer eucalyptus peppermint and blue mallee. Use the synergistic oil or make your own formula and massage twice a day:

BRONCHITIS ESSENTIAL OILS

Benzoin	**Eucalyptus radiata**
Frankincense	**Red thyme**
Eucalyptus peppermint	**Marjoram**
Eucalyptus blue mallee	**Ginger**
Eucalyptus globus	**Nutmeg**
	Clove

BRONCHITIS SYNERGISTIC OIL

Cinnamon	2 drops
Nutmeg	2 drops
Ginger	2 drops
Red thyme	10 drops
Eucalyptus	10 drops
Benzoin	4 drops

Diluted in 2 tablespoons vegetable oil

Although it may sound a bit strange, putting essential oil onto a tissue and into one's socks is an extremely effective measure in the treatment of bronchitis. Tear a tissue in half and on each piece put 2 drops of red thyme essential oil and arrange these in the sock so that the tissues are against the soles of your feet. Change the tissues twice a day—in the evening they should be placed in your bedsocks and worn overnight.

Bronchitis becomes chronic when the bronchi become narrowed by the overproduction of mucus and the tiny air sacks of which the lungs are composed are distended. The cause is still not really understood although pollution and open fires do certainly have a negative effect. Chronic bronchitis can develop into emphysema, but this is not to imply that bronchitis is not in itself a dangerous condition—in Britain over twenty thousand people die of it each year.

Rest is extremely important and you must not exert yourself for any reason whatsoever. Breathing exercises are the only "action" you should take while the condition lasts. You must stay out of cold air and keep yourself warm, especially in the hands and feet. Diet should be attended to: cut out all dairy products (except eggs), white flour products, and sugars, as these are mucus-forming. Also avoid toxins as far as possible, including coffee and tea. You can, however, have a little brandy to cheer yourself up: dilute 1 drop of eucalyptus oil in a little brandy then add to a cup of hot water to which you have added some honey and lemon. This soothing drink is very popular in Switzerland in the treatment of bronchitis. The Chinese—a very phlegmatic race—use ginger as a cure for bronchitis. Put a wineglassful of brandy (in place of the Chinese rice wine) in a clean bottle with about 1 tablespoon grated, fresh ginger and leave to stand for a week. Strain and add the brandy liquid to a glassful of honey and blend them together well, and bottle. Dilute 1 teaspoon of this in a cup of hot water for an excellent preventative drink throughout the winter or in the treatment of bronchitis. It will certainly keep colds at bay as well. Instead of a piece of ginger, you could substitute 6 drops of essential oil of ginger, leaving it to infuse for a week.

As well as your ginger or eucalyptus drink, take a lump of sugar with 1 drop of eucalyptus oil three times a day, and massage with the synergistic blend or essential oils recommended for acute bronchitis, adding the following oils:

ADDITIONAL OILS
FOR CHRONIC BRONCHITIS

Ravensara	**Cedarwood**

Pneumonia ◆◆◆◆◆◆◆◆◆◆◆

Pneumonia can result from a lowered resistance to infection following another illness, and in the maturing years this may just be a common cold. Antibiotics are prescribed with great success and should be taken no matter how much you may dislike doing so. This is one of those conditions where a symbiosis of different methods of treatment are brought into play. There are bacterial pneumonias and viral ones, the latter being less serious. The site of infection is the lungs.

Bed rest is essential, as is drinking plenty of fluids and keeping your feet and hands warm. Use essential oils in bedsocks, as outlined on page 288, replacing the thyme with 2 drops of essential oil of ginger. Inhalations are an extremely good way to speed recovery from pneumonia:

PNEUMONIA: FOR INHALATIONS

Ravensara	**Niaouli**
Tea tree	

Also make a body rub oil which can be used all over the body, except for the face, using the following:

PNEUMONIA: BODY RUB
ESSENTIAL OILS

Niaouli	**Eucalyptus**
Tea tree	**Oregano**
Eucalyptus lemon	**Thyme**
	Ravensara

FORMULA

Eucalyptus lemon	10 drops
Niaouli	10 drops
Thyme	5 drops
Ravensara	5 drops

Diluted in 2 tablespoons vegetable oil

Try to keep your diet as healthy as possible—eat fresh foods and drink plenty of honey-and-lemon water and herbal teas such as nettle, rosehip, and peppermint.

High Blood Pressure ◆◆

Certain specific diseases cause high blood pressure or hypertension, notably those of the kidneys, but for many people with this condition there is no apparent cause. Although in itself high blood pressure need not lead to any problems, it is a well-established fact that those with it do not live as long as those without it. This is in part due to the complications that can arise from it, including strokes, angina, and thrombosis. High blood pressure can cause hardening of the arteries and the loss of elasticity which leads to arteriosclerosis. In very bad cases it leads to heart failure and kidney disease. The causes of hypertension are still unclear, and so treatment is therefore limited to the high blood pressure itself, rather than to any underlying cause. Since symptoms may be nonexistent, or as vague as headaches, tiredness, and dizziness, the only way to keep track of blood pressure is to have it checked regularly.

Anyone who has high blood pressure needs to look at ways to reduce any stress, slow down on activities, rest, and lose weight if he or she is carrying too much for the poor old heart to handle.

Dietary changes are particularly important. Eat fruit, vegetables, fish, poultry, pulses, and grains. Use olive oil, spices, onions, garlic, and ginger, and eat raw food whenever you can. Make your own muesli (see page 356 for the recipe). Do not eat animal fats, sugars, refined wheat, red meats, and dairy foods, and cut out salt entirely. Cut down on coffee and tea, but two glasses of wine or a glass of beer each day won't hurt you. Exercise is very important—don't overdo things though. Take supplements such as vitamin A in the beta-carotene form, vitamins C and E, selenium, geranium, and the remarkable co-enzyme CoQ10.

Many of the essential oils have a profound effect on the cardiovascular system. Use them in your bath and start to have daily massages, always moving in the direction of the heart—from foot to thigh, for example. Ask a friend or your partner to massage your back—and perhaps you could return the favor (for we all need a little help from our friends). The massage should be gentle and with a rhythmic flow.

ESSENTIAL OILS FOR HYPERTENSION

Clary-sage	**Lavender**
Hyssop	**Marjoram**

Massage once a day.

The following massage formula is especially designed for the over-sixties with high blood pressure:

MASSAGE OIL

Hyssop	5 drops
Marjoram	10 drops
Geranium	15 drops

Diluted in 2 tablespoons vegetable oil

BATH SYNERGISTIC BLEND

Marjoram	15 drops
Lavender	5 drops
Geranium	10 drops

Blend together in these proportions and use 4 drops per bath

Atheroma and Arteriosclerosis ◆◆◆◆◆◆◆

These two conditions affect the arteries and are often associated. Arteriosclerosis is the better known of the two but it generally follows on from atheroma, which is the deposit of cholesterol and other fatty deposits on the lining of an artery. Arteriosclerosis refers to the thickening and hardening of arterial walls. These are dangerous conditions because they affect the efficient flow of blood: clots of blood may get stuck to the arterial walls, causing a thrombosis. Coronary thrombosis is brought about by a clot in the arteries supplying the heart, and a stroke results from a thrombosis in the arteries supplying the brain. Loss of efficiency in the blood flow may also cause all manner of serious problems from angina to kidney failure.

Ideally both these conditions should be treated by an aromatherapist, but there are things you can do to help yourself. Follow the diet outlined in the section on high blood pressure and include lecithin granules in your homemade muesli. Carry out some gentle daily exercise. Swimming is ideal, so why not take advantage of retirement and get to the swimming pool before anyone else arrives. Do some deep, yoga-style breathing each day, and—it goes without saying—stop smoking *now.*

Follow the massage and bath routine using these essential oils:

ESSENTIAL OILS FOR USE IN THE TREATMENT OF ATHEROMA AND ARTERIOSCLEROSIS

Juniper	**Ginger**
Rosemary	**Birch**
Black pepper	**Red thyme**
Lemon	

ATHEROMA AND ARTERIOSCLEROSIS MASSAGE OIL

Ginger	8 drops
Rosemary	10 drops
Lemon	10 drops
Red thyme	2 drops

Diluted in 2 tablespoons vegetable oil

ATHEROMA AND ARTERIOSCLEROSIS
BATH SYNERGISTIC BLEND

Lemon	10 drops
Black pepper	5 drops
Red thyme	5 drops

Blend together in these proportions and use 4 drops per bath

Apply the oil to your whole body once a day and also use the bath synergistic blend daily.

Loss of Memory ◆◆◆◆◆◆

Have you ever gone to dial a number but forgotten who you were supposed to be calling by the time you picked up the phone? Or walked into another room to fetch something, and forgotten what it was by the time you got there? Experiences such as these are common to us all, so don't start to panic just yet. Forgetfulness affects children, teenagers, and adults, as well as many in their maturing years. Lapses in concentration account for much of this, having too much on your mind or thinking of three things at once. Unfortunately there is no magic oil to bring back memory, but the essential oils can help concentration which, in turn, makes memory less difficult. Try using the following essential oils in equal proportions in one of the room methods—a diffuser or plant-spray would be simple and effective:

FOR CONCENTRATION

Basil	**Ginger**
Cardamom	**Black pepper**

In equal proportions

If you think of your brain as an electrical circuit that can short when switching from one circuit to another you can get an idea of what happens when the mind goes blank or gets confused. Fortifying the brain with the food it needs is very important. This is a very complex subject, as you can imagine, but certain vitamins, minerals, and micro-nutrients do seem to have a profound effect on brain function, notably vitamins C and E, selenium, and zinc. Pernicious anemia is reversed by taking vitamin B12 and iron treatments, and lack of potassium, which accounts for memory loss in some people, is easily remedied with potassium tablets. Lecithin is another important compound but taken in high doses it can cause digestive problems, so 25–30 grams of phosphatidyl choline is thought to be the better option.

Alzheimer's disease is a very disturbing disease which leads to mental deterioration in all areas so that the patient becomes unable to communicate in any way. It affects people in the prime of their lives and is therefore called "presenile dementia." One of the interesting aspects of recent research into this disease has been the discovery that tangles of nerve fibers are built around a central deposit of aluminosilicates which, as the name suggests, contain aluminum. This has led to the speculation that heavy metal poisoning may be involved in the development of the condition. It is now thought that the aluminosilicates that are a major component in aerosol sprays could be responsible for the aluminum deposits found in the brains of those with Alzheimer's disease. The aerosol sprays that we use in our daily lives may be causing untold damage, not only to the ozone layer because of the CFCs, but to human brains on account of the aluminosilicates.

However, research into Alzheimer's is still in its infancy, and therefore I would suggest it a wise precaution to avoid aluminum in any way whatsoever. This means aluminum cooking pots should be thrown out, and as aluminum salts are added by the water department to our drinking water, that should be treated with circumspection—especially since groups of Alzheimer's patients have been found to be living in areas where more than usual amounts of aluminum are added to the water supply. You might make inquiries of your local water department, but it may be simpler to start drinking bottled spring water and filtering water to be used in cooking. Although that won't solve all the problems, it will help. Aluminum already in the body can be reduced by taking vitamin C, calcium, and magnesium.

Watching the destruction of the intellect of a person close to you is a heartbreaking experience. Living with someone who has become a stranger, who cannot remember experiences you have shared or even recognize you, may seem an entirely hopeless task, but massage can help to bring back the closeness and reintroduce a method of communication when there is no other. This is not a therapeutic massage, just a means by which love can be conveyed, and so a gentle body massage or a foot or hand massage will suffice. The essential oils used in your massage oil will not only be pleasing to the Alzheimer's sufferer's senses, and your own, but may also possibly rekindle memories. Any essential oils may be used but if the sufferer is your mother and she always wore, for example, lavender perfume, lavender oil may be the perfect choice. Who is to know what the Alzheimer's sufferer, locked away inside her brain, will experience when given an olfactory memory jerk? Cast your mind back to the aromatic likes of the sufferer and try to re-create them now. Good choices are the citrus essential oils of lemon, grapefruit, and orange plus the spices such as coriander and cardamom, nutmeg, and ginger, because these also stimulate the gastric juices and touch upon the primeval sense of feeding and survival. Try to establish a communication pattern based on appetite, smell, memory, love, and trust.

In newly diagnosed and less advanced cases of Alzheimer's you can be more adventurous and utilize the gentle fragrances of flowers—lavender, rose, geranium, and neroli would be good examples, perhaps used in conjunction with the spices mentioned above or basil, rosemary, and hyssop. Make a massage oil using the essential oils and use them in a full body massage, hand or foot massage, or on the very important neck and shoulder area. Use 5 drops per 1 teaspoon of base vegetable oil in the following proportions:

Rose	5 drops
Geranium	5 drops
Basil	2 drops
Lavender	10 drops
Rosemary	2 drops

Trembling ◆◆◆◆◆◆◆◆◆◆◆◆

Trembling that is unrelated to a physical disorder such as Parkinson's disease (see below) can be helped by rubbing the body with the following oil:

Narcissus	2 drops
Nutmeg	4 drops
Lemon	2 drops

Diluted in 2 teaspoons vegetable oil

If the trembling is more pronounced in the upper body put the oil over your arm, across your chest, down the other arm, and over both hands. If the trembling tends to be in the lower portion of your body, put the oil—about the size of a quarter—in the palm of your hand and rub it over your lower back, hips, legs, and feet. You also need to get it all down your spine and about four inches on either side and to do this you may need someone to help you. If this is not possible, do what you can. Narcissus oil is expensive so if you cannot buy it in the very small quantity that you need, substitute chamomile German.

Parkinson's Disease ◆◆◆

This is a disorder of the basal ganglia group of cells in the brain which transmit conscious messages to the nerves and muscles. When the ganglia degenerate voluntary movement becomes impaired, sometimes in just some muscle groups, and in other cases, in many. Each case is unique depending on the extent of the degeneration of nerve cells. It is most characterized by the uncontrollable twitching of muscles. The muscles also stiffen, making movement difficult.

The essential oils are very helpful to Parkinson's sufferers because many of the oils work on the central nervous system and can bring great relief. Massage prevents muscles stiffening and maintains mobility. Warm, fragrant baths are often a cure for the depression that often accompanies the condition, when sensual pleasures are diminished.

If you have Parkinson's massage yourself as often as possible, as best you can. Better still, ask someone to massage you, and if you can manage to visit an aromatherapist once a month that will make all the difference.

Use the following essential oils in baths and massage oils:

ESSENTIAL OILS TO ALLEVIATE MUSCLE STIFFNESS AND WORK ON THE CENTRAL NERVOUS SYSTEM

Rosemary	**Marjoram**
Lemon	**Nutmeg**
Hop	**Lavender**
Basil	**Geranium**
Orange	**Valerian**
Bergamot	**Thyme**

PARKINSON'S BATH FORMULA

Orange	5 drops
Bergamot	5 drops
Lavender	10 drops

Blend together in these proportions and use 4–6 drops in a bath

PARKINSON'S GENERAL MASSAGE OIL

Nutmeg	5 drops
Valerian	2 drops
Geranium	5 drops
Rosemary	18 drops

Diluted in 2 tablespoons vegetable oil

PARKINSON'S MASSAGE OIL FOR MUSCLE STIFFNESS

Marjoram	10 drops
Basil	5 drops
Rosemary	10 drops
Lemon	5 drops

Diluted in 2 tablespoons vegetable oil

Arthritis ◆◆◆◆◆◆◆◆◆◆◆◆◆

This is a term which applies to several diseases of the joints, the three most common of which are rheumatoid arthritis, osteoarthritis, and gout. Pain is the common characteristic and millions of people suffer varying degrees of it. As these are degenerative diseases the pain tends to creep up slowly and it is easy to say to oneself, "It's a little bit worse today" without thinking that tomorrow it's going to be unbearable. People get used to the pain, but it is crucial to stop these conditions in their tracks.

Aromatherapy provides one of the most effective treatments for arthritis, not only in retaining the mobility of the joints but in giving pain relief and helping to ease inflammation and swellings. In all cases of arthritis, however, the first area of attack must be diet which, when changed, can in some patients completely transform their condition.

Diet

In many cases dietary changes stop arthritis in its tracks. You may be one of the lucky ones whose arthritis is the result of a food allergy, but there is only one way to find out—and that, unfortunately, means cutting out a lot of goodies. The following regime must be carried on for at least six weeks, longer if you can. Even if you do not instantly change your diet to the one below, start now writing down the date and time of your attacks and the foods you ate previously. You must be thorough about this. "Tea" should read "tea, milk, sugar" if those things apply. In some people a crippling effect can be felt just half an hour after eating the guilty food, in others it may be weeks afterwards. Obviously for this latter group of people identifying the cause will be a problem, but keep a food diary and you may see a pattern emerging.

Cut all the following from your diet: red meat, including pork; alcohol; tea, coffee; dairy products; all sugar; refined flour and products (biscuits, cakes, white bread); chocolate and drinking chocolate; fried foods, including stir-fried; peanuts; lemons, grapefruit, oranges, limes; gravy; root vegetables, including potatoes; tomatoes; and all preservatives and additives including natural ones.

You may eat lots of fish, including tinned; plenty of green vegetables; salads; pulses; nuts; seeds, such as sunflower and pumpkin; whole grain bread; chicken; grapes, apricots, and peaches. Drink filtered or bottled water, dandelion coffee, and herbal teas.

Simple meals can be made quite quickly without dipping into the freezer section at your local store. Try spinach with a poached egg on top with whole grain toast, or poached cod with herbs served with steamed broccoli and green beans. A large tuna salad mixed with all your favorite allowed ingredients is a good standby, and chicken stuffed with chestnut and whole grain bread stuffing makes a healthy alternative to roast beef, Yorkshire pudding and roast potatoes covered in lashings of gravy. If you really crave something sweet, drink a cup of hot water in which you have dissolved a teaspoon of honey.

Take 1000mg per day of vitamin C, 250mg per day of vitamin E, B-complex, and beta-carotene. Cod liver oil is also beneficial. Take at least 2 teaspoons with 5 drops of evening primrose oil or borage seed oil added; this can be taken in milk or orange juice, and should be sipped slowly. If you are allergic to cod liver oil, substitute halibut oil.

For the first two weeks, treatment is the same for all types of arthritis, including gout. This concentrates on detoxification, and takes the form of daily baths. To each bath add two handfuls of Epsom salts and one of rock salt, then add 4 drops of the following synergistic blend:

ARTHRITIS STAGE 1
BATH SYNERGISTIC BLEND

Fennel	30 drops
Cypress	16 drops
Juniper	10 drops

These quantities are enough for fourteen days.

During the two-week period of the preliminary bath treatment, toxins in the form of crystalline substances are dissolved by the body and passed out through the urine and feces. Do not follow any other treatments during this time, even those using essential oils.

After this two-week period the different forms of arthritis are treated individually.

Rheumatoid Arthritis

The causes of this condition are uncertain and there are many suspects. Often it follows a viral infection or other illness. It could be related to the glands and hormones, or possibly be due to a defect in the auto-immune system whereby the body starts to treat its own cells as invasive material. Whatever the cause, rheumatoid arthritis is extremely painful. It is caused by inflammation of the fibrous connective tissue around joints—usually the wrists and knuckles, although any joint may be affected.

It can lead to deformity and loss of mobility in the joints. It is easy to recognize by the shiny tight skin around and over the affected areas, swelling around the joints, and stiffness in the poor sufferer's hands, feet, and limbs.

Treatment is in three stages, the first of which has already been described above, which lasts for two weeks. The next two stages also take two weeks each, and throughout the total six-week period you should continue with the diet outlined previously.

RHEUMATOID ARTHRITIS
STAGE 2 ESSENTIAL OILS

Chamomile Roman	**Peppermint**
	Niaouli
Chamomile German	**Calendula**
	Tagetes
Lavender	**Eucalyptus (all)**
Yarrow	**Angelica**

As with stage one, add two handfuls of Epsom salts and one handful of rock salt to a daily bath, as well as 4 drops of the formula below:

RHEUMATOID ARTHRITIS
STAGE 2 BATH SYNERGISTIC BLEND

Lavender	10 drops
Eucalyptus peppermint	30 drops
Chamomile Roman	16 drops

These quantities are enough for fourteen baths.

Also massage morning and night over the whole of the body with the following oil:

RHEUMATOID ARTHRITIS
STAGE 2 MASSAGE OIL

Chamomile German	8 drops
Lavender	10 drops
Peppermint	2 drops
Eucalyptus	8 drops

Diluted in 2 tablespoons vegetable oil

Carry out the stage two treatment for two weeks, and then progress to stage three. These are the essential oils to use:

RHEUMATOID ARTHRITIS
STAGE 3 ESSENTIAL OILS

Ginger	**Chamomile German**
Black pepper	
Rosemary	**Chamomile Roman**
Lavender	
Eucalyptus	**Frankincense**
Tagetes	

The baths taken during the two weeks of stage three alternate daily between the formula already given in stage two (but omit the Epsom salts) and the following formula. Again, use 4 drops per bath:

RHEUMATOID ARTHRITIS
STAGE 3 BATH SYNERGISTIC BLEND

Ginger	8 drops
Rosemary	15 drops
Frankincense	5 drops

These quantities are enough for seven baths.

During stage three massage the affected joints only. Use the following oil and the stage two massage oil on alternate days:

RHEUMATOID ARTHRITIS
STAGE 3 MASSAGE OIL

Rosemary	8 drops
Lavender	7 drops
Frankincense	10 drops
Ginger	5 drops

Diluted in 2 tablespoons vegetable oil

After the six-week treatment, move on to the maintenance program that follows.

Osteoarthritis

This is a degenerative disease in which the cartilage wears away leaving exposed bone and causing the formation of rough bone deposits. It mainly affects the hips, knees, and fingers and is often the result of overuse in earlier years. It can start innocently enough with just an ache and stiffness, but it gets progressively worse as time goes on until one day a disconcerting creaking can be heard coming from the joint. It is very important to keep the affected area in action so as not to allow immobility to set in. Stage one treatment has already been outlined; that lasts two weeks, as does stage two for which these are the essential oils:

OSTEOARTHRITIS
STAGE 2 ESSENTIAL OILS

Cedarwood	**Ginger**
Sandalwood	**Lavender**
Pettigraine	**Rosemary**
Cypress	**Black pepper**
Pine	

OSTEOARTHRITIS
STAGE 2 BATH SYNERGISTIC BLEND

Pettigraine	10 drops
Ginger	30 drops
Rosemary	16 drops

Put two handfuls of Epsom salts and one handful of rock salt in the bath, then add 4 drops of the synergistic blend. These quantities are enough for fourteen baths.

As well as taking a daily bath you need to apply the following formula to the affected areas twice a day:

OSTEOARTHRITIS
STAGE 2 MASSAGE OIL

Ginger	13 drops
Black pepper	8 drops
Cedarwood	4 drops
Cypress	5 drops

Diluted in 2 tablespoons vegetable oil

Stage three of the treatment also lasts two weeks, and these are the essential oils:

OSTEOARTHRITIS
STAGE 3 ESSENTIAL OILS

Lavender	**Ginger**
Black pepper	**Nutmeg**
Rosemary	**Marjoram**
Sandalwood	**Cypress**
Pettigraine	**Pine**
Birch	

The baths taken during stage three should alternate daily between the formula already given for stage one and the formula below. Again, use 4 drops per bath:

OSTEOARTHRITIS
STAGE 3 BATH SYNERGISTIC BLEND

Black pepper	5 drops
Rosemary	15 drops
Marjoram	8 drops

These quantities are enough for seven baths.

During stage three massage only the affected joints. Alternate daily between the massage formula in stage two and the one that follows:

OSTEOARTHRITIS
STAGE 3 MASSAGE OIL

Sandalwood	15 drops
Ginger	5 drops
Nutmeg	10 drops

Diluted in 2 tablespoons vegetable oil

After this six-week treatment, move on to the maintenance program below.

If your arthritis developed during or after menopause add geranium and rose essential oils to your treatment. If your arthritis, of whatever form, gets worse during periods of stress add to your blend those oils which are helpful in combating stress—you will find relevant lists in several sections of this book.

Maintenance Program

The treatments above for rheumatoid and osteoarthritis may be repeated when needed. In the interim periods massage as needed with one or a combination of the oils below. Also use them in the bath—4 drops per bath.

ARTHRITIS MAINTENANCE OILS

Rosemary	**Eucalyptus blue mallee**
Chamomile Roman	**Ginger**
Chamomile German	**Marjoram**
Eucalyptus peppermint	**Thyme linalol**
	R1*
	Lavender

*Works extremely well in osteoarthritis and rheumatoid arthritis and may be used in any rheumatic condition.

Other Similar Disorders

If you are suffering from ankylosis or spondylosis follow the treatment as for osteoarthritis; if you suffer from lupus erythematosus follow the rheumatoid arthritis treatment.

Gout

Although it has for centuries been something of a joke, gout is actually a very serious and painful condition. The problem is caused by an overproduction of uric acid which causes the precipitation of crystals and these gather around joints, often at the base of the big toe or in the fingers. Hereditary biochemical problems are much more likely to be the cause than guzzling port and cheese.

The pain of gout can be unbearable and is often accompanied by a burning sensation and swelling. It is dangerous largely because the crystals can damage the kidneys, but their effects may be experienced all over the body, from the ears to the knees and, of course, the feet.

Follow the diet outlined for all arthritic conditions and take the baths and massage treatment outlined for rheumatoid arthritis. In addition to the essential oils recommended in that section, you can use the following in stages two and three:

ADDITIONAL ESSENTIAL OILS
FOR THE TREATMENT OF GOUT

Basil	**Pine**
Birch	**Thyme**

Dyspepsia (Indigestion) ♦♦♦♦♦♦♦♦♦

Indigestion is painful, and it can be crippling. It is brought on by a variety of things including worry, stress, rushing food and not chewing, or lack of muscle tone in the stomach walls. Persistent indigestion should be seen by your doctor.

If you eat slowly and chew thoroughly, to the point of boredom, this in itself is often all that is needed to cure indigestion and the flatulence that often accompanies it. And as these are your leisurely years, why not make eating a slow pleasure instead of the rushed event of your previously rushed years. Also make sure that dentures are fitted properly because if they are not you might be swallowing large pieces of food along with large gulps of air. Massage your upper abdomen area between meals with the following oils or blends, chosen from whichever category is most appropriate and using 30 drops per 2 tablespoons of base vegetable oil. Or try the tea remedy.

GENERAL

Aniseed	**Coriander** (15 drops)
Peppermint	**Ginger** (15 drops)
Cardamom	
Dill	
Fennel	

Tea: 1 drop peppermint diluted in 1 teaspoon honey, and dissolved in a cup of warm water

A TONIC (WEAK MUSCLE TONE)

Lavender	**Rosemary** (15 drops)
Cypress	**Cardamom** (15 drops
Fennel	
Peppermint	
Coriander	

Tea: 1 drop peppermint diluted in 1 teaspoon honey, and dissolved in a cup of warm water

NERVOUS

Ginger	**Spearmint** (15 drops)
Aniseed	**Lavender** (15 drops)
Vetiver	
Dill	
Peppermint	

Tea: 1 drop spearmint diluted in 1 teaspoon honey, and dissolved in a cup of warm water

Gastric Flatulence ◆◆◆◆

Flatulence can be organic, associated with a disease—the most usual cause is gallstones or a disease of the gallbladder—or functional, with no disease present. Food allergies can also result in flatulence, often with a strong odor, and the simple remedy is to cut out those foods which cause the problem. But functional flatulence is by far the most usual and is most commonly caused by swallowing air with each mouthful of food or unknowingly taking in air during the day—both of which can easily become a habit. Also, intestinal fermentation of the starches in carbohydrate foods leads to swelling as gases are formed. However the excess air or gas gets there, the result is that the abdomen swells as the intestines distend and discomfort is felt in the stomach. Sometimes the pressure is so great that the swelling extends under the ribcage causing palpitations and shortness of breath and even, in some cases, a pain similar to angina pectoris.

The cure for functional flatulence is simply to change eating habits and be aware of swallowing air. Don't attempt to belch as this only results in taking in yet more air. Cut down on cellulose and starchy foods such as potatoes, wheat, peas, pulses, onions, and carrots. After your meal sip a glass of hot water containing a pinch of bicarbonate of soda and 1 drop of either peppermint or spearmint essential oil. This works for the intestinal tract as well as for the stomach.

ESSENTIAL OILS
TO TREAT GASTRIC FLATULENCE

Coriander	**Spearmint**
Dill	**Cardamom**
Eucalyptus peppermint	**Peppermint**

If you are experiencing pain, make up a small amount of massage oil and rub over the whole of the abdomen in a clockwise direction

Cardamom	2 drops
Peppermint	3 drops

Diluted in 1 teaspoon vegetable oil

Constipation ♦♦♦♦♦♦♦♦♦

One of the causes of constipation is a weakness in the anus area and it can reach a stage where the feces becomes impacted and needs to be removed by a doctor. Feces left in the rectum become dried and hardened and as time passes they become more difficult to pass. This often causes spurious diarrhea, a watery discharge caused by irritation of the rectum.

Dietary changes may be needed and bulking agents such as fiber added to meals. A tiny sliver of soap inserted into the rectum often helps, as do glycerine suppositories. Plenty of water is recommended, and dried, stewed fruit.

Massaging around the lower abdomen following the intestinal tract often shifts impacted feces. Before massaging, however, drink a cup of hot water to which is added 2 teaspoons of honey in which you have mixed 1 drop of ginger and 1 drop of fennel essential oil. Sip the drink slowly, then wait for ten minutes before massaging with the following oils. Massage in a clockwise direction over the stomach as deeply as you can without causing discomfort, then over the hips and lower back, and down the spine to just above the anus. Do this three times a day.

ESSENTIAL OILS

Patchouli	**Fennel**
Rosemary	**Ginger**
Sandalwood	**Cardamom**
Black pepper	

FORMULA

Patchouli	15 drops
Black pepper	5 drops
Cardamom	5 drops

Diluted in 2 tablespoons vegetable oil

Hemorrhoids (Piles) ♦♦♦

Piles are often the result of straining with constipation. Eating live yogurt is helpful as the bacterium it contains promotes the healthy flora in the intestinal tract. Also bathe the area with a warm washcloth onto which you have put 2 drops of the following synergistic blend of oils. Apply the washcloth to the anal area for a few minutes and repeat three or four times, twice a day.

PILES APPLICATION
SYNERGISTIC BLEND

Patchouli	2 drops
Myrrh	10 drops
Cypress	5 drops

Use 2 drops per application

Bunions ♦♦♦♦♦♦♦♦♦♦♦♦♦♦

Bunions are a deformity of the first joint of the big toe and usually affect both feet. The joint is continually irritated by any pressure, including the wearing of shoes. The difficulties presented by bunions include finding a pair of shoes that will fit. Treatments are usually surgical but these may cause further trouble. A special bunion clinic has been established in London by Dr. Khan, who claims to be able to cure this painful condition with various natural products including marigold essences. Not surprisingly, it is called The Marigold Clinic.

Aromatherapy uses a type of marigold known as tagetes and although no claim is made to correct the joint, it does ease the swelling and pain felt in the area. The treatment is in two parts. These are the essential oils to use:

BUNION ESSENTIAL OILS

Tagetes	**Carrot**
Chamomile German	**Calendula**

BUNION OIL

Tagetes	1 teaspoon
Jojoba oil	1 teaspoon

Blend together well

Make up the bunion oil above and apply 3 drops to the foot, paying particular attention to the bunion itself and the ball of the foot. Then apply some of the foot massage oil below to the whole of the foot and toes, using gentle massaging movements over the whole area. Do this whole procedure twice a day.

FOOT MASSAGE OIL

Tagetes	10 drops
Carrot	5 drops
Chamomile German	15 drops

Diluted in 2 tablespoons vegetable oil

Corns and Calluses ◆◆◆

Corns are treatable with tagetes or calendula essential oils. As calendula is very expensive, why not make your own? All you need is some common marigolds, as many heads as possible, which you put into a dark glass jar which you have almost filled with almond or safflower oil. Leave the jar in the sun for at least forty-eight hours and then strain the contents through a paper coffee filter, squeezing out as much of the previous oil from the flower heads as you can. Repeat the whole procedure, using the same oil, up to seven times if possible. If you can't get the marigolds to make this oil, add 10 drops of calendula to 2 tablespoons vegetable oil, or 30 drops of tagetes to 2 tablespoons, and use that instead.

Rub the oil gently over corns and skin three times a day. This is excellent for general care of the feet, for example, after corns and calluses have been removed. Alternatively, use the following for a single treatment:

Tagetes	5 drops
Carrot	5 drops

Blend together well

It will take a few days to soften corns. Bathe the feet daily in a bowl of water which contains two handfuls of salt and two teaspoons of cider vinegar. Dry the skin and then rub either of the oils above into the hard skin and the corns. How much you use will depend on the area to be covered. Repeat this every day until the corn shows signs of softening, usually after three to four days, and rub the dead skin away with a pumice stone or metal nail file. Afterwards continue to use the oils on the area.

Nails and Nail Beds ◆◆◆

Nails and nail beds often become diseased and thickened in the maturing years and are prone to fungal infections. If a fungal infection is present use tea tree essential oil neat on the area. If a fungus is not apparently the cause of the problem, massage the following oil around the nail and nail bed:

Tea tree	5 drops
Tagetes	5 drops

Diluted in 2 teaspoons vegetable oil

♦ CHAPTER 13 ♦
FRAGRANT CARE FOR YOUR HOME

THE FIRST THING to greet your guests as they enter your home is the aroma, and the impression it creates may be more enduring than that made by the fixtures and fittings. This unique aroma fingerprint says a great deal about all who live in the house—whether there are smokers and pets, what kind of food is cooked there, and so forth. Estate agents are becoming increasingly aware of the importance of aroma and some advise their clients to create a homey atmosphere when prospective purchasers are due by baking bread, putting fresh coffee on to brew, or lighting the wood fire. If you are trying to sell your house, you might like to note that a few drops of clary-sage or lemon essential oil will make viewers feel at ease and often they will say, "The house just has a lovely relaxed atmosphere, we don't know why." But you do!

But every day is special to you and your family, and the essential oils provide the most natural way to give your home a delightful aroma. You have an infinite choice and can blend unique aromas that set your own aroma style for your home. Essential oils, however, have more to offer than their fragrances. You can choose oils which are antibacterial or antiviral when illness is around, that can lift the atmosphere when depression overhangs the house or you can tailor-make the aroma to suit the season of the year or a particular celebration. By the time you have read this chapter, you will have discovered a hundred new ways to enhance your home. Essential oils are so useful, beneficial, enjoyable, and versatile that you will wonder what you ever did before you came to know about them. Your only problem will be in deciding whether to keep them in the first-aid box, the garden shed, the kitchen, utility room, bathroom, or bedroom!

Air Fresheners ◆◆◆◆◆◆◆◆

You need never worry again about what the chlorofluorocarbons in your commercial aerosol of air freshener are doing to the earth's ozone layer, or what the chemicals it contains are doing to your family's health. Essential oils provide a far better option all around and I'm sure you will agree once you use them. You can use them in any of the room methods (see page 13), including the plant-spray method: use about 8 drops to 2½ cups water and spray as finely as possible into the air and towards curtains and carpets. Velvet, silk, and some wood should be avoided, as water stains could occur. By sheer force of gravity carpets will receive the aroma molecules, but those with pets may want to pay this area special attention. There is usually one room in the house that gets the brunt of breakfast's burned toast and it would be a nice idea to keep a sprayer permanently there so that you have an alternative to opening the windows every time there is an aroma leak from the kitchen.

Several types of rings are sold for using essential oils on light bulbs and you can also put the oil directly onto the bulb in a standing lamp—but do be careful not to use too much as the oils are inflammable. Use 1 drop maximum per bulb. Once the oil is in place, the bulb can be turned on when required to release the aroma molecules into the atmosphere by its heat.

The inflammable nature of essential oils means that you can turn a log fire into an aromatic event. Use cypress, pine, sandalwood, or cedarwood and simply put one drop onto each log before placing it on the fire. This can be done in advance so that your friends will think your wood is specially imported from the sandalwood forests of Mysore, India!

Diffusers are an extremely easy and effective way of giving an aroma to a room. Make sure you wipe them clean before applying each new oil or formula. A bowl of boiling water with a few drops of oil floating on top will leave a lingering scent all over the room if placed centrally. Remove it when the heat has gone, and be careful to put it out of the reach of children and animals if they are about. A cotton-wool ball or tissue with 4 drops of essential oil can be tucked behind a radiator in winter, or put as many drops as you like in a humidifier. You don't want the effect to be too overpowering, so prepare your room method with the door closed, then leave the room and reenter a couple of minutes later so you can get a true idea of the aroma level in the room. See "Methods of Use," page 11, for further information.

Hallways ◆◆◆◆◆◆◆◆◆◆◆◆◆

Because all the doors of a house or flat open onto the hallway, this is where the aromas from every room mingle to form the aroma fingerprint that is unique to your home. Since hallways often have no windows, the aromas linger and permeate the place—the stale air wafts up the stairs and landings, which may also be windowless, and hangs there like an aroma smog. And yet hallways are often neglected: we might put a potpourri in the living room, but do we think of placing one in the hall? It is this neglected area of the home that greets our guests and, let's not forget, the family as they wend their weary way home from the polluted outside world.

Hallways need something pleasant and fresh, rather than the spice and herb aromas of the kitchen or the more heavily scented oils we might use elsewhere. The citrus oils of lemon, lime, bergamot, and grapefruit are particular favorites for the hall. Good mixers with these are geranium and lavender; lavender is better in the morning, giving an uplifting aspect, while geranium is preferable in the afternoon when things are calming down after the rush of the day. Geranium is an excellent choice too when guests are due because it makes them feel good before they even sit down. If someone in the house has a cold or flu, add 2 or 3 drops of either rosemary or niaouli to the citrus base. Using a total of 8 drops of essential oil in 2½ cups of water in a plant-spray will keep the hallway smelling fresh for several hours. Spraying the carpet in the hall and stairs will also help freshen up the whole area.

Hallways take a lot of traffic and are very prone to gathering dust and scuff marks. Washing down paintwork is a job made more enticing by the uplifting aromas of the essential oils—and the knowledge that they are performing antiseptic, disinfectant, and other useful roles. For this put a few drops of essential oils in the water or one drop on your cloth. You can even aroma-coordinate your choice of oil with what you use in the air freshener spray.

Try to coordinate your choice of oils, not only with the time of the day and occasion, but also the season of the year. In summer use a light, refreshing essential oil or mix, and in the winter use one that warms. For example:

SPRING/SUMMER

Lime	**Pettigraine**
Lemon	**Lavender**
Geranium	

AUTUMN/WINTER

Orange	**Frankincense**
Nutmeg	**Cypress**
Benzoin	

The following synergistic blends provide lovely evocative fragrances:

SPRING/SUMMER
SYNERGISTIC BLEND

Lemon	10 drops
Geranium	4 drops
Pettigraine	3 drops
Sandalwood	2 drops

AUTUMN/WINTER
SYNERGISTIC BLEND

Orange	8 drops
Frankincense	3 drops
Benzoin	3 drops
Geranium	4 drops

Bacteria Busters ◆◆◆◆◆◆◆

The majority of essential oils are antiseptics and bactericides, which means they inhibit the growth of bacteria, clearly a major concern in the home. In whichever method you use them, they not only make your environment smell delightful but make it safe as well. The essential oils listed below have other properties, too—some are antifungal and antiviral. The following have been chosen for their price as well as their power:

BACTERIA BUSTERS

Cinnamon	**Pine**
Clove	**Niaouli**
Lemon	**Thyme**
Eucalyptus	**Grapefruit**
Lavender	**Lime**

Although most essential oils have a therapeutic life of about two years (as a perfume they will last forever and a day), the disinfectant qualities of eucalyptus oil actually improve with its age. If you have some that are too old to incorporate in body or skin care, keep them by the sink in the kitchen or bathroom and use 2 drops on a cloth to wipe the surface down, then squeeze it out and let the water run down the pipe to kill the bacteria lurking here.

The Kitchen ◆◆◆◆◆◆◆◆◆◆

The kitchen produces many smells, from fresh baked bread to malodorous boiled cabbage. We all have a rubbish area and perhaps too this is where the wet coats and overalls get hung up and where the muddy boots are left to dry. The cat litter tray or dog's bed is often located in the kitchen, although this really isn't a good idea. There are innumerable sources of aroma in the kitchen and yet kitchens are often badly ventilated, so that not enough air circulates to clear away the bad or unpleasant aroma molecules.

Essential oils are about cleansing the air, rather than merely masking bad smells. Another huge advantage is that when used correctly they are harmless, so while it is best, from the point of view of taste, to avoid spraying food, no harm will come to it if you do—or to the baby if he happens to be sitting in the high chair. Indeed many oils are used as preservatives and thyme, for example, will prevent fungi molds. You could even take a tip from the French butchers who spray their shops with essential oils so that they will prevent meat putrefaction—not, as you may have thought, to cover up the smell of rotting meat.

As well as water from the cooking steam, there are tiny molecules of fat in the atmosphere which are released in roasting, frying, and grilling. What we need here are essential oils that are capable of wrapping themselves around the fat molecules, deodorizing them, and leaving the kitchen as fresh and appetizing as the food you prepare there. The following oils make an excellent air spray used on their own or in combinations, to your taste:

KITCHEN AIR SPRAY ESSENTIAL OILS

Rosemary	**Lavender**
Lemon	**Lime**
Eucalyptus	

When washing out the fridge, freezer, or oven, add 1 drop of lemon or of the fruit essential oils—lime, grapefruit, bergamot, mandarin, or orange—to the final rinse water. This will deodorize without permeating the fridge or whatever with an aroma, whereas the herb oils are too powerful to use in this way.

For washing down surfaces use one of the following, 1 drop directly on the cloth or 7 drops in the rinse water. Use this when wiping down work surfaces, cupboards, sinks, tiles, or paintwork:

FOR WASHING KITCHEN SURFACES

Eucalyptus	**Pine**
Lavender	**Cypress**
Lemon	**Lemongrass**
Lime	**Thyme**
Grapefruit	**Palma rosa**

Bergamot is just one of the other oils that could be added to the above list, and, as proved by Professor Rovesti in experiments in Milan, it has antidepressant properties too—which brings us to washing the floor! Use any of the above, approximately 4 drops to each pint of water in the final rinse.

Here is a synergistic blend which I always have made up and ready to use. It is extremely effective, being disinfectant and antibacterial, and leaves a delightful fragrance. Use it for all kitchen surfaces, including the floor, and also in a spray around the kitchen: 8 drops in 2½ cups of water. Keep the blend in a clean, brown glass bottle and store away from light and heat.

THE CLEAN KITCHEN
SYNERGISTIC BLEND

Lavender	8 drops
Lemon	10 drops
Eucalyptus	5 drops
Bois de rose	8 drops
Palma rosa	3 drops

Mix together in these proportions

Aroma preferences vary not only from person to person but from country to country and time to time. In Venezuela commercial floor cleaning products contain ten times the amount of pine fragrance that a similar product would contain in the United States. In the West, the aroma of pine is being replaced by the lemon and floral fragrances. All too often, however, we think of a chemical smell as one that must be good for us and dismiss an aroma as charming as an essential oil as being ineffective. If you have any doubt about the effectiveness of essential oils, relax. There is a mass of literature to prove it, and some commercial products have natural essences as their effective ingredient although they may cover up their smell with a repellent chemical one so we will think it's good for the job and buy it.

Dish towels used to be boiled—and not only to keep them white. Since modern washing machines rarely reach boiling point, one needs to kill the many microbes that accumulate on dish towels by another method. Simply soak them in a bowl of boiling water to which you have added 1 drop of eucalyptus, thyme, tea tree, or lavender. Leave them to soak for a while before washing in the machine as usual.

You can also use essential oils in the dishwasher. Before putting the detergent into its compartment add 2 drops of lemon oil to the measuring spoon and stir it in.

Most dishwashers, however, are human, and most of those have to wash piles of dishes, day in and day out. So remorseless are most domestic tasks that many women (for it *is* mostly women) enter their kitchens with a feeling of deep dread—"Here we go again." The sheer boredom associated with these repetitive jobs is made worse by the isolation; we are standing in the kitchen once more, dishwashing, ironing, cleaning, washing clothes, putting the shopping away, or preparing food while the rest of the family can be heard laughing at the television in the other room.

These days vast amounts of synthetic lemon are added to our dishwashing liquids, but why not use the real thing? With the natural aroma of essential oils you get not only the fresh smell and the cleanliness connection we have learned from the advertisers but the emotional effect as well—in the case of lemon, the zing. How about lime or grapefruit for a sparkling morning, lavender to give you a gentle lift at midday, geranium for a soothing afternoon and, for real indulgence, rose or jasmine dishwashing liquid last thing at night. It might even make your partner keener to do his bit at the sink! Simply add 10 drops of your chosen essential oil to the bottle of dishwashing liquid, shake well, and allow to settle. If you find the whole business of dishwashing depressing, the obvious choice for you is bergamot which has antidepressant properties. As I'm not crazy about dishwashing myself, my own formula contains some of this lovely oil:

SPECIAL FORMULA
DISHWASHING LIQUID

Lime	5 drops
Bergamot	3 drops
Lavender	2 drops
Orange	1 drop

Add to a bottle of 3 ounces of liquid and shake

Most essential oils lose their medicinal and beautifying therapeutic properties after about two years but save them to put, 2 drops at a time, down the drain. This will ensure a nice fragrance when the hot water runs down. Also use them in the water to wash windows and trash cans, both inside and out.

For all these chores, the essential oils make working in the kitchen a safer and altogether more pleasant experience.

The Utility Room ♦♦♦♦

There's nothing new about giving the laundry the aromatic treatment. Our Elizabethan ancestors dried their clothes and bed linen on rosemary or lavender bushes to infuse them with the smell and scented the washing water with orris root. We have many more possibilities, because although most of us haven't seen a rosemary bush big enough to hang our double sheets over, we do have a multitude of essential oils which can be used in the wash, the dryer, or drawers and wardrobe where we keep our clothes. And it is not just about making clothes smell sweet, as we shall discover.

If you have a washing machine put 3–5 drops of your chosen essential oil into the softener compartment. If hand-washing, put 2 drops in the final rinse water and swish it around. Avoid the resinous oils, and some of the heavier oils such as rose which tend to cling to the clothes in the wash but are fine to use when drying or storing clothes.

To add delicious fragrance to your wash try lemongrass or lavender. If you prefer a more exotic perfume, try ylang-ylang or neroli. If winter colds or flu have struck the household, put eucalyptus, rosemary, or pine in the wash. These oils are especially beneficial on bed linen to relieve coughs and catarrh throughout the night. If whooping cough is in the house, use hyssop and peppermint. If insomnia is the problem, marjoram, chamomile, or orange blossom will help to aid sleep if used when rinsing the bed linen or nightwear.

To infuse clothes with an essential oil when putting them through the tumble dryer, simply add 2 drops onto a piece of material no larger than 4 inches square and pop it in with the clothes. Here are some oils you might like to try:

FRESH

Lavender	**Bergamot**
Rosemary	**Pettigraine**

FLORAL

Geranium	**Neroli**
Palma rosa	**Bois de rose**

ROMANTIC

Ylang-ylang	**Jasmine**
Rose	**Vervaine**

You may also like to utilize the essential oils when ironing. You can either put 1 drop of essential oil in a plant mister and spray the clothes before ironing, or put a drop on a damp linen cloth and place that between the iron and the material. You could also put the essential oils directly into the water compartment of your steam iron, but essential oils are not water soluble and could leave a residue in the iron.

Essential oils can be left to infuse the clothes while they are in the drawer or closet. Put a drop on little pieces of natural material or cotton-wool balls and place them between the clothes. Here is a lovely synergistic blend:

CLOTHES SWEETENER

Bois de rose	4 drops
Geranium	2 drops
Lemon	3 drops

Mix in these proportions

To keep moths away from your clothes use 2–3 drops of one of the following oils. These are particularly useful when coats and woolens are stored away during the summer months:

MOTH REPELLENTS

Lavender	**Rosemary**
Lemongrass	**Citronella**
Camphor	

Small cotton-wool balls with essential oils on them can also be put between the clothes in drawers. Drawer liners made with the essential oils are much nicer than their chemical aroma counterparts and very simple to make. Cut paper to the size of the drawer—blotting paper or other absorbent types of paper are best—and dot with the essential oils. Then brush over the orris root powder, which acts as a fixative, shake off and place in the bottom of the drawer. Which oils you use, and how much, is entirely up to you and rather depends on the size and contents of the drawer. Rose in the ladies' underwear drawer would be appropriate, for example, and a relaxing, calming oil like chamomile for the children's nightwear drawer, and a stimulating one such as grapefruit or basil for the school clothes drawer. When colds are around, get your family to use handkerchiefs that have been left in a drawer with an antibacterial or disinfectant oil.

Shoes are often kept in the utility room. To freshen them up inside, put 2 teaspoons of bicarbonate of soda into an egg cup and add 2 drops of lemon, lavender, or rosemary. Mix this as well as you can, sprinkle it into the shoes and leave overnight. Tap it out in the morning and your shoes will be as fresh as new.

Sneakers can get pretty pungent even if you don't have a foot odor problem. Follow the method above but use 2 drops of the following synergistic blend of oils to each teaspoon of bicarbonate of soda. By morning, they won't seem the same wild things you left there:

SNEAKER TAMER
SYNERGISTIC BLEND

Sage	2 drops
Rosemary	5 drops
Lavender	3 drops

Mix in these proportions

The Living Room ◆◆◆◆◆

Most living rooms get pampered with an assortment of perfumed products from furniture polish to air fresheners, dusting powders for the carpets to upholstery cleaners. These products aren't aroma coordinated and, more important, they all contain chemicals. They are not the best option because all their functions can be taken over by natural products which have been enhanced with essential oils.

In years gone by people put aromatic grasses under their rugs and mats so the aroma would be released to freshen the room as they walked on them. Today most of us have wall-to-wall carpeting and we need something else. A carpet freshener powder, which can be used in exactly the same way as the commercial products, can be made by using essential oils in conjunction with talc*, kaolin, bicarbonate of soda, or borax powder. For each tablespoon of one of these base powders, you will need 1 drop of your chosen essential oil—use one of the less expensive ones. Simply add the essential oil to the powder in a blender and mix it in well. How much you make depends entirely upon your requirements. Once made, store in a sealed jar or sealable plastic bag. Leave it overnight in a drawer or closet for one night before using

* This should be plain, unperfumed talcum powder available from good pharmacies.

for the first time. Then sprinkle it on your carpet, leave for a few minutes, and vacuum it up.

To stop the odor that builds up from the dust and dirt in the vacuum cleaner, you can put a teaspoon of the carpet cleaning powder in the bag, which will fragrance the air as it is sucked through the machine. A more effective method, however, is to add 6–8 drops of essential oil on a cotton-wool ball and pop it in the bag. Replace it with a new fragrance, if you wish, each time you change the bag, or empty it out—whichever is applicable to your machine. An even simpler method is to place the drops of essential oil directly onto the bag, just by the air outlet, but this isn't a good option for nonreplaceable bags because you may wish to change the aroma later. Try the essential oils of lemon, orange, lavender, or pine to eradicate that dustiness which so often makes vacuuming the sort of job that you feel you want to take a bath after!

It is difficult to get windows absolutely perfectly sparkling—there always seem to be a few streaky marks left after you have finished. To get rid of these, screw up a sheet of newspaper, put a drop of lime, grapefruit, or lemon essential oil on it and polish the windows again. The essential oil soaks into the newspaper and combines with the print to give a sparkling finish which also releases a fresh and subtle fragrance when the sun shines on the glass.

The so-called "old-fashioned" furniture polishes you can buy today are usually made with synthetic lavender fragrance and all manner of chemicals. The only old-fashioned thing about them is the packaging. Beeswax polish is the best, which is why French polishers and antique restorers insist upon it. It is really quite easy to make, and certainly well worth the trouble. These are the ingredients:

"THE REAL THING" FURNITURE POLISH

8 ounces beeswax
2½ cups turpentine
2½ cups water
2 ounces pure soap flakes (or grated pure soap)
10 drops or more of essential oil

The beeswax should be plain and unrefined, not the white refined type. You can get this direct from beekeepers, or from hardware or health food stores. Using the bain-marie method, melt the beeswax, take it off the heat and add the turpentine. This shouldn't be too cold so don't bring it in from the freezing garden shed just when you want to use it; make sure the bottle has been standing at room temperature for a while. Put this mixture to the side. In another pot boil the water and melt the soap in it. Leave this until it is cool but still retains some of its warmth and then add it very slowly to the pot with the beeswax and turpentine mixture. This should be done with great patience, trickle by trickle, stirring all the time. Now add the essential oil of your choice. After blending all the ingredients together well, pack the polish in old, flat tins or small ice cream cartons—the type with their own lids. Use as ordinary polish—you only need a small amount at a time, and the smell and shine will reward your efforts. (A little white spirit will remove marks from some woods, including pine, before polishing.)

The fruit of the lemon has long been used to polish copper, and essential oil of lemon works equally well. Simply put 1 drop on a soft cloth and buff the copper for a clean, gleaming polish.

The living room is the place to prove to yourself that you can do without all those commercial sprays. Use a plant mister spray with water and essential oils to freshen up furniture, curtains, and carpets. As this is where your family and friends spend most of their time, you will want to choose a nice relaxing essential oil or formula. Use the spray, diffuser, light bulb, radiator, or humidifier method or add the oils to your potpourri (don't buy synthetic potpourri revivers). Make your own blend of oils or use this tried and tested formula:

THE RELAXING LIVING ROOM SYNERGISTIC BLEND

Geranium	8 drops
Clary-sage	3 drops
Lemon	5 drops
Bergamot	3 drops

Mix in these proportions

And if you want something to rouse your family out of their Sunday afternoon lethargy, try this:

THE STIMULATING LIVING ROOM SYNERGISTIC BLEND

Grapefruit	8 drops
Lavender	4 drops
Lime	4 drops
Basil	2 drops

Mix in these proportions

The Bedroom ♦♦♦♦♦♦♦♦

The bedroom is the place to sleep or play—that's up to you. When aroma and romantics come together we have "aromantics," which is such a big subject that another book has been devoted to it. If romance is on your mind, ylang-ylang, rose, jasmine, palma rosa, and clary-sage are all very appropriate.

To keep your bedroom smelling romantic at all times make up a special mix to use separately from the general house formula. Spray it in the air and on the carpets.

THE ROMANTIC BEDROOM SYNERGISTIC BLEND

Palma rosa	8 drops
Ylang-ylang	1 drop
Clary-sage	2 drops
Nutmeg	2 drops
Lime	4 drops

Mix in these proportions

For general bedroom use, ideal scents are chamomile, geranium, lavender, or lemon. A diffuser will help you to sleep if you place a drop of one of the relaxing oils such as chamomile or clary-sage on it. Bed linen can be washed, dried, or stored with essential oils—see page 306. And palma rosa works just as well as lemon on your windows—see page 308.

Wardrobes can benefit from fragrance too—place cotton-wool balls in the corners with a favorite smell on it, or one to keep the moths away—see page 307. In the same section you will find how to make drawer liners and these can also be put at the bottom of the wardrobe. You don't want the aroma of the essential oils to permeate the clothes hanging in the wardrobe as this will interfere with the effect of your various perfumes, so aim for a subtle aroma just to keep the air fresh.

The Bathroom ♦♦♦♦♦♦♦

As with the kitchen, the main concern in bathrooms is to clear bacteria and viruses, especially if the toilet is in the bathroom. Use a "Bacteria Buster" in the final rinse water when you wash all the surfaces in a bathroom, including the bath, sink, and toilet—not only to kill germs but to give the whole place a nice fragrance. Use one of these essential oils, or one of the synergistic blends that follow, in the air spray and window cleaning methods. Electric diffusers should not be used in the bathroom but you can buy metallic rings which are fixed to downward hanging light bulbs and these can be kept stocked with the essential oils so that there is a permanent source of antibacterial aroma. Another method which is particularly appropriate for toilets that are separate from the bathroom and therefore probably without surfaces to hold receptacles for releasing the aroma molecules involves the toilet paper itself. Put a couple of drops of the concentrated blends below on the cardboard ring inside the toilet paper roll before placing it in the holder. The cardboard soaks up the essential oil and gently releases the cleansing aroma molecules, keeping the whole area clean and fragrant. Here then are two excellent disinfectant and antibacterial synergistic blends for use throughout the bathroom:

BATHROOM SYNERGISTIC BLEND 1

Bergamot	5 drops
Lavender	10 drops
Cinnamon	5 drops
Lemon	10 drops
Citronella	10 drops

BATHROOM SYNERGISTIC BLEND 2

Oregano	5 drops
Sage	10 drops
Thyme	10 drops
Lemon	20 drops

Mix in these proportions

Since electric diffusers can't be used in the bathroom that gives you an excuse to get a candle heated one, and there's nothing nicer than relaxing in a warm bath with candlelight gently flickering and the aroma you have chosen wafting through the air.

Making Your Mark in a New Home ◆◆◆◆◆◆◆

Moving into a new home is always an exhausting business. What looked to be in good shape when viewed with all the furniture in place, suddenly looks very grubby with marks where pictures hung and dust piled up in corners that were hidden by sofas and wardrobes. Not to mention the same in the house you are leaving. One is always faced with an enormous cleaning task and more often than not, with a huge decorating one.

Standing in the empty shell of a house we may also become aware for the first time of its atmosphere. A part of what constitutes "atmosphere" is the aroma of a place. Each inhabitant puts his or her aroma imprint on a building and in older houses we may be subconsciously picking up the aromatic habits of many generations. One company which specializes in industrial humidifiers and dehumidifiers was asked to dehumidify a centuries-old church that had been badly water damaged from a leaking roof. After their equipment had been in place for a few days a powerful aroma of incense began to pervade the church. The vicar was most surprised because it was an incense that hadn't been used for centuries. Like a sponge, the building had soaked up the aroma over the years and was now releasing it under the effect of the special dehumidifying equipment. It is not so easy for most of us to release the aromatic imprint from a house we have just acquired, but we can put our own imprint down on top of the rest, and with such force that it will overlay all those that have gone before. When you move in to a new house, even before you put the furniture in place, go around with a water spray containing your favorite essential oils and change the odorous pattern to your own. Do this for several consecutive days until the place begins to feel like your own space.

A great deal of controversy accompanies the idea that buildings act as a sort of recorder of the conversations and events that have taken place in them. If the thought patterns and actions of the inhabitants were on a positive vibration, so the theory goes, this positivity will be embedded in the very walls. On the other hand, if bad thoughts, actions, and vibrations inhabited the place they too will be stuck in the bricks and mortar and will be contributing to the bad atmosphere. It's going to take someone a long time to prove or disprove this theory and while we're waiting why not err on the side of caution and take the idea seriously. All you have to do is fill the house with wonderful vibrations (a little frankincense helps too!), so put on whatever music you think has "good vibrations." Have a housewarming party and invite all your friends, especially those who laugh at the top of their voices. Let the walls shake with the knowledge that you have arrived!

Papers and Inks ♦♦♦♦♦♦♦

Most people's mail consists of brown envelopes full of bills and junk mail which just clutters up the house. How refreshing then to receive a party invitation or a letter packed with gossip from a friend—and how much more uplifting it would be if the letter released charming aroma molecules when opened up. It's almost guaranteed to turn a gloomy Monday morning into a special, lovely day.

Making perfumed paper is extremely easy with the essential oils. To infuse a whole box of paper and envelopes, cut into small pieces a paper tissue, a cotton handkerchief, blotting paper, or gauze—you only need half a dozen or so pieces about an inch square—put a drop of essential oil on each piece, and place them in different places between the sheets of paper or envelopes. Seal the box tightly, or if you don't have a box put them in a plastic bag and seal, and leave for at least twenty-four hours.

Which essential oil or blend of oils you use is entirely up to you. Try lemon oil on lemon- or cream-colored paper, orange oil on peach-colored paper, lavender on lavender paper, and so forth. Remember though that the aroma will henceforth be associated subconsciously not only with you but with the nature of the news you send, so don't send perfumed letters with bad news in them or the recipient of that letter will relive the emotions they felt on reading the news every time they smell the same aroma in the future. Send only good news in perfumed letters.

Lovers have traditionally sent each other perfumed letters, not only because it's a caring, loving gesture, but because the perfume when smelled again by the recipient will automatically remind him of the sender. But why not send an antidepressant bergamot letter to a friend who is having a hard time?

Perfumed inks have the same effect as perfumed paper. Just add to the bottle 10 drops of essential oil for each 1 teaspoon of ink.

Rolls of paper towels and toilet paper can be made aromatic—and antibacterial—using a method similar to that recommended for notepaper. This time place the rolls in a shoe box or large cardboard box that you can close tightly with adhesive tape and put a tissue to which you have added the essential oil in with them. Try lemon or pine essential oils. Also, see page 310 for the method of placing the essential oils onto the cardboard inner roll. Do not use essential oils on paper napkins as this will detract from the aroma of your food.

Perfumed Pillows and Sachets ◆◆◆◆◆◆◆◆◆◆◆

Once upon a time, sleeping beauties laid their pretty heads on pillows perfumed with sweet smelling rushes and soporific dried hops. Households used to make wide use of herbs in pillows and sachets, for both their fragrance and medicinal value. Day pillows would release a portion of their fragrance each time someone leaned back on them, and sachets were slipped into drawers, cupboards, shoes, and boots to keep them all sweet smelling. Even today, these items are on sale in numerous stores.

Making your own perfumed pillows and sachets not only saves you a great deal of money, but using the essential oils increases their effectiveness and makes reviving them very easy. All you need is a piece of material stitched along three sides, whatever size you choose, some fresh dried herbs or spices, and the oils. It is of course the essential oil contained in the raw product that gives dried herbs and spices their aroma but you can enhance this by leaving the herbs in a plastic bag overnight with the essential oils so they can be absorbed. How many drops of oil you add depends upon the size of the pillow or sachet you are making and the strength of your dried product. When using the essential oils it is not necessary to use dried herbs—any stuffing will do. For sleep pillows use chamomile, lavender, neroli, marjoram, valerian, nutmeg, or hop. Day pillows can have their fragrance matched to the fragrance you like to use in individual rooms, for example lemon, geranium, or clary-sage. Stuff the pillow and sew the fourth side.

With creativity and imagination you can make marvelous tailor-made presents for family and friends. And reviving them is so easy. Just add the oil neat on the outer material or, if this is delicate, open a little of a corner seam and drop the oil onto the stuffing.

Potpourris and Pomanders ◆◆◆◆◆◆◆◆◆◆◆

To keep a potpourri smelling sweet you need to close it up some of the time, otherwise the fragrance will gradually fade. Synthetic refreshers are sold for the purpose, but it seems a great shame to put chemicals on beautiful flowers, herbs, or spices when the essential oils can do the job naturally.

There are several different types of potpourri. The classical one we all know is made by putting dried flower petals in an open bowl. Wet potpourris are made with fresh, damp petals which, because they aren't too pretty to look at, are placed in a container which is partially closed—usually the lid is peppered with holes through which the aroma can escape. Then there are the herbs and spice potpourris. With all these varieties, you can buy the ingredients separately and blend them together as you choose, or make your own.

Flowers often have no aroma when dried and are used for their beauty and color only. Put them together with a few drops of your chosen essential oil in a plastic bag and leave it sealed for a few days so the aroma can penetrate the petals. The floral fragrances are obviously the ones to go for or try one of these synergistic blends, depending on the type of flowers you have and the additional decorative items you choose to mix them with:

FLOWERY SYNERGISTIC BLEND

Bois de rose	3 drops
Geranium	4 drops
Grapefruit	1 drop
Pettigraine	1 drop
Palma rosa	2 drops

ORIENTAL SYNERGISTIC BLEND

Sandalwood	3 drops
Patchouli	2 drops
Benzoin	1 drop
Nutmeg	2 drops
Ylang-ylang	2 drops
Lime	1 drop

Blend the essential oils together and add to the potpourri ingredients drop by drop until the desired strength is reached. Leave them together in a sealed bag so that the aroma can penetrate.

Wood shavings should always be saved, because dyed and dried they make a very attractive addition to any potpourri. Dilute the dye, place the shavings in it, take out and dry. Orris root powder makes a good fixative. Cleaned and dried fruit stones —plums and peach especially—can be added to potpourris, either natural or dyed. Dried leaves too can look very beautiful. Whole nutmegs look attractive and if you put a drop of nutmeg oil on them and store in a plastic bag for a day or so their aromatic quality will be much intensified. The same applies to cinnamon sticks and cinnamon oil and cloves and clove oil. Other additions to a spicy potpourri could be the peel of orange, lemon, or lime (there is a special kitchen tool which cuts the peel into lovely curly shapes). These can also be enhanced by leaving in a plastic bag with their appropriate essential oils. Here is a synergistic blend you might like to try with a spicy potpourri:

SPICY SYNERGISTIC BLENDS

BLEND 1

Nutmeg	2 drops
Clove	1 drop
Cinnamon	2 drops

BLEND 2

Lemon	4 drops
Basil	2 drops
Orange	3 drops

A potpourri to repel moths can be made with wormwood, southernwood, rosemary, sage, lavender, and mint. Enhance it with the essential oils of lavender, lemongrass, rosemary, and citronella.

Pomanders are traditionally made by sticking cloves into a citrus fruit and rolling it in powdered spices. Again, these can be much enhanced in fragrance and preservative value by rolling the fruit in the appropriate essential oils.

Making Your Own Soaps ♦♦♦♦♦♦♦♦♦♦♦♦♦♦♦♦

Making your own soap is a bit of a messy job, but it's well worth the trouble. Not only are you ensured of using the purest of ingredients on your skin, and of having the exact fragrance you want, but with all the permutations there are in terms of ingredients and shape, you can be sure of having a unique product for your efforts.

Which essential oils you use to fragrance the soap is up to you, and you can have a lot of fun making blends. Here are three formulas you might like to try; they each contain enough essential oil for 9 ounces of grated soap:

MORNING FRESH

Grapefruit	4 drops
Lime	2 drops
Lemon	1 drop
Basil	2 drops
Lavender	2 drops

GENTLEMAN'S SPICE

Nutmeg	1 drop
Bay	2 drops
Lime	6 drops
Clary-sage	2 drops

COUNTRY LIFE

Lavender	6 drops
Geranium	2 drops
Chamomile Roman	1 drop
Rosemary	3 drops

Use as your base grated, one hundred percent pure soap. Excellent additions would be oatmeal, almond meal, avocado oil, olive oil, jojoba, or carrot oil. Bring to a boil an amount of water that is half the volume of the grated soap you intend to use. Put this in a bowl over a pot of boiling water on the stove, or in a bain-marie if you have one, and add the grated soap. Stir until the soap is fully melted (it becomes quite sticky and sloppy). Take it off the heat and leave until it is starting to set, then add your chosen essential oils. Mix again very well. You can scoop out the soap and mold it by hand to the shape you want or put it into pre-prepared molds. You can use old soap boxes for the traditional shape of soap or any small carton or container of your choice, so long as they are well oiled or lined with greaseproof paper. Leave until well set and then turn out the soap. If the soaps are intended as presents, wrap them in colored tissue paper before they go in the wrapping paper.

Fragrant Candles ◆◆◆◆◆

Making candles is a hobby many people enjoy, and with the advent of candle-making kits it is relatively easy to do. To perfume the candles all you have to do is add 30–60 drops of essential oil to 8 ounces of candle wax and follow the instructions with your kit. Even if you don't want to go to the trouble of making your own candles, a good effect can still be made by placing 3 drops of essential oil on the wax by the wick just as the candle has been lit and is beginning to melt the wax.

Choose which essential oil to use not only for its fragrance but for its other effects. Use relaxing essential oils for that special evening for two, stimulating ones to get the conversation going during the pre-dinner drinks, and soothing ones with the after dinner brandy. Later still, you might want to bring out the aromatic candles. . . .

All the essential oil candles have a very subtle effect and are not overpowering like chemical candle fragrances. The ultimate in hostess attentiveness must be coordinating the fragrance of your candles with the color of your candles and decor, and when you really get the hang of it, you can match the oils with the personalities of your guests—try putting a relaxing candle next to the person who always hogs the conversation and a stimulating one next to the introverted guest.

Unwanted Visitors ◆◆◆◆

Essential oils are not about murdering insects and small animals on a mass scale but about deterring them from entering or staying in our living space. The other great advantage of using the oils for this purpose is that we do not have to spray inside the house with chemicals which pollute the air we breathe and endanger the health of our family and friends.

Creepy-Crawlies

Essential oils are altogether a better way of dealing with the creepy-crawlies that fly innocently through our open windows, or are attracted by our central heating in winter and the cool nooks and crannies when the summer sun is blazing down.

Lavender oil is reputedly an antidote to the bite of the black widow spider, and when a consignment of imported grapes brought an invasion of them to my hometown in southeast England, I can assure you that I had a big bottle by me at all times. And I strap the bottle to my person to make quite certain I don't lose it when I go to California. But Britain is a pretty harmless place as far as creepy-crawlies go, unless you count the sight of a flight of baby blowflies escaping from their former life as maggots in the trash can.

Insects have a very short life and, like tourists, they come and go at particular times of the year, in waves. One week the place is full of spiders and another week it's daddy long-legs. Because we have a fair amount of information about their movements and likes and dislikes, with a little planning it's fairly easy to ensure that the insects run along and bother someone else. You will find a lot more information about creepy-crawlies in Chapter 18, including the chart which lists each particular insect's dislikes in terms of essential oils, but here is a good general list for use in the house:

ESSENTIAL OILS
CREEPY-CRAWLIES HATE

Lavender	**Cinnamon**
Citronella	**Thyme**
Peppermint	**Rue**
Lemongrass	**Basil**

To deter insects from coming in through the windows make paper strips—from a roll of paper towels for example—or cut lengths of cotton ribbon, put a drop of essential oil on each one and hang them above the window. One fashion-conscious young bachelor I know has made an arrangement of gray and black ribbons above his window that looks more like a work of art than the very effective insect deterrent it is. But anything, however makeshift, looks better than the sticky flypaper one can buy—I don't know what is worse, looking at this insect graveyard or breathing in the chemicals that make it such a disaster area for the poor little creatures. The essential oil version, however, gives out a lovely fragrance to the whole room as the warm breeze wafts in on a summer's evening.

Flies and moths particularly dislike lavender oil, while peppermint keeps mosquitoes away. Moths have an aversion to the citrus oils too. Either of these blends will do a good job of keeping most insects on their side of the window frame:

UNWANTED VISITORS

BLEND 1

Citronella	10 drops
Peppermint	3 drops

BLEND 2

Lavender	5 drops
Citronella	5 drops

These blends and the other essential oils can also be placed on cotton-wool balls and popped in the nooks and crannies or sprayed around the room. Peppermint oil keeps ants at bay and is well worth using if the ants have decided that your house is a big attraction. Just drop the oil neat around their likely entrance places, doors and windows, and watch them run. To keep blowflies and all the rest from turning your trash can into a maternity ward for themselves, soak strips of material in an essential oil and water mix and hang inside the can. The citronella and peppermint formula above would work well, or use the very effective rue* essential oil—although it doesn't have a particularly nice aroma and might not go down too well in the house. But whatever oil you use will be a far better option than spraying pesticides in your living space.

*Rue should only be used for this purpose.

Mice

From below, a few tiny field mice running around inside the roof sounds like a cavalry of giant rodents. And they can be particularly disturbing during the night. To discourage any rodent from entering your house, use spearmint or peppermint—fresh or dried plant, or essential oil to water and alcohol. Perfume is the strongest formulation and should comprise 15 to 30 percent essential oil. This placed strategically around the house and roof should discourage them from turning your residence into theirs.

♦ CHAPTER 14 ♦
THE STILLROOM

IN THIS CHAPTER we shall be looking at how the essential oils can help us to revive the Elizabethan institution of the domestic stillroom. This is not about distilling alcoholic drinks, but about making your own eau de colognes and perfumes. Doing this can be as easy or as difficult as you like. While it is true that the most exclusive and expensive perfumes can be composed of a hundred, two hundred, or even more compounds, and can take the perfumer—Le Nez, or "the nose," as he is known in France—up to two years and more to design, it is also true that some of the most successful perfumes are made from just two or three essences. We shall be seeing too how to make essential oils themselves. You will find that it really is not very difficult to take care of all your aromatic requirements without going further than your very own stillroom.

The ingredients in a bottle of store-bought perfume or cologne costs about ten percent of the retail price—the rest is your contribution to packaging, advertising, sales profit, and tax. With the money you save on making your own you can afford to buy some of the really exotic essential oils which could set you back considerably. But don't panic, you need only a drop or two of jasmine, for example, to infuse a bottle of really luxurious perfume and, unlike many a store-bought preparation, you can be sure you are buying the real thing. Indeed, maintaining natural purity is one of the advantages of making your own because store perfumes are a cocktail of natural and chemical components. Besides the essential oils, the modern perfumer uses a whole array of ingredients which not only cut costs but cut out the uncertainties of dealing with natural products—

elements like weather and transport which, if adverse, can mean he is without his basic ingredients. To bypass uncertainty, the modern perfumer must be less of an artist and more of a chemist and his shelf of ingredients will include things as unromantic as dimethyl-benzyl-carbonyl-butyrate and phenyl-ethyl-dimethyl-carbinol. You, on the other hand, do not have to worry about maintaining the same standard of product year after year, and can instead enjoy the slight variations that occur with each year's harvest. Nor do we have to worry about chemical preservatives because you won't be putting your bottle on a store shelf for an unknown period of time before it is used. Finally, you will not be trying to create an aroma that appeals to millions of purchasers, just one that appeals to you and, perhaps, your lover.

The strength of your aromatic liquid depends upon the ratio of essential oil to water and alcohol. Perfume is the strongest formulation and should comprise 15 to 30 percent essential oil with the remaining 85 to 70 percent being between 90 to 95 percent alcohol and 10 to 5 percent water. This is shown more clearly on the chart that follows:

TYPE OF AROMATIC LIQUID	PERCENTAGE OF ESSENTIAL OIL	THE BALANCE: PERCENTAGE OF ALCOHOL
Perfume	15–30	90–95
Eau de perfume	8–15	80–90
Eau de toilette	4–8	80–90
Eau de cologne	3–5	70
Splash cologne	1–3	80

The essential oils should be used neat—that is to say, they shouldn't be diluted in vegetable oils or anything else. Perfume always contains a percentage of water, even if this is as little as 5 percent of the whole, and you should use distilled water (available from pharmacies) or plain, bottled spring water. Ideally, the alcohol should be pure pharmaceutical but this is impossible to buy at present in Britain, although it is available elsewhere. Kitchen perfumers should therefore use vodka—the higher the proof the better. Brandy is another alternative, but it does have a strong smell which can ruin a delicate combination of aromas or one that has a low concentration of essential oil. If you want to add color, use a high quality, natural, vegetable food dye. You will also need some small sterilized bottles to put your creations in and, although they look nice, clear cut-glass ones will be a quick death for the delicate liquids they contain because they attract perfume's number one enemy—the sun. Finally, you will need a notebook to record the exact formulations, in drops, of essential oils that you use when making your concentrate. Just one extra drop of this or that can completely change the aroma of the whole, and when you create a masterpiece you are going to kick yourself if you cannot remember whether it was 3 drops of neroli and 1 of bergamot or 1 of neroli and 3 of bergamot. Make notes all the way, so you know your failures as well as your successes.

Making Your Own Perfumes ♦♦♦♦♦♦♦♦♦♦♦♦♦

First, decide the strength of perfume you are going to make. Eau de perfume is lighter than perfume but lasts longer than eau de toilette, which is best put in an atomizer and sprayed on several times during the day.

In the lists that follow I separate feminine oils from masculine oils although you should in no way feel constrained by these guidelines. You will see that some oils, in any case, appear on both male and female lists. Feel free to follow your own nose and intuition—you are the creative artist here, not me or any perfuming tradition. Only you know what you like and who you are trying to please. Do, though, start with a general idea of what you want—is it something spicy, citrony, floral, or seductive? It helps too to know the form that all perfume-making follows, and this is like a musical form of base notes, middle, and top notes, with "fixative" or "bridging" elements between them. The musical analogy is most appropriate to perfume-making, for it is a symphony or concerto of aromatic elements, no different in essence from the artistic blending of notes. The best perfume designers take their work as seriously as do the great musical composers or painters, with the general form, the first impact, the subtle undertones, the highlights, and background melodies, all playing their part in making the whole a beautiful composition. There has to be contrast, light and dark, highs and lows, movement between all the contributing parts, and, above all, harmony.

Perfumes are dynamic and change with people and with time. Not only do they react differently with different skin, and so cannot be said to be just one, specific smell; they also evaporate and as they do so, the aroma changes. The speed with which a particular component evaporates is its volatility—if it is fast, it's a top note; not so fast, a middle note; and if it is slow, it's called a base note. The fact that essences with different rates of evaporation are incorporated into a single perfume accounts for the fact that it will smell differently on your skin when first placed there, a few minutes later, and later on in the day.

It is the harmonious blending of these three stages of volatility that makes a good perfume. If it simply changes dramatically and smells quite different as time passes, the perfume isn't "hanging together"—it isn't integrated into one harmonious whole. This is why a perfume needs "bridges" or "fixatives" to hold it together.

You might by now be thinking that the whole prospect of making a good perfume sounds too complicated. But don't be put off. With a little experience and your aromatic good taste, you will soon get the hang of it. The hero (or antihero) of J. K. Huysman's *Against Nature,* Des Esseintes, enjoyed making perfumes and, above all, imitating the aroma of particular flowers. Here, he was after the aroma of the sweet pea: ". . . after trying various combinations he finally hit on the right tone by mixing the orange blossom with tuberose and rose, binding the three together with a drop of vanilla." Vanilla was his bridge between the three elements. Benzoin and heliotrope are other effective bridges, while lavender and bois de rose are good bridges between the citrus and floral essences.

Sweet pea is one of the flowers that has defied all attempts to extract its scent, from before the time *Against Nature* was written in 1884 right up to the present day. However, new techniques for analyzing the aroma molecules emitted by a flower into its charmingly called "headspace" mean that certain long-standing challenges to the perfumer will doubtless be overcome. In the future we shall have sweet-pea perfumes that are, if not distillations of the real thing, chemical reconstitutions made by putting together the dozen or more elements that can be identified by headspace analysis. One difficulty of perfumery is the fact that certain flowers change aromatically as they are picked; an unpleasant sort of stress perspiration called stress metabolites is produced and it is unlikely that these will ever be stabilized sufficiently to be made into perfume. Reproducing these aromas will probably always have to be done by chemical analysis and reconstitution or, in the old-fashion way, by mixing various natural essences in an attempt to capture the real thing.

Perfumery may be as simple as using a natural essence mixed with alcohol and water to make a liquid that carries the perfume of one flower. It may be that you wish to create the aroma of a flower that cannot, for one reason or another, be distilled and need to blend other essences to re-create it. Or, and this is where the grand symphonies of perfumery come into play, you wish to create a picture, not of one flower, but of a field of flowers. This is when you need to sit down and let your imagination play to conjure up aromatic images of vitality and complexity and interaction. It could be that you have in mind an Alpine mountain in spring, or an English garden in summer, or an autumnal aromatic scene or, perhaps, something more exotic—a Balinese flower festival, a Caribbean night, or an Eastern delight. The choice is entirely yours, and with the vast array of essential oils any aromatic image is possible. But, above all, have fun and enjoy the challenges and sheer pleasure of making your own perfumes.

When making a perfume, first establish your base note, or combination of base notes, then your middle note or notes, then the top notes. Often the same essential oil will be used as a middle or top note. Add your essential oil concentrate to the alcohol and water base in a large bottle. Swirl the mixture around gently until it is well diffused and leave it for at least four to six weeks before pouring through a paper coffee filter and bottling.

Feminine Notes ♦♦♦♦♦♦♦

Here is the recommended list of base notes for feminine perfumes or colognes. As you can see, these are usually roots, gums, or resins:

FEMININE OILS:
BASE NOTES

Balsam de Tolu	**Myrrh**
Balsam de Peru	**Oakmoss**
Benzoin	**Olibanum**
Cedarwood	**Opoponax**
Cinnamon	**Patchouli**
Frankincense	**Sandalwood**
Guaiacwood	**Styrax**
Heliotrope	**Tonka bean**
Labdanum	**Vanilla**
Melilot	**Vetiver**

Next we have the oils which are found in either base or middle notes; they could make good bridges between the two—depending upon your overall formula, of course.

FEMININE OILS:
BASE OR MIDDLE NOTES

Cedarwood	**Patchouli**
Cinnamon	**Sandalwood**
Frankincense	**Styrax**
Heliotrope	**Vetiver**
Myrrh	

FEMININE OILS:
MIDDLE NOTES

Carnation	**Nutmeg**
Cassia	**Orchid**
Clary-sage	**Oriental rose**
Clove bud	**Palma rosa**
Geranium	**Pimento berry**
Ginger	**Pine needle**
Hyacinth	**Rosa centifolia**
Jasmine	**Rose**
Jonquil	**Rosewood (Bois de rose)**
Lemongrass	
Linden	**Thyme**
Marjoram	**Tuberose**

Mimosa	**Violet flower**
Narcissus	**Ylang-ylang**
Neroli	

FEMININE OILS:
MIDDLE OR TOP NOTES

Bay	**Neroli**
Cassis	**Nutmeg**
Clary-sage	**Palma rosa**
Hyacinth	**Rosewood**
Marjoram	**Thyme**
Mimosa	

Top notes are the most volatile—that is to say, they evaporate the most quickly and are, therefore, the ones you smell first of all. They gradually evaporate and leave the middle notes which eventually fade and reveal the base notes. You could think of the whole process as a love affair: the top notes represent the excitement of love at first sight, the middle notes (or "heart notes" as they are known in the perfume trade) grow on the heart, and the basic notes make it a long-lasting affair. One reverses this order when actually making the perfume, so that the top notes are your final flourish, so to speak. Use several essences, or just one, from each list to formulate your own perfume—and, we hope, love affair!

FEMININE OILS: TOP NOTES

Angelica	**Galbanum**
Anise	**Juniper berry**
Armoise	**Lavender**
Basil	**Lemon**
Bergamot	**Lime**
Cardamom	**Mandarin**
Chamomile Roman	**Marigold**
	Neroli
Coriander	**Pettigraine**
Cumin	**Spearmint**
Estragon	**Tagetes**

The exact formulas of the world's most famous perfumes are a closely guarded secret but we do know a little about them. Joy, from Jean Patou, advertised as "the costliest perfume in the world," contains rose and jasmine—but what else and in what proportions remains a fact locked away in a Swiss bank. Arpège, by Lanvin, is a blend containing rose, jasmine, iris, lily of the valley, vetiver, and sandalwood—and more besides. Jicky, a perfume that suits both men and women with its sporty scent, contains lavender, lemon, and bergamot—and that's as much as we know. But perfumes are usually composed of several ingredients and their base, middle, and top notes are themselves quite complex concoctions. Here are some of the components of the base, middle, and top notes of some popular perfumes to give you an idea of what makes that most mysterious of product, a perfume, a success:

BASE NOTES

Vetiver	**Vanilla**
Sandalwood	**Balsam de Peru**
Benzoin	**Balsam de Tolu**

Chamade by Guerlain

In perfumer's terms this would be called a "sweet balsamic" note

MIDDLE NOTES

Jasmine	**Orris root**
Rose Maroc	**Carnation**
Ylang-ylang	**Tuberose**

Femme by Rochas

A "sweet, floral, spicy" note

Jasmine	**Rose**
Narcissus	**Carnation**
Jonquil	**Tuberose**

Mink and Pearls by Jovan

A "narcotic, floral" note

Rosewood	**Cinnamon**
Rose	**Ylang-ylang**
Jasmine	**Ginger**
Carnation	

Royal Secret by Monteil

An "exotic, floral" note

TOP NOTES

Lemon	**Mandarin**
Bergamot	**Rosewood**

Shalimar by Guerlain

A "citrusy, fresh" note

Bergamot	**Mandarin**
Lemon	**Neroli**

Bal de Versailles by Despres

A "fresh" note

Hyacinth	**Narcissus**
Galbanum	**Lemon**
Bergamot	

Norell by Revlon

A "green and fresh" note

Although no perfumers will give away the formula of their product, they are prepared to offer a few clues while keeping the exact proportions hidden away in their vaults. Here are some of the vital ingredients of some very popular makes; these would be contained in the top, middle, and base notes:

SHALIMAR by Guerlain

Lemon	**Orris root**
Bergamot	**Vetiver**
Mandarin	**Opoponax**
Rosewood	**Vanilla**
Patchouli	**Benzoin**
Rose	**Balsam de Peru**
Jasmine	

OPIUM by St. Laurent

Orange	**Cinnamon**
Pimento berry	**Jasmine**
Bay	**Orris root**
Carnation	**Benzoin**
Rose	**Patchouli**
Ylang-ylang	**Frankincense**

NO. 5 by Chanel

Bergamot	**Orris root**
Lemon	**Ylang-ylang**
Neroli	**Vetiver**
Jasmine	**Cedarwood**
Rose	**Vanilla**
Lily of the Valley*	

*This is not available as a natural essential oil.

Masculine Notes ♦♦♦♦♦♦

When making colognes for men follow the same procedures as for making perfume, although the concentration of essences will be far less.

MALE OILS: BASE NOTES

Bay	**Oakmoss**
Benzoin	**Olibanum**
Cedarwood	**Sandalwood**
Cinnamon	**Styrax**
Frankincense	**Tonka bean**
Moss	**Vanilla**
Myrrh	**Vetiver**

MALE OILS:
BASE TO MIDDLE NOTES

Bay	**Patchouli**
Cedarwood	**Pimento berry**
Cinnamon	**Sandalwood**
Myrrh	**Vetiver**

MALE OILS: MIDDLE NOTES

Angelica	**Mandarin**
Anise	**Marjoram**
Artemisia	**Neroli**
Basil	**Nutmeg**
Caraway	**Oregano**
Cardamom	**Orris root**
Carnation	**Pepper (black)**
Carrot	**Peppermint**
Clary-sage	**Pettigraine**
Clove	**Pine**

Coriander	**Rose**
Cumin	**Rosemary**
Galbanum	**Rosewood**
Geranium	**Sage**
Ginger	**Tarragon**
Jasmine	**Thyme**
Juniper	**Ylang-ylang**
Lavender	

MALE OILS:
MIDDLE TO TOP NOTES

Angelica	**Nutmeg**
Basil	**Oregano**
Bay	**Pepper (black)**
Caraway	**Pimento berry**
Clary-sage	**Rosemary**
Coriander	**Rosewood**
Lavender	**Tarragon**
Marjoram	**Thyme**

MALE OILS: TOP NOTES

Anise	**Lime**
Artemisia	**Mandarin**
Bergamot	**Neroli**
Cedar leaf	**Orange**
Cumin	**Peppermint**
Galbanum	**Pettigraine**
Juniper	**Sage**
Lemon	**Verbena**
Lemongrass	

And here are some of the ingredients of some famous male colognes:

BASE NOTES

Tonka bean	**Cedarwood**

E.D.C. Imperial by Guerlain

Vanilla	**Heliotrope**

Royal Spice by Royale Lyme Ltd.

Cedarwood	**Vetiver**

Pour Homme by Weil

MIDDLE NOTES

Lavender	**Carnation**
Juniper	**Jasmine**
Pine	

Halston 1-12 by Halston

In perfumer's terms a "green resinous" note

Jasmine	**Carnation**
Vetiver	**Geranium**
Patchouli	**Orris root**
Cinnamon	

Kouros by Yves St. Laurent

A "floral, woody" note

Clary-sage	**Basil**
Orange	**Geranium**
Jasmine	

Monsieur by Givenchy

A "fresh" note

Jasmine	**Pine**
Carnation	**Thyme**
Cinnamon	

Devin by Aramis

A "spicy, resinous" note

TOP NOTES

Lavender	**Anise**
Lemon	**Lime**
Pettigraine	**Mandarin**
Bergamot	

Tuscany by Aramis

A "citrusy, fresh, herbaceous" note

Lavender	**Bergamot**
Rosemary	**Lemon**

Pour un Homme by Caron

A "lavendaceous, fresh" note

Bergamot	**Artemisia**
Lavender	**Pettigraine**
Basil	**Lemon**

Pour Homme by Gucci

A "fresh, herbaceous" note

These are the essential oil ingredients of some of the most popular male perfumes and colognes:

PACO RABAN

Laurel (bay)	Geranium
Bergamot	Rosewood
Lavender	Cinnamon
Rosemary	Pine
Pettigraine	Tonka bean
Clary-sage	Cedarwood
Carnation	

ARAMIS

Orange	Jasmine
Bergamot	Ylang-ylang
Pimento berry	Patchouli
Lemon	Sandalwood
Carnation	Vanilla
Cinnamon	Olibanum
Rose	Benzoin

GEORGIO

Orange	Orris
Bergamot	Rose
Pimento berry	Cedarwood
Carnation	Benzoin
Cinnamon	Olibanum
Patchouli	Vanilla

You can see from the preceding lists that fragrances one might consider to be exclusively "feminine" actually feature very strongly in male preparations. The difference between male and female fragrances does of course depend largely on the ingredients, and by scanning the male and female lists you can see where these differences lie. But another important factor is the proportion of each oil used, and to come to a fragrance that perfectly suits you will be a matter of experimentation. Although the marketing of male products relies heavily on macho images such as the martial arts and predatory animals, the fact of the matter is that the products themselves contain delicate ingredients such as lavender, bergamot, lemon, lime, orange, jasmine, carnation, and geranium. As with the female products, these are, of course, used in addition to synthetic and animal products, which by making our own we are going to do without.

Making Eau de Cologne ◆◆◆◆◆◆◆◆◆◆◆◆◆◆

First make your concentrate using the information that has gone before or following one of these formulas:

EAU DE COLOGNE FORMULAS

FORMULA 1

Bergamot	10 drops
Rosemary	2 drops
Lemon	10 drops
Orange	20 drops
Neroli	2 drops

FORMULA 2

Rose	4 drops
Lemon	2 drops
Orange	2 drops
Basil	1 drop
Neroli	1 drop
Pettigraine	1 drop
Bergamot	2 drops

FORMULA 3

Palma rosa	10 drops
Orange	8 drops
Pettigraine	3 drops
Lime	2 drops
Geranium	1 drop

Pour your essential oils into 2½ ounces of 100 percent proof vodka, stirring slowly but long enough to ensure complete dispersal. Leave it to stand for forty-eight hours and then add 2 tablespoons spring water and, again, stir slowly but enough to ensure a thorough mixing is taking place.

The mixture should be left to stand now for at least another forty-eight hours, but the fragrance will be much stronger if you follow the procedures of the perfume trade and leave the liquid for four to six weeks. After letting the liquid mature, for however long you decide that shall be, pour it through a paper coffee filter and bottle. If you find the aroma too strong, the eau de cologne can be further diluted by adding more spring water and mixing well.

Making Your Own Essential Oils ◆◆◆◆◆◆◆◆◆

Home stills can often be bought and will save you a great deal of trouble. With these stills you can make floral waters and small quantities of essential oils, but although the quantity may be small it will go a very long way, and quality, which is of utmost importance, can be ensured. Also, you can produce essential oils which may not be readily available commercially. Depending on the flower or herb, the raw material you require may be enormous or quite small, and depending on the exact procedures you follow, the strength of the finished product can be varied to suit your requirements. You will see from the various procedures that follow that there are also other ways of making essential oils and flower- or herb-infused vegetable oils, but whichever method you choose remember that organically grown raw materials are a far better option than those grown with the usual pesticides and fertilizers, so even if you do not plan to start making your own oils just yet, do begin right now to think about ways of growing your raw materials organically—see "Gardens for the Future," page 365. This is especially important if you plan to use your finished products therapeutically, but in any event, making your own oils gives you tremendous scope for concocting your own cosmetic lotions and potions.

Do-It-Yourself Still

Here is a method of making essential oils and fine floral or herb waters at the same time. You will need a large, enamel kettle—you can find these in Chinese emporiums—and about five feet of plastic hose to fit the spout. Fill the kettle with the flower or herb you wish to distill and then pour in as much bottled water as it can hold. Put it on the stove and attach the hose to the spout. Put a low table next to the stove—it should be a little less than half the height of the stove—and put on it a bowl filled with ice. Finally, place a jug on the floor, near the table. Now bend the hose so that the bend rests in the ice, and put the end of the hose into the jug on the floor.

Boil the kettle and then turn down the heat so that it stews but doesn't quite simmer, and leave it for an hour or so. The steam leaving the kettle spout will contain molecules of essential oil; this will cool in the ice, and the water that drips into the jug on the floor will contain particles of essential oil along with water particles. When the process has finished, the essential oil will float to the top of the water in the jug. Allow a little time for this to happen, and then use an eye dropper to take it off carefully. These droppers are available from pharmacists, or use the dropper from a new dropper-bottle, also available from any pharmacist for a few cents. The liquid remaining in the jug will be a fine flower or herb water.

Pomades

This is a two-part procedure that will leave you after stage one with a pomade—a perfume-infused fat which can be used in creams or, mixed with other essences, as a cream-perfume. If you continue through stage two, essential oil can be extracted from the pomade.

Spread two equally sized pieces of glass with a "Flora" type of vegetable fat. This is not margarine but pure sunflower oil blended with vegetable fat which is high in essential polyunsaturates. You may have to shop around a bit to find this product, which is the vegetable version of lard, but it is worth it to avoid using the animal fat products routinely used by commercial perfumers. Lay in rows on top of the fat the flowers whose oil you wish to extract. Jasmine has traditionally been extracted in this fashion, as has tuberose, but you might equally try carnation, narcissus, lilac, and stocks. Put one sheet of glass on the other, fatty sides together, cover and leave overnight. Keep changing the flowers daily until you run out of them, or until you have a heavily perfumed fat.

To extract the essential oil you need to blend the pomade with four times its volume of alcohol. Leave this sealed in a jar for several weeks and then skim off the fat and evaporate the alcohol very slowly in a bain-marie on the stove. You will be left with the essence.

Infused Oils

There are two methods of infusing vegetable oils with the aroma of flowers or herbs. Put the flowers or herbs of your choice in a large cooking pan with a lid and add half their volume of a good odorless vegetable oil. Heat the pan, with the lid in place, to a temperature of 150° Fahrenheit. At this temperature the cells containing the odoriferous molecules burst and these are taken up by the oil. Strain and then bottle the oil.

Alternatively, pack a jar tightly with your chosen flowers or herbs and cover them with the vegetable oil; seal the jar very tight and put it outside in the sun for a few weeks, bringing it in at night. Strain and then bottle the oil.

These infused oils can be used on their own or as a base in which to dilute essential oils.

♦ CHAPTER 15 ♦

SWEET-SCENTED CELEBRATIONS

THERE ARE MANY special events to celebrate throughout the year, and invariably special aromas are associated with them. Traditional practices involving natural aromatic substances determined the legacy that we enjoy today, but the practicalities of city life have largely eroded the possibility of bringing into our homes the natural products that gave us the original aromatic connection. However, in the essential oils we have a mobile, compact, and thoroughly modern method of re-creating the aromatic impact of old.

When using the essential oils around the house during a celebration, aim for an aroma that is evocative without being overpowering. Gently build up an aroma picture that reflects the occasion, using several methods at the same time, or making one special celebratory blend.

Christmas ♦♦♦♦♦♦♦♦♦♦♦♦

The association of a particular aroma for the individual very much depends on where he or she was brought up and lives. In America, Christmas is evoked by the aroma of bay berry because traditionally at this time candles with this fragrance are burned in memory of the first settlers who used the wax from the bay berry to make their candles.

The aroma of pine evokes memories of happy childhoods to North Americans and northern Europeans alike because of the tradition in these areas of festooning a pine tree or similar resinous conifer with decorations, lights, sweets, and presents. But it isn't always easy to recapture that aroma of pine when Christmas trees are made of plastic and tinsel, and real ones are coated with preservatives to stop the needles dropping in the modern, centrally heated home, so that even if they are present, the resins that were once gently released from the needles can no longer escape to perfume the air—and Christmas just doesn't seem quite the same. But with nature's essential oils the evocative aroma of Christmas need not be lost. Simply spray the tree with a mixture of 1 cup water and 6 drops of essential oil of pine, or put a few drops of pine oil on a piece of absorbent material and tuck it around the trunk of the tree.

THE CHRISTMAS ESSENTIAL OILS

SPICES	CITRUS
Cinnamon	**Mandarin**
Clove	**Orange**
Bay	**Tangerine**
TREES	RESINS
Pine	**Frankincense**
Cedarwood	**Myrrh**

Frankincense and myrrh were presented to baby Jesus in their resinous form—which is still burned in churches from Addis Ababa to Athens today while the essential oils are produced by steam distillation of the crude gum. Unless you want your house to smell like a church it is better not to use frankincense too liberally and myrrh is a bit heavy and acrid—so they are both best used in blends of essential oils. You could, for example, add 1 drop of frankincense to this blend to give it a spiritual edge:

CHRISTMAS HOUSE SPRAY

Pine	4 drops
Mandarin	2 drops
Cinnamon	1 drop

Diluted in 1¼ cups water in a plant-spray

There are many combinations of oils that work equally well at Christmas, so just experiment. Mandarin, tangerine, and orange are fresh smelling and Christmasy and a good choice when visitors are due. Celebratory cakes and breads all contain spices and their aromas suffuse a home with a hospitable glow. The spice essential oils of cinnamon, clove, and bay will add this warm hint to your blends. With even very small quantities of essential oil, it is easy to build up an aromatic image of the season.

When making Christmas logs for the fire you will need only one drop of essential oil per log and only one oil-log per fire. Surprisingly perhaps, this one drop will be enough to provide an aromatic boost to the Christmas ambience. You can use any old wood that happens to be around, but the fire will smell like the wood from which the particular oil was extracted. Simply put 1 drop of a "Firewood" oil onto the log and leave enough time for the oil to soak through before putting it on the fire. The essential oils are inflammable so unless the oil has been given time to soak into the wood a little, you might see more sparks than you bargained for! It is a good idea to prepare several logs at the same time and use them as needed.

FIREWOOD OILS

Sandalwood	**Frankincense**
Cypress	**Myrrh**
Cedarwood	

Candles add a lovely touch of warmth at Christmas and can be made aromatic very easily with the essential oils. Light the candle and wait until the wax begins to melt and then add 1 drop of essential oil to it, just by the wick. Bay is a good choice—especially for traditionally minded Americans. Pine and mandarin also work well on candles to evoke the atmosphere of Christmas.

CHRISTMAS CANDLE BLEND

Mandarin	4 drops
Geranium	1 drop
Cinnamon	1 drop

Here is a blend which works well at Christmas. The mandarin will evoke memories of Christmas while the geranium will put people in a good mood and the cinnamon will whet their appetites. This formula can also be used in a room spray—these quantities to 2½ cups water.

Decorations are an integral part of celebrations and the essential oils can be incorporated into them very easily. Today, pine cones are usually bought in stores rather than picked up fresh from the forest floor, and can be dry and without aroma. This is easily rectified by putting the cones in a large plastic bag with a cotton-wool ball to which you have added 2 drops of pine oil. Seal the bag and leave overnight, and in the morning the cones will be gently suffused with their natural aroma. They can be decorated with ribbons which have been infused with the essential oils of the season. Simply add 6 drops of a Christmas essential oil to 1 cup of water, swish the ribbons around in this and dry them. Holly and ivy decorations can be tied in ribbons infused with bay or a citrus essential oil, which will contribute to the "aroma picture" of Christmas by releasing their gentle aroma. Ribbons for the mistletoe, however, might be more exciting infused in one of the sensual oils.

Oranges studded with cloves are a classic Christmas decoration, as well as an ingredient in certain Christmas punches. We know from experience that a clove-orange used as a decoration won't go bad because clove is a natural preservative, but you can boost the aromatic effect by rolling the oranges beforehand in orange and clove essential oils—and then the oranges will last forever! But why not branch out on this theme: with the essential oils it couldn't be easier. Try adding a drop of cinnamon to the clove-orange essential oil boost. And how about mandarin clove-balls, rolled in mandarin and clove oil; or lemons, limes, and grapefruit, all rolled in their respective oils to ensure maximum aromatic effect.

Store your aromatic decorations separately—by aroma—in sealed plastic bags and their impact will last from year to year. "Christmas" will jump out of the bags when the season rolls around again.

Old-fashioned traditional presents are always welcome and can easily be made by yourself. Indeed, making a whole variety of essential oil presents is literally child's play, and a more creative way to keep the children busy in the weeks leading up to the big day would be difficult to find. There are many suggestions for present-making throughout this book and the Christmas oils can be incorporated into them to make a truly seasonal gift. Besides making your own table decorations of small pine cones impregnated with pine oil, arranged with holly and aromatic ribbons, why not make a few extra to give away.

But first, of course, you have to make your scented wrapping paper. Simply place 2 drops of oil on a cotton-wool ball and leave it in a sealed bag with the wrapping paper overnight. Use a different aroma for different members of the family. Try cedarwood or frankincense for the men, geranium or cinnamon for the women, and lemon or mandarin for the children.

In England, Christmas isn't Christmas without mince pies and even the most traditional recipe for the sweet, spiced mincemeat can be enhanced with a drop of essential oil of orange or lemon. The combination of spices and fruit oils works deliciously and the aroma as the pieces cook will draw everyone to the kitchen.

The essential oils that have been distilled from spices are excellent in various Christmas cakes and desserts. Ginger essential oil in the Christmas pudding or spice cake releases a heavenly aroma and does what you would expect to the flavor —spices it up! Try any of the following in your seasonal dishes:

SPICE OILS FOR CHRISTMAS COOKING

Cinnamon	**Ginger**
Mace	**Nutmeg**
Clove	**Cardamom**

The essential oils can be used in place of the spices in mulled wines too, and there is nothing more welcoming to a winter-chilled guest. Here is just one recipe; the amounts given are for 4 cups of red wine:

Cinnamon	1 drop
Clove	1 drop
Orange	2 drops
Mandarin	2 drops

Blend together in 2 tablespoons honey

Slowly heat the 4 cups of red wine in a nonmetallic pan, add the flavored honey, and stir well while still on the heat. When the wine starts to bubble take it off the heat and serve. Merry Christmas!

Saint Valentine's Day ◆◆◆◆◆◆◆◆◆◆◆◆◆◆◆◆◆◆

When you send a scented Valentine's card, the fragrance is your signature. All you have to do is make sure that you are wearing the same fragrance when you next see your sweetheart for your intentions to be clear. Old lovers can be sent a fragranced Valentine card to ensure that the memory of you lingers on. But do make sure you send a fragrance they will associate with you for the aroma memory to do its trick.

Fragrance and the sense of smell cause a quicker reaction in the brain than any other sense, so when you greet your lover in the evening, make sure you convey your romantic intentions as soon as you open the door. Spray the atmosphere and have arranged around the room scented candles —pink for love. For Valentines with serious matters of the heart in mind, here are the essential oils to use:

SENSUAL OILS FOR SAINT VALENTINE'S DAY

Rose Bulgar	**Jasmine**
Rose Maroc	**Ylang-ylang**
Egyptian rose	**Geranium**

Over your romantic candle-lit dinner, share a bottle of aphrodisiac wine. The recipe for East-West Aphrodisiac Wine in my *Aromantics* (Pan Books, U.K.) is guaranteed to make this year's Saint Valentine's a memorable one! And then exchange presents. Rose-flavored Turkish delight is a traditional gift of romance, but whether the Eastern ladies of the harem incorporated this aphrodisiac flavoring into the sweets to please their Sultan or themselves remains a mystery. You can enhance store-bought Turkish delight by putting 2 drops of rose essential oil on a small gift card and popping it into the box where the aroma molecules will be absorbed by these most sensual of sweets.

Ylang-ylang is a well-known aphrodisiac aroma and it can very simply be infused into chocolates or other sweets to make a special gift. Buy your lover's favorite sweet, something not itself aromatic but bland, like fudge or plain chocolates. Put the loose sweets in a pretty container along with a small piece of absorbent paper on which you have placed a drop of ylang-ylang essential oil and leave them so that the flavor is absorbed. Decorate the sweets with crystallized flowers and package them attractively, wrapped with a big red bow perhaps.

Then you can show each other your appreciation of your gifts by giving each other a romantic massage, using the oils below:

LOVERS' MASSAGE OILS

BLEND 1

Rose	10 drops
Ylang-ylang	2 drops
Lemon	8 drops
Palma rosa	10 drops

Diluted in 2 tablespoons vegetable oil

BLEND 2

Jasmine	10 drops
Nutmeg	5 drops
Black pepper	5 drops
Mandarin	10 drops

Diluted in 2 tablespoons vegetable oil

Or perhaps a bath and bed is all you have in mind, in which case how about using these oils:

LOVERS' BATHS

BLEND 1

Rose	2 drops
Palma rosa	3 drops

BLEND 2

Ylang-ylang	3 drops
Grapefruit	4 drops

The morning after Saint Valentine's night send your lover into the harsh reality of the day with an aide-memoire tucked in their pocket—an aromantic hankie suffused with the perfumes of lovers such as rose, jasmine, or ylang-ylang. As your lover reaches for their key or pen and the aroma wafts up to meet their nose, memories of you will be conveyed in the silent aromantic message of love.

Easter ◆◆◆◆◆◆◆◆◆◆◆◆◆◆◆◆

Whether baking hot cross buns or spice or simnel cake, essential oils in the cooking will add an extra dimension to their taste and a seasonal aroma to your home. Even store-bought hot cross buns can be made extra specially spicy and fruity if you store them in a bag or tin with a half a teaspoon of cinnamon powder to which you have added 1 drop of orange essential oil. Or the essential oil can be put on a small piece of clean, natural material and popped into the container.

Kits for making chocolate eggs, rabbits, and chicks are widely available and made even more delicious if you add to the chocolate the essential oils of orange, lemon, grapefruit, or lime.

Easter is all about life renewing itself and the house will be full of the spring flowers of daffodils, tulips, and crocuses. These do not produce essential oils, but the fresh smelling and spring evoking hyacinth and narcissus do. In your home air sprays aim for a light, fresh aroma or follow my recipe:

SPRING FLOWERS BLEND

Palma rosa	3 drops
Geranium	1 drop
Bois de rose	2 drops

The spicy flavor associated with Easter can be achieved by adding 2 drops of coriander to the above blend. Use these essential oils in any of the room methods around your home. A drop of bois de rose put on a log half an hour before it goes on the fire will give a subtle, fresh aroma to the house.

Gifts may be wrapped in paper that has been left with scented tissues between it. At Easter, use the essential oils of vanilla, cinnamon, lemon, bois de rose, or palma rosa.

Halloween ◆◆◆◆◆◆◆◆◆◆◆

On October 31st each year the witches and spooks have their day. Children love Halloween parties—all that dressing up and game playing bring forth peals of laughter and squeals of delight. Little witches need special cakes and biscuits, of course, and you can make "magic" ones by simply flavoring your favorite recipe with a very small amount of geranium or sandalwood.

The traditional Halloween activities of trick or treat and bobbing for apples—getting an apple out of a bowl of water with just the mouth—can be supplemented with a show of drama and magic. Get a piece of charcoal (the type that is sold in special stores that stock burning incense), place it in a heat resistant dish, light it, and when it has begun to burn put two or three drops of essential oil onto it. Billows of aromatic smoke will issue forth, impressing even the most blasé of little witches or warlocks. Use a heavy oil like patchouli or benzoin or one of the woods, such as cedarwood. These can be lightened up with melissa or verbena. Whatever you do, don't use rue or myrtle—after all, you do want that knock at the door to be a *pretend* witch, don't you? And to scare the witches and spooks away, use frankincense.

Provided that there is adequate adult supervision, candles, which give a magical effect to any decoration, can be fragranced with cedarwood or galbanum or something similarly deep and mysterious.

Fragrant witches' brooms can be made by tying twigs into bundles. Soak the twigs first in a strong woody fragrance such as pine or cypress, or a rooty one like vetiver, diluted in water. These make good souvenir presents for the guests good and bad alike.

ESSENTIAL OILS FOR HALLOWEEN

Cedarwood	**Melissa**
Cypress	**Verbena**
Pine	**Benzoin**
Galbanum	**Patchouli**
Orange	**Sandalwood**
Mandarin	**Vetiver**

Other Celebrations ◆◆◆◆

There are many annual events—New Year's Eve, midsummer festivals, birthdays, and anniversaries—which may be enhanced and made memorable by the use of essential oils. Why not establish your own aroma traditions, to enhance the occasion and act as a reminder and reinforcer of other times spent in having fun and giving thanks. Use your favorite blend in the room methods or on your body, or both, on your birthdays, to mark out the aromatic landscape and say "This day is mine." The same goes for weddings and wedding anniversaries. Make a special blend for the bride and groom and give them the formula so that they can use it in the future on their anniversaries, when it will stimulate clear memories of the happiest day of their lives. On the big day itself, the formula may be used on candles, as a room fragrance at the reception or put on an artificial flower to be taken home as a memento. No doubt you can think of other ways in which to use the unique powers of essential oils to make celebratory days special and ordinary days into celebrations.

Setting the Mood ◆◆◆◆◆

Parties seem to have a life of their own. There are those which fall flat on their faces despite sumptuous food, copious drink, and the largest of high tech hi-fis, and those that are a total wow with just a bowl of potato chips, a few beers, and an old radio. What makes the difference is difficult to define but the answer lies not in the refreshments or surroundings so much as in the people present and their combined mood.

You will already know from other sections of this book that the mood-inducing effects of essential oils are one of their interesting properties, and as you will already have guessed they can have a profound effect upon a group of people gathered at a party. Which particular oils you use depends upon the type of party you are having and the mood you want to create, but with a little experience you will know just the combinations you need to blend an aroma for a jumping Saturday night, a relaxed conversational Sunday afternoon, or a special romantic party for two. These are the oils I suggest you choose from:

RELAXANTS

Geranium	**Jasmine**
Sandalwood	**Ylang-ylang**
Clary-sage	**Hyacinth**
Rose	**Jonquil**
Frankincense	**Narcissus**

STIMULANTS

Grapefruit	**Coriander**
Melissa	**Cardamom**
Mandarin	**Ginger**
Orange	**Black pepper**

FOR ROMANTIC TOUCHES
(Use in small amounts)

Benzoin	**Oakmoss**
Vanilla	**Tonka bean**
Balsam de Peru	**Patchouli**
Ylang-ylang	**Jasmine**
Rose	

These lists could be very much longer but I have only included the oils that are readily available. Each oil is rather like each individual guest in that it has its unique personality to contribute to the whole.

Geranium: Relaxes, creates a good mood; use in small amounts.
Clary-sage: Euphoric, rather masculine, relaxes and encourages conversation; use in small amounts.
Sandalwood: Relaxes and encourages conversation.
Rose: Romantic, special, extravagant.
Ylang-ylang: Oriental, rather heady.

By blending together 2 drops of clary-sage, 2 drops of geranium, and 1 drop of sandalwood you would have a good basis for a warm, relaxed, and happy evening with free-flowing conversation. Add in grapefruit and lemon to refresh and stimulate. Use any of the room methods including heat sources, candles, and flower bowls. In each of these, use 2–4 drops of essential oil and renew as needed. The aroma will act as an olfactory reminder to your guests that it is party time and work through their limic system to bring relaxation and fun, and by taking the little time and forethought necessary to blend the perfect combination of oils for a particular gathering you will ensure that everyone comes away feeling they've had a great time.

Unfortunately, there are people who consider it heroic to go to work or to social engagements when their health is below par, especially during the winter months when colds and flu are so common. And they are common precisely because people go around spreading their viral infections to others. But you can take precautions to ensure that any unwelcome microbe guest gets well and truly dealt with by the antibacterial and antiviral essential oils. Here then are the viral and bacterial bouncers:

THE ANTIVIRAL AND ANTIBACTERIAL PARTY OILS

Lemon	**Clove**
Bergamot	**Pine**
Geranium	**Lavender**
Melissa	**Clary-sage**
Cinnamon	**Rose**

When you use a blend of the above essential oils in the room methods during parties nobody need know that you are protecting them from germs because these essential oils smell so very pleasant. Your guests can just carry on enjoying themselves oblivious to the realistic precautionary measures you have taken on their behalf. There are many possible combinations, but for Christmas parties you might like to try equal parts of cinnamon, clove, and pine. This provides the appropriate seasonal aroma while creating a flu-free zone in your home. Use 2–4 drops of the protective essential oil blends in the room methods, or 6 drops in a plant-spray before the guests arrive. It can also be used when washing the bathroom and toilet. This avoids the smell of disinfectant while providing effective action against bacteria. Here is a formula which gives a terrific aroma while working hard to ensure that your guests have a safe and happy time:

THE BACTERIA BUSTERS PARTY FORMULA

Lemon	3 drops
Bergamot	5 drops
Cinnamon	1 drop
Clary-sage	1 drop
Geranium	5 drops

Toilets can be kept hygienic and fresh smelling for the duration of the party if you prepare a box of essential oil tissues and ask your guests to wipe the toilet seat when they have finished, as a courtesy to the next user. Place 10 drops of essential oil in different places throughout the box of tissues and leave the box sealed overnight so the aroma molecules can permeate all the tissues.

Party Punches ◆◆◆◆◆◆◆◆

Party punches can be hot or cold, alcoholic or nonalcoholic, and essential oils used for their flavoring and aroma make these easy-to-serve drinks very interesting. The oils we use fall into three groups:

ESSENTIAL OILS FOR PARTY PUNCHES

SPICES

Cinnamon	**Coriander**
Clove	**Cardamom**
Nutmeg	

CITRUS FRUITS

Lemon	**Orange**
Lime	**Tangerine**
Mandarin	**Grapefruit**

FLOWERS/HERBS

Geranium	**Rose**
Melissa	**Neroli**
Verbena	

All these essential oils are suitable for inclusion in punches of any type. Hot punches are a wonderfully warming drink after skiing or walking or to greet guests coming in from the cold. But even a simple bottle of wine can be transformed into an extravaganza with a little imagination and the essential oils. The recipes that follow are merely an indication of what can be done.

Hot or Cold Orange Wine

1 bottle red wine
2 cups orange juice
1 drop **coriander** essential oil
1 drop **geranium** essential oil

If served hot, add sugar to taste. If served cold, add ice cubes in which marigold petals have been frozen.

Mandarin Grog

In this variation of the traditional grog recipe, mandarin and mandarin essential oil are substituted for oranges:

6 ounces water
1 bottle red wine
1 bottle port
7 ounces vodka (or brandy)
2 drops **clove** essential oil
1 drop **nutmeg** essential oil
6 drops **mandarin** essential oil
2 mandarins (washed)
2 ounces blanched almonds (flaked)
2 ounces raisins
2 ounces prunes
2 ounces raw cane sugar

Put the water, vodka, essential oils, fruit, and sugar in a large nonmetallic pan. Bring to a boil, then simmer on a low heat for thirty minutes. Add the wine and port and bring to a boil. Take the pan off the heat and allow to stand for at least eight hours. Strain, add the almonds, and reheat, then serve.

Fruit Punch

4½ pounds sliced fruit
4 teaspoons honey
1 bottle brandy
6 bottles white wine
Lemonade to taste
2 drops **melissa** or **lemon** essential oil
Lemon balm and mint

Put the fruit—peaches, apricots, oranges, apples, etc.—in a large bowl, with a few springs of lemon balm and mint. Add the brandy (which does not have to be the best quality) and the honey, and leave to stand overnight. Put in the essential oil and the white wine, then add lemonade to taste and ice cubes in which sprigs of lemon balm and mint have been frozen. Stir well and serve.

Rose Punch

1½ wineglasses brandy
6 bottles rosé wine
1 tablespoon grenadine
6 ounces fresh strawberries (or tinned)
2 quarts lemonade
8 drops **rose** essential oil

Dissolve the essential oil in the brandy and mix with the wine and grenadine. Puree the strawberries, blend in with the lemonade and add this to the wine mixture. Serve with ice cubes in which you have frozen rose buds (wash them beforehand) and decorate the whole beautiful creation by floating your best rose in the bowl.

Overindulgence ♦♦♦♦♦♦♦

Hangovers

Good hospitality is all very well but it can certainly take its toll. Too much alcohol leads to dehydration and results in the miserable sensations which every one of us has surely experienced at least once—nausea, headache, and loss of equilibrium. "Never again," we say, meaning it! To a greater or lesser degree the body is having to cope with poisoning. In this respect there is quite a lot we can do to ensure that we don't feel so bad the next time we have a party. Wines and beers vary enormously in their chemical content. Some are organic, in that their ingredients were not cultivated with chemicals nor were chemicals added in their processing; while others are practically pure chemical. Good quality organic drinks will do far less damage—in terms both of your head the morning after, and of your liver over a longer period of time. You can now buy organic wines at most large food chain stores, but if you can't find them go for the more expensive bottles and most certainly avoid those labeled "From more than one country."

Other preventative measures against hangovers include drinking plenty of water before you drink alcohol, as this slows down the absorption rate and allows the body to cope better. Before going to sleep, take at least 1000mg of vitamin C. (A higher dose, up to 2000mg, will be more effective but may cause diarrhea.) Do not drink black coffee as this will make things worse. Drinking plenty of water after the event will certainly help because it provides something to flush the toxins out of the body, but as the poisons are released you will feel tipsy again until urination and defecation flush them out.

These are the essential oils which will help return the body to its pre-alcoholic state:

THE MORNING AFTER ESSENTIAL OILS

Juniper	**Carrot**
Sandalwood	**Fennel**
Grapefruit	**Rosemary**
Lavender	**Lemon**

You can make your own blends from this list, using a total of 6–8 drops in a bath or 4 drops in an inhalation. The oils do have slightly different effects and you can see their differences by looking at the two formulas below: the first is sedative, the second stimulating.

Apart from flushing the toxins out of the body by the usual elimination methods, sleep is the best remedy for a hangover. For the lucky ones who can take it easy during the morning and even the afternoon after the night before, here is a relaxing blend of oils that will help your body deal with the onslaught that last night went by the name of fun.

THE GENTLE APPROACH
HANGOVER CURE

Fennel	5 drops
Lavender	3 drops
Sandalwood	5 drops
Lemon	10 drops

Blend and bottle, ready for the next emergency

Use 8 drops in a bath, rub 2 neat drops around the liver area, and 2 neat drops on the back of the neck. Drink plenty of water with honey dissolved in it as well as eating a spoonful of honey into which 2 drops of carrot oil have been blended.

For those who have to battle through the rush hour and get to work in the morning after a heavy night of drinking, or get the children organized for school, here is a formula that will give you the necessary stimulation. It also has a diuretic effect. Use in the same way as the formula above, and also drink water and take honey, as above:

THE WORKER'S HANGOVER FORMULA

Grapefruit	10 drops
Rosemary	7 drops
Fennel	4 drops
Juniper	3 drops

Blend and bottle in these proportions

Overeating

It happens every Christmas. We swear that this year we will not pig out and will ignore the table piled high with all manner of goodies. We'll give the boxes of chocolates to the local hospital. We'll just keep it simple—no nuts or candied fruits, no mince pies or Christmas pudding and brandy butter. Really this is all a waste of time because we'll do exactly what we did last year, which is overindulge, and then spend weeks feeling guilty and sick!

The essential oils can no more miraculously dissolve away copious amounts of food than they can turn back the clock. What they can do is facilitate digestion. They do this best in honey teas, but this is a method for adults only. Mix 1 or 2 drops of essential oil into a teaspoon of honey, pop it into a mug, pour hot water onto it, and stir. Sip the drink slowly. These are the essential oils to use:

OVEREATING ESSENTIAL OILS

Lemon	**Spearmint**
Ginger	**Cardamom**
Cumin	**Dill**
Coriander	**Caraway**
Peppermint	**Mandarin**

But why not be realistic and prepare the following formula ready for the party season:

THE PIGGING OUT FORMULA

Mandarin	10 drops
Peppermint	2 drops
Ginger	2 drops
Lemon	5 drops
Coriander	3 drops

Blend together in these proportions and use 1–2 drops in honey tea

Making Presents ◆◆◆◆◆◆

There are many formulas and items made with essential oils described throughout this book that would make ideal presents. Essential oil soaps, bath oils, perfumes, candles, and writing paper make very special presents because in this hurried age the time that goes into their making is a gift in itself. Children who are always looking for something new to do can amuse themselves for hours making presents for family and friends and they don't need the excuse of a birthday or Christmas to give someone a nice surprise.

Scented Beads, Pendants, and Mobiles

Although making papier mâché is child's play, with a little flair and imagination it can be formed into really beautiful objects. When you include essential oil in the making process, the result is lovely aromatic items. Those worn close to the body exude their fragrance in response to body heat, while mobiles gently release their aroma molecules as they are waved by the breeze. How strong the aroma is will depend upon the amount of essential oil you use, and there are four opportunities for adding in the essential oil during the making process: in the flour and water base; to the newspaper itself; on the finished object before it is left to dry; and in the paint used to decorate. By all means, use the fragrant oils in each of these steps.

When making beads, add 1 drop of oil to each bead after it has been rolled into shape. Pendants can be made by molding papier mâché into shapes—how about a heart infused with rose oil and hanging them on pretty ribbons. Mobiles can be of any shape: birds and animals are popular with children. To put the hole into all these, use a warm knitting needle before the papier mâché dries. Of course, papier mâché can be formed into any shape whatsoever, and the beads, brightly colored and smelling divine, can just be piled into a dish to make a very attractive gift.

Bookmarks

All that's needed to make bookmarks is a few bits of colored or decorated paper and most, if not all, children have made a few in their time. They can be made that bit more special, however, if you place a drop of essential oil onto them and pop them into a plastic bag, sealing it and leaving overnight for the aroma to infuse the paper. A bead—a papier mâché or a spicy one—can be strung with ribbon from the top so that it hangs out from the pages of the book.

Spicy Beads

The following recipe makes a paste which is rolled to make small round beads which can be made into necklaces or earrings. The warmer they get, the more they smell. Here I use geranium essential oil but the choice is entirely up to you—use a single oil or a blend of oils to create your own unique fragrance.

1 ounce powdered benzoin (the gum variety)
1 ounce powdered acacia (the gum variety)
½ ounce powdered orris root
½ ounce powdered cinnamon
½ ounce powdered clove
2 drops vanilla essence
½ teaspoon grated nutmeg
2 tablespoons glycerine
10 drops **geranium** essential oil, or essential oil of your choice

Mix all the ingredients together except the essential oils, which should be added in last. This gives you a paste which can be rolled into little balls. Leave them to dry, and when dry enough to handle, make a hole in them and thread them onto a hot metal darning needle. Put them on a tray and leave them to dry.

Neck Pillows and Padded Coat Hangers

These can be made into memorable presents simply by putting a couple of drops of essential oil on them. Rosemary or lavender would make good choices for the pillows and lavender or lemon for the hangers.

Shoe Bags

Shoe fresheners can be made very easily by using essential oils with dried leaves. Crush any type of dried leaf, add 2 drops of essential oil to each handful of leaves, mix well, cover, and leave to dry. Sage oil is a deodorant and a good choice for men who wear sneakers that could sneak off by themselves, while lemon, lemongrass, and lavender would be good choices for the more delicate high heels of the ladies. Put the leaves into small, pretty cotton bags.

Hanging Bags

To keep flies and other flying insects away, use the dried leaf method above to make little bags which can be hung by ribbons. Use lavender, thyme, sage, or citronella essential oils.

Fragranced Wood

Fragranced wood can be used either to freshen and perfume drawers or purely decoratively. Any dried wood will soak up the essential oils, and if the objects are to be used for decoration they can be colored as well. Put the essential oils into a dish of water, colored with food dye if you wish, and let the wood soak in this. Dry it and use your imagination to create interesting, natural set-pieces. Flower arrangers will undoubtedly be able to utilize this method to make permanent shows with dried flowers, grasses, and herbs. If you live by the sea, walking by the shore at low tide may reveal some beautiful worn pieces of wood. But even very small creations can be most impressive—and with the essential oils, aromatically satisfying too.

♦ CHAPTER 16 ♦
COOKING WITH ESSENTIAL OILS

NATURE'S ESSENTIAL OILS can be used in so many ways in the kitchen that it is difficult to know where to begin. Indeed, there is no dish whose flavor is not enhanced by the addition of essential oils, and no limit to the number of new possibilities for culinary delight they open up. Using them is so simple, too. A pepper steak is made into a gastronomic great by mixing a drop of lemon essential oil to the pepper before spreading it on the steak. Vanilla ice cream can be transformed into a Cordon Bleu fantasy by whisking with it any number of essential oils—try ginger, peppermint, or rose.

As flavorants and aromatics essential oils are widely used in the food processing industry, a fact boasted of by advertisers proclaiming that "real fruit essences" or "real oil of . . ." are included in the product. They perhaps more than any of us know that modern large-scale commercial production methods rob the ingredients of much of their natural strength. Essential oils are used to replace the nature that technology took out. But as well as this, the food industry uses the essential oils to create totally new inventions, such as spearmint gum, peppermint drops, or chocolate oranges. If you had a model for making the segments, you too could use orange essential oil to make chocolate oranges, or how about a chocolate lemon, lime, grapefruit, mandarin, or tangerine? When you use essential oils in the kitchen, there is no end to the interesting tastes you can create.

Essential oils for the kitchen come in four main groups—herbs, spices, citrus

THE ESSENTIAL OIL COOKING CHART

	MEAT	CHICKEN	FISH	EGGS	CHEESE	VEGETABLES	RICE
Lemon		◆	◆	◆	◆	◆	◆
Orange	◆	◆	◆	◆	◆		◆
Grapefruit		◆	◆			◆	◆
Lime	◆	◆	◆			◆	◆
Mandarin	◆	◆	◆	◆	◆	◆	◆
Rose		◆		◆	◆		◆
Geranium				◆	◆		◆
Jasmine		◆		◆	◆		◆
Lavender	◆	◆	◆		◆	◆	◆
Ylang-ylang		◆					◆
Cinnamon	◆	◆					◆
Nutmeg	◆	◆		◆		◆	◆
Clove	◆						◆
Cardamom			◆		◆	◆	◆
Coriander		◆	◆				
Peppermint						◆	
Mellisa		◆	◆	◆	◆	◆	◆
Basil	◆	◆	◆		◆	◆	◆
Anis			◆			◆	◆
Dill			◆			◆	◆
Cumin	◆	◆	◆		◆	◆	
Fennel		◆	◆		◆	◆	◆
Ginger	◆	◆		◆		◆	◆
Black pepper	◆	◆	◆	◆		◆	◆
Marjoram	◆	◆	◆				
Rosemary	◆	◆					
Parsley	◆	◆	◆	◆	◆	◆	◆
Thyme	◆	◆					
Sage	◆	◆					

THE ESSENTIAL OIL COOKING CHART

PASTA	DESSERTS	PASTRIES	BREAD	CAKES	SORBETS	ICE CREAM	FRUIT
◆	◆	◆	◆	◆	◆	◆	◆
◆	◆	◆	◆	◆	◆	◆	◆
◆	◆	◆	◆	◆	◆	◆	◆
◆	◆	◆	◆	◆	◆	◆	◆
◆	◆	◆	◆	◆	◆	◆	◆
	◆	◆	◆	◆	◆	◆	◆
◆	◆	◆	◆	◆	◆	◆	◆
◆	◆	◆	◆	◆	◆	◆	◆
◆	◆			◆	◆	◆	◆
◆	◆	◆	◆	◆	◆	◆	◆
◆	◆	◆	◆	◆	◆	◆	◆
◆	◆	◆	◆	◆	◆	◆	◆
◆	◆	◆	◆	◆	◆	◆	◆
◆	◆		◆				◆
◆	◆		◆	◆			◆
	◆	◆		◆	◆	◆	◆
◆					◆	◆	◆
◆							
			◆				◆
◆			◆				◆
			◆				◆
◆							
	◆	◆	◆	◆	◆	◆	◆
◆							

fruits, and flowers. They can be used in soups and starters, in marinades and sauces, with red and white meat dishes, with fish and vegetables, in salad dressings, and in breads, biscuits, cakes, desserts, and confectionery.

The herb essential oils make a delicious contribution to casseroles, either used in a marinade for the meat before cooking or simply added to the pot. These are very strong oils so be careful not to overpower your dish. To enhance the flavor of stir-fry vegetables just one drop of an herb essential oil is sufficient. Added to a bread mixture, the herb oils create marvels—try sage or rosemary bread.

The citrus essential oils may be used in salad dressings, marinades, sauces, and desserts. They also work very well with both fish and poultry: added to a wine marinade lemon adds an excellent flavor to beef. Lemon butter works wonders with vegetables and fish, giving the food a special zing. And talking of butters, try ginger butter on green beans or peas—it must be tasted to be believed!

The purity and clarity of flavor obtained with essential oils is, however, just one of their advantages. They help in the digestion of meat, and although their nutritional value is unknown, they are powerful, pure natural products containing vitamins, nutrients, and trace elements which will certainly do you more good than anything to be found in artificial flavorings. The essential oils also provide natural preventative care with their antibiotic and other medicinal values, as well as having a psychological side to them. Make a geranium soufflé to cheer yourself up; geranium leaves have been used in cooking for hundreds of years, and besides giving you a lift this delicate soufflé tastes sensational.

Not least among the advantages of the essential oils is the fact that they are very economical to use. A few drops of essential oil of lemon will be much cheaper than whole lemons and gives as good a flavor, and you can make an orange-chocolate sauce for ice cream using essential oil that will be far more flavorsome than if it was made with an orange alone. And as you will probably have many of the essential oils in the house already, you can experiment with new culinary ideas without going to any extra expense. Never use too much essential oil: the idea is to enhance the natural flavors of real food, or put flavor into bland packaged foods. Aim for a subtle taste enhancement.

All I aim to do in this chapter is give you some suggestions to get you started on cooking with essential oils. New ideas will come to you as, for example, with the basic mayonnaise recipe, which can easily be converted into countless dips, sauces, garnishings, or dressings.

Dips ◆◆◆◆◆◆◆◆◆◆◆◆◆◆◆◆◆

Basic Mayonnaise

1 egg yolk
½ teaspoon Dijon mustard
¼ teaspoon salt
¼ teaspoon ground black pepper
1 teaspoon wine vinegar
3 ounces (approx.) olive, vegetable, or nut oil

Put the yolk in a bowl and add all the ingredients except the oil. Mix and then start to trickle the oil in very slowly, whisking the mixture continuously with your other hand. Use a fork or hand whisk, gently and always in the same direction. How much oil you use will depend on the size of the egg and how hot or cold the weather is, but carry on adding it very slowly until the sauce is the desired consistency. The type of oil you use will depend on the flavor you want.

Garlic and Lime Dip

4 tablespoons basic mayonnaise
2 cloves crushed garlic
4 drops **lime** essential oil

Crush the garlic with the drops of lime on a board, then mix well with the mayonnaise.

Tomato and Lemon Dip

4 tablespoons basic mayonnaise
1 teaspoon tomato puree
4 drops **lemon** essential oil

Whisk the mayonnaise and tomato puree until it is an even orangy-pink. Add the lemon and mix well. To make the dip more spicy, add 2 drops of Tabasco and freshly ground black pepper.

Fennel Dip

4 tablespoons basic mayonnaise
2 drops **fennel** essential oil

Mix together well. This is an excellent sauce for all fish, but especially oily fish such as herring.

The sauce can easily be adapted to make Fennel and Fish Pâté by mixing with any flaked fish and chopped capers. Garnish and serve with whole grain toast.

Salad Oils and Vinegars ♦♦♦♦♦♦♦♦♦

You can buy the essential oil of herbs for cooking purposes already combined with vegetable oils. To prepare your own, combine 1 drop of essential oil to 2 teaspoons vegetable oil. Use a bland oil such as soya bean, sunflower, or safflower.

The citrus oils of lemon and orange, tangerine or lime, even grapefruit, can be included in salad oils. Use 100 drops of the essential oil or oils of your choice in 4 cups of vegetable oil, shake well and use in your usual way.

Fragrant vinegars play an important part in essential oil cuisine. Essential oils are incorporated into the vinegars at the rate of 1 drop per 2 teaspoons of vinegar.

Use rose or geranium vinegar in dips, vinaigrettes, sauces, and salad dressings; lemon vinegar on fish and fatty meat dishes.

Vinegars store well, but shake them well before use.

Butters, Spreads, and Cheeses ♦♦♦♦♦♦♦♦♦♦

Essential oils may be incorporated into butter to top potatoes, meat, and pastas. The butter stores well and can be frozen.

Leave 4 ounces butter in room temperature until soft, place in a bowl, and add 1 drop of your chosen essential oil, stirring well. Refrigerate and use when needed.

Use 1 drop of essential oil in 8 ounces fromage frais or creamed cheese. Try rose and mandarin fromage frais over strawberries in summer, or orange and grapefruit creamed cheese on a watercress salad.

Appetizers ◆◆◆◆◆◆◆◆◆◆◆

Russian Eggs

6 hard boiled eggs
1 teaspoon chopped green olives
1 teaspoon chopped chives
3 tablespoons basic mayonnaise (see page 344)
1 teaspoon chopped onion
A dash of Tabasco
¼ teaspoon freshly ground black pepper
1 teaspoon chopped parsley
2 drops **lemon** essential oil
1 drop **grapefruit** essential oil

Cut the eggs in half and remove the yolks. Put into a bowl and add all the ingredients except the parsley. Mix well until it forms a paste and spoon back into the egg whites. Arrange on a bed of lettuce and sprinkle the parsley over them.

Orange and Ginger Prawns

1 pound uncooked prawns (king if possible)

Marinade
2 tablespoons soy sauce
2 tablespoons sherry
2 tablespoons vegetable oil
1 clove garlic, crushed
1 small orange, squeezed
2 drops **ginger** essential oil
2 drops **orange** essential oil

Mix all the marinade ingredients and pour over the uncooked prawns. Leave for 1–2 hours. Remove the prawns from the marinade and stir-fry with 1 teaspoon of marinade until cooked. Add the remaining marinade and cook for another 5 minutes.

Serve on a bed of watercress, decorate with orange slices or nasturtium flowers.

Chicken Mint Balls

¾ pound minced chicken meat (or soya substitute)
1 egg, beaten
1 small onion, chopped
2 tablespoons crumbled bread
1 tablespoon parsley
¼ teaspoon cinnamon
¼ teaspoon allspice
Salt and freshly ground black pepper
1 drop **spearmint** essential oil

Stir the onion, parsley, spearmint, cinnamon, allspice, salt, and pepper into the egg, then add the minced chicken and the bread. Stir to an even consistency and place in the fridge until needed.

Roll into bite size balls and fry quickly in a small amount of olive oil.

Serve with black olives and the following dip.

2 tablespoons chopped cucumber
1 cup yogurt
1 drop **spearmint** essential oil
1 drop **lime** essential oil

Combine ingredients and serve in a bowl in which you dip the chicken balls.

Savory Sauces ◆◆◆◆◆◆◆◆◆

Savory sauces can be used to enhance a plain dish or disguise leftovers, or they may just be eaten on their own with fresh chunks of whole grain bread. Once again, the versatility of essential oils can be used to advantage.

Blender Hollandaise Sauce

4 ounces hot melted butter (or substitute)
3 egg yolks
½ teaspoon salt and pepper
4 drops **lemon** essential oil

Put the egg yolks into the blender with your chosen essential oil, salt, and pepper. Blend. Slowly add the hot butter and continue blending for about 10 minutes.

Grapefruit or lime essential oil can also be used.

Green Sauce

2 tablespoons chopped parsley
2 tablespoons chopped watercress
1 tablespoon chopped onion
1 teaspoon chopped capers
1 small potato, boiled
1 clove garlic, crushed
1 tablespoon olive oil
1 teaspoon vinegar
Salt and pepper to taste
4 drops **grapefruit** essential oil
1 drop **orange** essential oil

Combine all the chopped ingredients and the garlic together. Mash the potato in another bowl and add all the oils and vinegar, salt, and pepper. Stir into a smooth paste. Now add the combined chopped mixture and continue stirring for a few moments.

Serve with cold meats, vegetables, and pasta. Green sauce can be added to yogurt and served over boiled or baked potatoes.

Lime and Mint Sauce

The combination of lime and mint add freshness of flavor to summer vegetables, pulses, and rice dishes.

4 tablespoons olive oil
1 teaspoon mustard
1 teaspoon chopped parsley
1 teaspoon chopped chives
1 tablespoon chopped mint
4 drops **lime** essential oil

Mix the olive oil and lime essential oil together. Add the remaining ingredients and blend well. Warm slowly over low heat if required hot.

Marinades ♦♦♦♦♦♦♦♦♦♦♦♦

In the days before refrigeration, spicing meats was a way of preserving food in preparation for the long cold winter ahead. These days marinating meat is no longer a necessity, but is used to add flavor and to tenderize cheaper cuts of meat.

Red Meat Marinade

Enough for 2 pounds of beef:

1 cup red wine
1 drop **thyme** essential oil
1 drop **marjoram** essential oil
1 drop **clove** essential oil
2 tablespoons olive oil
2 cloves garlic
1 chopped onion
A pinch of salt
¼ teaspoon whole black peppercorns
1 drop **orange** essential oil

Blend the thyme, marjoram, and clove oils in the olive oil.

Pour the red wine into a dish large enough to hold your meat and add the garlic, onion, and orange oil. Rub 1 tablespoon of the blended oil over the meat then place the meat in the red wine. (Keep the second tablespoon for another time.) Leave the meat covered for eight hours, turning once or twice.

Cook in your favorite way, using the marinade to make a sauce.

Fresh Tuna Marinade

Enough for 1 pound fresh tuna:

1 cup dry white wine
1 clove garlic
1 small onion, sliced
1 tablespoon olive oil
A pinch of salt
¼ teaspoon whole black peppercorns
1 drop **lime** essential oil
1 drop **fennel** essential oil

Pour the white wine into a dish large enough to hold the tuna and add garlic, onion, salt, and pepper. Mix the lime and fennel oils with the olive oil and rub this into the tuna, then place in the white wine. Leave covered for 3–6 hours. Grill or poach the tuna and use the marinade for a sauce.

Soups ◆◆◆◆◆◆◆◆◆◆◆◆◆◆◆◆◆◆

Avocado and Lime Soup

2 ripe avocados
1 small onion, chopped
5 ounces plain yogurt
5 ounces milk (or soya milk)
1 clove garlic, crushed
1 vegetable stock cube
1 cup water
A pinch of salt
Freshly ground black pepper
2 drops **lime** essential oil

Blend, by hand or in a blender, the avocados, onion, yogurt, milk, garlic, and lime essential oil.

Dissolve stock cube in the water and bring to a boil. Reduce to a simmer and slowly add the blended mixture, stirring all the time. Bring gently back to a boil and serve.

Basil, Tomato, and Potato Soup

1 pound chopped tomatoes
1 pound potatoes, peeled and diced
2 onions, finely chopped
2 ounces butter
2 cups water
1 teaspoon sugar
2 teaspoons yogurt
Salt and pepper
2 drops **basil** essential oil

Melt the butter in a pan, add the onion and cook until soft. Add tomatoes, cook until soft. Add water and bring to a boil. Now add the potatoes, sugar, salt, and pepper. Simmer for 15 minutes.

Combine the yogurt and basil essential oil, leave to stand. Sieve the soup and bring back to a boil. Stir in the yogurt and basil. Serve.

Mandarin and Carrot Soup

1 pound carrots, grated
1 large potato, grated
1 small onion, chopped
1 ounce butter
2½ cups vegetable stock
Salt and pepper
4 drops **mandarin** essential oil

Melt the butter in a heavy pan, add the carrots, potato, salt, and pepper. Stir and leave on a low heat for 10 minutes, covered. Add the stock and bring to a boil. Now add the essential oil of mandarin and reduce to a simmer for 10 minutes. Sieve and return to the heat, serving when thoroughly hot.

An easy way to use essential oils in soups is to combine them with the oil, butter, or margarine used to sauté meats or vegetables before turning into soup, or blend them with yogurt or cream before adding to the soup.

Vegetables ♦♦♦♦♦♦♦♦♦♦♦♦

Vegetables benefit from the addition of essential oils in vinegars, oils, butters, and sauces. The basic mayonnaise recipe (see page 344) can be adapted for many uses by the addition of purees and essential oils.

Potato Salad

2 pounds new potatoes
4 tablespoons basic mayonnaise
1 tablespoon chopped chives
1 small onion, finely chopped
5 drops **lemon** essential oil
1 drop **spearmint** essential oil

Boil the potatoes and leave to cool.

Blend the essential oils and use 2 drops of the blend, mixing with the mayonnaise, chives, and onions.

Pour over the potatoes, chill and serve.

Steamed Green Beans

2 pounds green beans
4 tablespoons basic mayonnaise
1 tablespoon flaked almonds
1 drop **ginger** essential oil

Steam the beans. Combine the mayonnaise with 1 drop of ginger essential oil and blend well. Pour over the beans and decorate with almonds.

Stir-Fry Vegetables

Any vegetables may be stir-fried using the essential oils. Ginger oil is excellent, as are the spices cardamom, cumin, and mace—1 drop to 1 tablespoon of cooking oil.

Steamed Vegetables

Steam your vegetables over water to which an essential oil of your choice has been added. Nutmeg, mace, and lemon are particularly good for cabbage and greens, but try the flower oils too, such as geranium and lavender.

Sweet Vegetables

Sweet potatoes, swedes, and beets can all be used with essential oils to make interesting and unusual dishes.

Tangerine or mandarin essential oils blend particularly well with sweet potatoes as a dessert.

Tangerine Sweet Potato

1 pound sweet potatoes
2 ounces butter (or substitute)
3 tablespoons brown sugar
1 tablespoon chopped walnuts
2 tablespoons rum or cooking sherry
6 drops **tangerine** essential oil

Boil and mash the sweet potatoes. Cream the butter and sugar and add the essential oil of tangerine and rum or sherry if desired. Pour over the potatoes and mash together.

Place in an ovenproof dish and sprinkle with walnuts. Heat in a moderate oven, and serve.

You may replace the essential oil of tangerine with that of mandarin if you prefer.

Lemon or Orange Pepper

Lemon pepper is a delicious substitute for conventional pepper. Use it in any dish that you feel would be enhanced by a zing of lemon—fish and salads are special favorites of mine.

Put 1 ounce of coarsely ground pepper into a small bowl and add 2 drops of lemon oil. Mix together and bottle for at least three days before use.

Orange pepper is made in exactly the same way, using orange oil instead of lemon.

Fish ◆◆◆◆◆◆◆◆◆◆◆◆◆◆◆◆◆◆

White fish steaks can be brushed with a prepared cooking oil before grilling. Lemon, fennel, dill, grapefruit, and lime essential oils are all interesting additions to the flavor of white fish. Using 1 drop of essential oil to 1 tablespoon of vegetable oil, prepare your cooking oil with the essential oil of your choice. Then simply brush your fish steak with the oil and grill in the normal way. Turn the steaks and repeat the process.

Fatty fish such as mackerel are exceptionally good with essential oils. Herring combines very well with essential oil of lemon and lime.

Baked Mackerel

2 mackerel, cleaned and prepared
1 grated apple
1 teaspoon chopped parsley
1 tablespoon fresh bread crumbs
1 small onion, cut in rings
1 glass apple juice
3 drops **orange** essential oil

Combine the apple, parsley, and essential oil of orange with the bread crumbs. Stuff the mackerel with equal amounts of stuffing and place the onion rings on top of the stuffing. Put the fish in an ovenproof dish and pour the apple juice over the fish. Bake for 20 minutes in a medium hot oven.

Lemon Sole and Almonds

2 fillets of sole
1 tablespoon vegetable oil
3 drops **lemon** essential oil
1 tablespoon flaked almonds
Salt and pepper

Blend the vegetable oil, essential oil of lemon, salt, and pepper together and brush over the fillets on both sides. Drain off excess oil, sprinkle with almonds, and grill.

Meat ◆◆◆◆◆◆◆◆◆◆◆◆◆◆◆◆◆

When cooking red meat, the essential oil should be combined with vegetable oil and brushed over the meat: 1 drop of essential oil to 1 tablespoon of vegetable oil is sufficient. Many essential oils are sold in this fashion ready to add to stews, casseroles, and sauces. Rosemary, basil, thyme, sage, bay, paprika, coriander, cardamom, and marjoram can all be used for this purpose.

Soya protein may be substituted for meat in all the recipes.

Garlic Lamb

Soak 4 cloves of garlic in 1 teaspoon of olive oil and 1 drop of rosemary essential oil for 30 minutes. Using a sharp pointed knife, pierce the meat and insert the cloves of garlic. Depending on the cut, the meat may be roasted, grilled, or braised.

Spiced Garlic Beef

Soak 4 cloves of garlic in 1 teaspoon of olive oil and 1 drop each of orange, nutmeg, and cinnamon oils. Prepare as for the garlic lamb.

Minced Beef or Lamb

Minced beef or lamb dishes can incorporate various types of essential oils, as can soya protein recipes. Use 1 drop per 1 pound of meat. Add the essential oil to the cooking oil when starting the mince.

Honeyed Chicken

4 tablespoons honey
2 drops **lemon** essential oil
2 drops **orange** essential oil
1 glass white wine or cider
1 medium chicken
1 small orange
1 lemon
4 ounces plain yogurt
2 ounces butter (or substitute)

Add the oils of lemon and orange to the wine or cider and honey and store until needed.

Place washed whole orange and lemon inside the cleaned chicken. Smear the butter over the chicken and roast as usual for 45 minutes. Remove the chicken and brush the honey mixture all over the chicken. Return to the oven until cooked, basting frequently.

After removing the chicken from the roasting dish, strain the remaining liquid into a small saucepan and place over a low heat. Stir in the yogurt and add salt and pepper to taste.

Grilled Chicken

4 tablespoons honey
2 teaspoons mustard
2 drops **lemon** essential oil
2 drops **orange** essential oil

Stir all the ingredients into a smooth paste and brush over the chicken before grilling.

Desserts ◆◆◆◆◆◆◆◆◆◆◆◆◆◆

The essential oils of flowers can do much to enhance the fragrance and taste of desserts.

Rice Pudding

By the addition of essential oils you can lift a traditional rice pudding out of the ordinary and into the extraordinary. Try adding 1 drop of palma rosa to your favorite recipe.

Egg Custard

Baked egg custards and other sweet egg dishes respond particularly well to the flavors of orange, tangerine, and mandarin. Add 1 drop per 1 cup of liquid.

Chocolate Mousse

Add 1 drop of peppermint, lime, mandarin, lemon, orange, or ylang-ylang essential oils. For a romantic mousse, use 1 drop of rose or 1 drop of lime essential oil to 2½ cups of mousse.

Soufflé

The beauty of using essential oils in soufflés is that you can achieve the flower fragrance without the risk of the soufflé sinking. Use 1 drop of your chosen oil per 2½ cups of liquid.

Crêpes

Add 2 drops of essential oil, fruit or flower, per 2½ cups of batter.

Dessert Sauces

Use 2 drops of essential oils per 1 cup of liquid for a sauce to transform any pudding.

Custards

Use 2 drops of essential oil per 1 cup of custard.

Fruit Puree

Use 1 drop per 1 cup of puree. The essential oils of geranium, rose, and orange complement the flavor of apple.

Frozen Desserts ◆◆◆◆◆◆

Sorbets

Here we are looking at a strongly flavored dessert sorbet, not the palate cleanser served between courses. This citrus sorbet also makes a wonderful addition to a hot summer's day.

Citrus Sorbet

2½ cups water
6 ounces sugar
1 egg white
Fruit as desired
2 drops **lemon** essential oil
2 drops **grapefruit** essential oil
2 drops **lime** essential oil

You can use fruit or not for this recipe, as you please. I prefer to use fruit for its texture: it may be any fruit I happen to have. Strawberries are excellent, as are raspberries, black currants, lemon, or grapefruit.

Boil the sugar, water, and essential oil for 10 minutes. Cool, then partially freeze. Remove from the freezer and beat the mixture until soft and mushy. Beat the egg white until stiff. Add your fruit, if required, to the frozen mixture and fold in the egg white. Refreeze for about 4 hours.

Any essential oil can be used in a basic sorbet mix. When using the flower oils, try decorating with petals. Tangerine or mandarin sorbet is delicious served in its own fruit shells.

Ice Cream

Making your own ice cream ensures that you get exactly what you want. You can cheat if you wish though by buying ready made ice cream and mixing in the essential oil of your choice: to a half pound block add 2 drops of essential oil. Tangerine or mandarin make an interesting combination with chocolate ice cream. And how about peppermint or spearmint?

An old-fashioned ice cream mix was made from a custard, using large amounts of cream, eggs, and sugar, much too rich for the taste of most of us today. Here are two recipes, one traditional and one modern.

Traditional

6 eggs
1 cup castor sugar
2½ cups cream
6 drops essential oil
3 ounces fruit or chocolate

Modern

4 egg yolks
¼ cup castor sugar
1 cup milk
5 ounces cream
2 ounces fruit or chocolate
6 drops essential oil

Beat the eggs or egg yolks with sugar, add a little milk or cream. Heat the remaining milk or cream, but do not boil. Take off the heat and stir slowly into the egg mix. When thoroughly mixed return to a low heat. If you are using the milk and cream recipe, gently fold the cream into the mixture when cool. For both versions now add the essential oils and fruit, or nuts, coffee, and anything else you would like to include at this point. Cool and freeze.

Geranium Cream

1 cup cream
4 tablespoons sugar
8 ounces cream cheese or fromage frais
4 drops **geranium** essential oil

Heat the cream, sugar, and geranium oil together; leave to cool. When the mixture is cold beat into it the fromage frais or cream cheese, then freeze. This cream may be eaten on its own or used to top cheese cakes or fruit.

Frozen Yogurt

Essential oils can be added to the yogurt before freezing. Use 1 drop per 1 cup of yogurt.

Cakes ◆◆◆◆◆◆◆◆◆◆◆◆◆◆◆◆

Since the essential oils will not clash with any of the ingredients they can be incorporated into any cake recipe. A plain sponge cake can be turned into an extravagant and exotic cake just by adding essential oils during preparation. During cooking much of the fragrance escapes, leaving a very subtle flavor.

If you want a stronger fragrance or flavor, use essential oils in the creams or toppings and they will permeate the whole cake. This recipe can be used with white or whole grain flour.

Vera's Sponge Cake

1 cup self-rising flour (do not use baking powder)
1 cup sugar
1 cup soft butter (or substitute)
4 eggs
2 tablespoons warm water
2 drops **orange** essential oil

Cream the butter and sugar. Add the eggs one at a time and beat well until mixture is stiff and uniform. Add the water and orange oil. Fold in the flour with a spoon. Divide the mixture and pour into two buttered and floured sandwich tins. Bake in the center of the oven at 350° Fahrenheit for 25 minutes.

Butter Icing

4 ounces soft butter (or substitute)
6 ounces sifted icing sugar
4 drops **orange** essential oil

Beat butter and sugar to a soft, fluffy cream. Add 4 drops of orange oil and beat well.

The cream may be used for filling and top icing, and any of the following essential oils may be substituted for the orange —rose, lemon, jasmine, geranium, or grapefruit.

Choco-mint Cake

6 ounces soft butter (or substitute)
6 ounces sugar
3 eggs
1 tablespoon warm water
4 ounces self-rising flour
½ teaspoon natural vanilla extract
6 drops **peppermint** essential oil
2 ounces chocolate or carob powder

Cream the butter and sugar, beat in the eggs. Add water slowly, then the flour. Blend in vanilla, peppermint oil, and chocolate or carob powder. Divide and pour into two sandwich tins. Bake for 25 minutes at 350°. Use peppermint filling with grated chocolate.

Emma's Carrot Cake

3 eggs
3 large carrots, grated
1 cup brown sugar
1 teaspoon orange juice
2 ounces ground almonds
2 ounces self-rising flour
3 drops **orange** essential oil

Separate the egg yolks and beat well. Place the grated carrots in a pan of boiling water and cook for 5 minutes; take off the heat and drain. Combine the carrot, egg yolks, and sugar, and mix well. Slowly add the orange juice and the orange essential oil, then the almonds and the flour. Beat the white of the eggs until stiff, and fold into the cake mix. Pour the mix into a greased cake tin and bake at 325° for about 40 minutes. Test with a skewer.

Bread and Pastry ♦♦♦♦♦

The essential oils may be added to bread dough just before baking. Use 1 drop per 4 ounces of dough. To make orange and cinnamon bread, for example, add 4 drops of orange and 1 drop of cinnamon oil to 16 ounces dough.

Included in a basic pastry mix, the essential oils add spice, citrus, or flower fragrance as desired. Use 1 drop per 2 ounces of pastry.

Flower and Herb Syrups ♦♦♦♦♦♦♦♦♦♦♦♦♦♦♦

These syrups are simply made and are reminiscent of Elizabethan times. They can be used in puddings and drinks, as toppings, and as remedies. Rose syrup, for example, can ease a sore throat, and peppermint helps indigestion. To make a true syrup, you need flowers as well as essential oils.

Flowers or herbs to fill a pint jar
3 drops essential oil
1 pound sugar
2½ cups water

Add your freshly picked flowers to the water, bring to a boil. Turn down the heat and simmer for 10 minutes. Leave to cool for a further 10 minutes, then strain and top up the water level to reach 2½ cups. Heat the sugar and water together, slowly stirring until the mixture thickens—the longer it cooks, the thicker the syrup. Add to the syrup the essential oils and a few more flowers for effect. Pour into jars and store.

Choose your flowers to complement the essential oil—lavender flowers with lavender essential oil, for example.

Honey and Sugar ◆◆◆◆◆

Fragrant honeys are useful in both the kitchen and the medicine chest. They can be used as drinks, spread on toast, or used in any recipe that calls for honey. In a pound jar of honey, stir 3 drops of essential oil. Flower petals can be added to clear honey for the effect.

Sugar absorbs fragrance very well. Do not drop essential oils directly into the sugar, but place 2 drops on a piece of paper towel and leave this in the sugar jar. Leave for at least twenty-four hours before using. Try ylang-ylang, lavender, lemon or orange.

Aromatic Petals ◆◆◆◆◆◆◆

Crystallized petals make wonderful decorations for cakes and desserts. Gum arabic is often used, but I like to use egg white, although this cannot be stored as long as other methods.

Beat the egg white until stiff, pour into an egg cup and add 1 drop of essential oil. Dip the clean petals in the mixture then place them on a wire tray to dry, sprinkling well with castor sugar.

Fragrant Flower Jams ◆◆◆◆◆◆◆◆◆◆◆◆◆◆◆◆◆◆

To make a flower jam, choose soft-petaled flowers or herbs (lavender and rosemary, for example, will leave tough particles in the jam).

1 pound flowers or herbs
1 pound sugar
5 ounces rosewater or orange flower water
2 drops essential oil

Heat the sugar and water until you have a syrup, then add the petals or leaves. Simmer for 5 minutes, then include your choice of essential oil. Leave the mixture to simmer gently on a low heat for 45 minutes, stirring occasionally. Pour into clean small jars and store.

Jams made of fruit can also have the essential oils incorporated into them. Some good combinations are strawberry and rose, raspberry and lemon, plum and orange, orange and neroli—the combinations are endless and need no more than a little imagination.

Jellies ◆◆◆◆◆◆◆◆◆◆◆◆◆◆◆◆

Jellies make an interesting accompaniment to all manner of meat, fish, and vegetable dishes. Flower jellies can be used in pies and cakes, or melted to use as topping, or in drinks. The following is a basic jelly which you can adapt as you please. Suggestions for accompanying dishes are listed below.

1 pound apples
1 pound sugar
1 cup water
Flowers or herbs to fill a pint jar

Cut the apple, including the peel, into small pieces. Place in a pan with the water. Simmer gently until reduced to a pulp. Strain the pulp in a jelly bag for 8–10 hours, measure the liquid and top up to 2½ cups with water. Add the sugar and stir over a low heat until the sugar melts, then add the flowers or herbs. Bring to a boil, stirring all the time—do not allow to burn. Continue boiling until the jelly starts to set, then add 3 drops of essential oil to complement the flowers or herbs used. Pour into jars and store.

Basil: cold meat, tomato dishes, pasta, salads
Fennel: fish, vegetables, poultry
Dill: fish, poultry, vegetables
Parsley: vegetables, grains, poultry, red meat
Rosemary: lamb, poultry, vegetables
Jasmine: fatty meats, oily fish, curries, desserts
Lavender: meat, vegetables
Melissa: poultry, fish, vegetables
Geranium: meat, rice, curries
Rose: meat, poultry, vegetables, rice
Spearmint: meat, vegetables

Bircher Muesli ◆◆◆◆◆◆◆◆

Authentic muesli is not the dehydrated cereal and fruits you will find in a packet on a supermarket shelf, but a delicate mixture of oats, grated fresh apple, nuts, and fruits, that is rich and creamy, with or without milk. For each person you will need:

- 1 tablespoon oats
- 3 tablespoons water or apple juice
- 1 tablespoon evaporated milk or soya milk
- 1 tablespoon grated or whole nuts
- 1 large grated apple with the peel
- 1 drop **lemon** essential oil

Soak the oats overnight in the apple juice or water, in the refrigerator. Before breakfast, grate the apple and add with the rest of the ingredients, sprinkling the nuts on top if you prefer.

Other fruits in season may be added, as well as yogurt, but the base is always the same.

The combination of apples and oats can help to lower cholesterol, as well as assist the body in the removal of heavy metals, such as lead and radioactive strontium. As part of a whole food diet, this recipe can help protect against arthritis and rheumatism.

Nut Milks ◆◆◆◆◆◆◆◆◆◆◆◆

Nut milks are delicious and nutritious. They can be used in cereals, in puddings, or as a base for drinks or sauces.

Almond Milk

- 2 tablespoons almonds
- 1 teaspoon honey
- 5 ounces water

Mix the almonds and the honey in a blender. Add the water and leave to stand for one hour. Strain.

The same recipe can be used for milks of sesame seed, pistachio, and hazelnut.

♦ CHAPTER 17 ♦ NATURAL HEALTH FOR DOMESTIC ANIMALS

BESIDES THE IMPROVED good health of your pets, there are additional advantages to be gained by using nature's essential oils in their care. Essential oils aren't expensive and you can often use an oil you happen to have in the house already—thus saving on veterinary charges and commercial pet care products. And pets provide living proof that the effectiveness of the essential oils isn't due to supposed psychological factors.

Dogs ♦♦♦♦♦♦♦♦♦♦♦♦♦♦♦♦♦♦

Dogs have a very good instinct for the essential oils and even seem to know what is good for them. If you put an oil that is digestive on one hand, and a pesticide oil on the other, a dog with a stomach upset will invariably come forward to lick the hand that will do him most good. Remember though that dogs have a much stronger sense of smell than humans, so generally aim to use a minimum quantity of essential oil and increase the quantities if and when necessary. It is thought that dogs have about 200 million olfactory receptors, perhaps twenty times the number we have.

The essential oils discourage the fleas, ticks, and other minute parasites for which dogs seem inevitable homes. If you shampoo your dog, one of the easiest ways to deal with this problem is to add 1 drop of either lemongrass or citronella oil to his shampoo. Large dogs like Great Danes will require 2 drops. Most dogs seem to like the aroma, and it gives them a nice fresh smell.

Fleas can be as much of a problem for the rest of the household as for your dog. Here is a remedy that will not only get rid of fleas and other parasites but will keep your dog's coat in good condition too. The essential oils don't disturb the natural oil balance of your dog's skin and coat and will do him nothing but good. Take an old steel brush and a piece of material the same size as the face of the brush. The material needs to be quite thick so a single piece of towel or sheet folded three or four times will do. Pull the material down over the teeth of the brush so that it lies about 1 inch above the base, depending on the length of your dog's hair. Prepare a bowl of warm water and mix in 4 drops of cedarwood or pine oil and soak the prepared brush in this before brushing your dog's coat. This treatment will disinfect the dog, condition the coat, and collect the parasites and eggs in the brush—which must be rinsed out thoroughly several times during the brushing, in the bowl of essential oil water.

If your dog is suffering seriously from fleas or other parasites, put 4 drops of cedarwood or lavender oil directly onto a piece of material, as above, and rub the material together to disperse the oil before putting it on the brush. Then use with plain warm water and rinse several times while brushing the dog. (See also Flea Collars, page 361.)

If your dog is cut or grazed, bathe the area in a water solution of thyme or lavender oil. Use 6 drops of either essential oil to half a gallon of water. The essential oils will help clean the wound as they are natural antibiotics and disinfectants, and you can rest assured that if the dog licks the wound afterwards he won't be taking in any unnatural substances.

It is very important to ensure that all dirt is removed from a cut, but as animals are difficult to confine to bed until healing is complete, you may have to keep attending to the wound. If an animal has a wound which has become ulcerous and weeps pus, the first stage in treatment is to draw away from the wound as much infection as possible. At this stage essential oils applied directly onto the wound would make it heal too quickly and if there was still infection inside this would clearly lead to further problems. So to draw out the toxins we use the cabbage leaf treatment (see page 96). Wrap an ironed leaf around the wound, secure firmly, and change the leaf four to six times in one day, or until all the toxins have been drawn off. Now wash the wound thoroughly in a solution of 4 drops of lavender oil to 5 ounces warm water. This is an extremely effective method of treating bad wounds and can be applied to any animal—dog or cat, horse or donkey, sheep or cow.

Dogs suffer from coughs, colds, and flu, just as we do, and the best essential oils for them in these circumstances are niaouli, tea tree, and eucalyptus. You can use two methods—one oil-based and the other water-based—but in either case, have respect for your dog's greater sense of smell and start treatment with the minimum quantity of essential oil, increasing the dose slowly if necessary. The following rub should be applied over the chest, all around the rib cage, around the throat and, most importantly, in a direct line from the ears into the shoulders. For the oil-based treatment, add 2 drops each of any two essential oils mentioned above to 2 tablespoons vegetable oil. Some people don't like the idea of putting oil on a dog's coat, and with long-haired pets one can see their point. So for them, make a "mother tincture" by adding 2 drops of essential oil to 1 teaspoon of alcohol (vodka, brandy, etc.) and then adding this to 6 teaspoons of water. You will need to make a large quantity because this, like the oil-based treatment, needs to be applied twice a day for three days. If your dog is very sick, eucalyptus oil can be used neat and applied lightly to the areas mentioned, for a few days only.

You should also treat the area where the dog sleeps to get rid of the bacteria and viruses lurking there. Blankets can be washed in the essential oils, and depending on the size of the blanket 5–6 drops should do the job. If you are washing the sleeping area, add 6 drops of essential oil to half a bucket of warm water. Alternatively, you can use an essential oil and water dilution in a plant-spray around the area. A good formula would be 6 drops of hyssop and 6 drops of eucalyptus oil to 2½ cups water.

Arthritis is as painful to dogs as to people, so be careful when treating them. Having said that, however, dogs generally love to be massaged and a dog with arthritis will both enjoy and benefit from the following treatment:

ARTHRITIC DOG TREATMENT

Rosemary	4 drops
Lavender	2 drops
Ginger	3 drops

Diluted in 2 tablespoons vegetable oil

Try to get the oil onto the affected joints by working through the coat and into the skin. Starting at the back, massage into the muscles in rhythmic movements working inward from the haunches. Cover the whole of the legs and also the vertebrae. Don't worry about this being messy—your dog will soon lick much of the oil off but by then the correct amount of essential oil will have penetrated the skin and got into the affected tissue and bone—and by the licking it will also reach the digestive system. The cabbage leaf method mentioned earlier will also help tremendously: apply the leaf while it is warm and replace after an hour, repeating several times. Half a teaspoon of white clay in your dog's water will help absorb toxins from the intestine.

Dogs often suffer from ear wax which becomes smelly and offensive. The wax needs removing and the ear deodorizing and disinfecting. One of the best essential oils to use for this is lavender. Dilute 3 drops of lavender in 1 teaspoon of witch hazel and insert at least 4 drops into each ear. This can be done by using a soaked piece of cotton wool if you do not have a dropper. Gently massage the whole ear and repeat this procedure daily to soften the wax. It can then be removed with cotton wool.

Dribbling and bad breath often indicate that the dog has dental problems. Dogs' teeth should be checked regularly and cleaned. Common baking soda (sodium bicarbonate) and essential oils provide a great way to keep teeth clean and fresh and help to remove tartar. If tartar is a problem, include dried food in your dog's diet.

DOGS' TOOTHPASTE
AND BREATH DEODORIZER

Baking soda	2 tablespoons
Clove	1 drop
Aniseed	1 drop

Make up the toothpaste and use as needed, with cotton wool rather than a toothbrush to avoid damaging the gums. Dampen the cotton wool, dip it into the mixture, and use on the teeth. Afterwards, give the dog a drink of water.

Bad breath that is not caused by teeth or gums indicates a stomach problem. Peppermint oil is excellent to use here, not because it's a mouth freshener but because it's an intestinal cleanser and an aid to digestion. Rub a drop of neat peppermint in a line from beneath the ears and into the shoulders.

Diet

Dogs and cats fed on tinned food may not be hungry but could well be deficient in vitamins and minerals. We can help them nutritionally by giving them bonemeal for calcium, kelp and alfalfa for beneficial minerals, dolomite for nerves and fretfulness, brewers' yeast for vitamin B and trace elements, and dried liver tablets. Cod liver oil two or three times a week will give the coat a shining gleam and provide vitamins A and D, but do not give more than 2 or 3 drops each time. Good health is very much a matter of good nutrition for animals, as it is for humans.

Cats ◆◆◆◆◆◆◆◆◆◆◆◆◆◆◆◆◆◆

Cats not only make good pets, they can also help our health. Studies by Dr. Erika Friedmann and others have shown that stroking a cat has a calming effect on the nervous system and lowers blood pressure. People who have had a heart attack lengthen their chances of survival if they own a pet. And cats love the attention too.

But no matter how much we love our cats, they can be aggravating, to say the least, when they ruin the furniture with their scratching. Cats who do this are working towards shedding their nails and making way for the new ones, and also adding their scent to yours. To prevent this, make a scratching post from any old piece of wood and put essential oil of valerian on it. The oil of valerian sends cats into the height of ecstasy, as does the root of the valerian plant. Cats adore cat mint too, and if you have a patch of it in your garden they will roll in it with great pleasure.

Treat arthritis and fleas in cats in the same way as described for dogs. Cats often get abscesses, usually as a result of a hectic night on the prowl. To treat an abscess put neat tea tree essential oil onto it to bring it to a head. As the cat licks the fur he will ingest the oil which will also help to clear the abscess up. After it has burst and all the pus has been discharged, apply lavender oil to speed up healing.

Cats suffer from coughs and bronchitis and these can be treated in much the same way as you would humans, massaging along the back and on the chest with 4 drops of eucalyptus oil once a day until it clears.

Canker of the ear is another problem that cats encounter, one form of which is eczematous, and the other due to a parasite. The scratching can cause a sore and infection can set in. The ear will feel hot and there could be a discharge of wax. Try to clean the ear if possible. To prevent a sore from forming from the scratching, warm a teaspoon of olive oil to which you have added 1 drop each of chamomile and lavender essential oils, insert a small amount into the ear, and also rub it around the ear. Canker is contagious and must be treated.

For any kind of bacterial or viral infection turn to the Bacteria Busters list on page 386 and use these oils on the chest, back, and neck of the cat, as you would for a child.

Cats will eat grass to induce the vomiting they need to bring up hair that collects in them as a result of their constant grooming. If your cat is off its food, a hairball could well be the problem. Two teaspoons of olive oil in its food will help it until the hairball is passed or vomited. To prevent a buildup of hair, add a small amount of olive oil to your cat's food on a fairly regular basis.

Mange is contagious and all the bedding should be treated or thrown out. Cover the cat as much as is possible in water to which

3 drops each of lavender and tea tree have been added. Chamomile essential oil could be used as well. Although the cat may not be too happy about the idea, try to coat the whole of its skin in this solution.

Flea Collars

Most commercially sold flea collars are made with highly toxic chemicals which can be absorbed through the skin of our pets, and us. Cats often cannot bear being near these as they try desperately to lick and groom the area surrounding the collar, only increasing the level of chemicals absorbed.

Fleas spend only about one-eighth of their life on an animal, so if the flea has gained entrance into your home via your pet the remaining seven-eighths of its life will be spent in your pet's bedding or on your carpet and furniture. Contrary to popular belief, fleas prefer walking to hopping about on their powerful legs, so spotting them isn't just a matter of waiting to see a little high-jumper.

An essential oil collar provides excellent protection against fleas and is very cheap and easy to make. Buy a soft material collar—a cheap one from a market will do—and soak it in the following mixture:

Alcohol	½ teaspoon
Cedarwood	1 drop
Lavender	1 drop
Citronella	1 drop
Thyme	1 drop

Mix with

4 garlic capsules

or

2 drops of the following mixture:
1 teaspoon vegetable oil in which
1 drop garlic essential oil has been diluted

If you are using the garlic capsules, break them open and add the contents to the mixture. Blend your ingredients together and pour it over the collar until fully absorbed. Leave to dry before putting around your pet's neck. It should be effective for one month.

Blood is the fleas' only food, but when garlic is detected in it they will leave well alone. Add 1 or 2 capsules of garlic to your pet's diet during spring and summer, depending on its size.

Rabbits ◆◆◆◆◆◆◆◆◆◆◆◆◆◆◆

In the wild, rabbits run about in clean fields and woods, but in captivity they often have to put up with urine-soaked straw under their feet in confined living quarters. It really is only fair to ensure that their cages are kept clean and fresh. Urine and feces that are allowed to rot cause bacteria and all their attendant problems, so clean your rabbit's cage out regularly and put the hay up off the floor, where it can be taken as feed. Dried herbs on the bottom of the cage stops maggots from breeding. Flies spread myxomatosis, a manmade disease that was devised to control the wild rabbit population. This is another reason to prevent flies and maggots in the cage.

Sniffles and cold affect rabbits. Use eucalyptus, peppermint, or tea tree on the fur—chest and back. Also wash the cage out in water that has had tea tree or eucalyptus added—this will also put an end to the fleas.

Canker can affect rabbits in the same way as cats and dogs. Apply to the affected ear a little olive oil to which 1 drop of lavender has been added. Tea tree can also be used and helps to prevent any infection from the scratching.

Hamsters ◆◆◆◆◆◆◆◆◆◆◆◆◆◆

Hamsters should be kept clean and dry. A jam jar placed on its side will often be used by the hamsters as a toilet and this can be cleaned out quite easily. Use essential oil to wash the cage, just as for rabbits. Hamsters seem to like the smell of lavender, which is handy because it is antiseptic and antibiotic and will keep the hamsters healthy. Add 2 drops of lavender oil to 2 quarts of water and swish this around the whole of the cage after you have washed it in the usual way.

If your hamster feels very hot and is panting, leave it alone. This can be rather difficult to do because the creature may look so ill as to be almost dead, but it will soon recover so don't panic. Hamsters store their food and this can rot, so use dried herbs and essential oils on the floor of the cage to prevent maggots.

Horses ◆◆◆◆◆◆◆◆◆◆◆◆◆◆◆◆

A horse's stable needs to be kept clean and dry, but this environment also provides a perfect place for a family of mice to make their home. To prevent this, wash the floor in the usual way and as a final rinse, wash down the whole stall with 1 gallon of water to which 15 drops of peppermint oil has been added.

Horses get worms, just as other animals do. To treat worms, include tansy leaves in the horse's feed and add 3 drops of thyme oil to each feed.

Flies are a problem in stables and it is said that a walnut tree planted nearby will keep them away. But that isn't always possible! To stop horses fretting with these annoying little insects, put 3 neat drops of lemongrass or citronella essential oil onto the brush you use to brush them down.

Hoof rot can affect all hoofed animals. The affected hooves should be treated with hot compresses.

Use 1 teaspoon of the following formula for each compress:

Chamomile	10 drops
Thyme	15 drops
Melissa	5 drops

Diluted in 3 ounces vegetable oil

It is also very important to wash down the stall with an essential oil mix:

Chamomile oil	2 teaspoons
Thyme oil	1 teaspoon
Lemongrass oil	40 drops

Add to 1 gallon water, then use 2 cups to 1 gallon water

Horses are often struck down with leg problems. Fractures of the leg are about the worst thing that can happen to a horse, but healing can be speeded up by compresses of ginger oil. Add 10 drops of ginger to 3 ounces olive oil. Heat the oil and add to a compress, which should be wrapped around the leg. Cabbage leaves are also helpful. Massaging the leg after the fracture has healed will strengthen the ligaments and help prevent calcification. This is the oil to use:

Thyme	20 drops
Rosemary	10 drops

Diluted in 3 ounces vegetable oil

Small-Scale Farming ◆◆◆◆◆◆◆◆◆◆◆◆◆◆

To wash down pens and keep flies away, refer to the section on horses. The following essential oils can be used in the care of farm animals.

TO KEEP INSECTS AWAY
FROM ANIMALS

Patchouli	**Tea tree**
Rue	**Lavender**
Lemongrass	**Thyme**
Citronella	**Peppermint**

TO KEEP RODENTS AWAY
FROM ANIMALS

Peppermint	**Patchouli**
Rue	**Garlic**
Spearmint	

Cows, Bulls, and Calves

Cows often need a tonic. Make up the following for them:

Fennel	10 drops
Chamomile	5 drops

Diluted in 3 ounces boiling water

When you have added the essential oils to the water, shake well and use 1 teaspoon mixed with more water in a plant-spray to spray the feed in winter.

The milk production of cows can be increased by adding to their feed the right herb or oil instead of these worrying hormones that the unwitting consumer must drink along with the milk. Hazelnut leaves are said to increase the butterfat content of the milk while also being very good for the cow's digestive system. Melissa (lemon balm) is also effective for an increased milk production. Use it dried in the feed or add 15 drops of melissa essential oil to 3 ounces boiling water and use 1 teaspoon of this, sprayed on the feed. Marjoram is also good for increased lactation, as well as preventing cows aborting. Put 10 drops of marjoram essential oil in 3 ounces boiling water and add 1 teaspoon of this to 1 quart of water in a plant-spray, and spray the cows' feed. Use this method after the birth as well, to help the uterus.

Diarrhea or scours in calves can be treated by adding 1 drop of chamomile oil to their feed. Bathe the abdomen with a large piece of old material which has been soaked in 4½ quarts of warm water to which 10 drops of chamomile oil have been added.

Goats

Goats' milk production is increased by adding 1 teaspoon of the following formula to their feed:

Fennel	7 drops
Dill	8 drops

Diluted in 3 ounces boiling water

Goats are prone to worms. Giving them large amounts of carrots will help, or spray the feed with 1 teaspoon of the following, diluted further in the plant-spray:

Carrot oil	10 drops

Diluted in 3 ounces boiling water

Sheep

Mice are a problem in lambing sheds, but as mice hate peppermint grow some around the sheds as a border. When washing the pens down use as a final rinse a gallon of water to which 5 drops of peppermint oil have been added. You can also drop neat peppermint oil onto the straw, all around the edges of the pen. The peppermint seems to relax the mothers and makes the pen a pleasant place to be in. After the birth, give the sheep a drink made by adding 1 drop of yarrow oil to a quart of boiling water and allow it to cool.

Bees

To make bees take to a new hive, blend the following essential oils together in a tablespoon of water, soak a piece of material in this, and use it to rub the inside walls of the hive. Melissa essential oil is also good for this purpose. All these essential oils can be used on their own.

Hyssop	1 drop
Fennel	1 drop
Thyme	1 drop

Natural Health Care for Pets ◆◆◆◆◆◆◆◆◆◆◆◆◆◆

ABSCESS Put 1 drop of tea tree on the abscess. Then when the pus is discharged, put on 1 drop of lavender. Clean with salt water.

ANAL SWELLING Apply the following to the area on cotton wool:

Chamomile	5 drops
Tea tree	5 drops

Diluted in 1 teaspoon vegetable oil

BAD BREATH Add 1 drop of dill or aniseed to the feed. If the cause is gingivitis, try to get the following onto the gums with a toothbrush:

Clove	1 drop
Lavender	1 drop
Myrrh	1 drop

Diluted in 1 teaspoon vegetable oil

BRONCHITIS Apply niaouli or eucalyptus on a warm piece of cloth to the back and chest. Preferably, use a blend of 2 drops of each.

BURNS AND SCALDS As for humans—cold water followed by neat lavender oil, as soon as possible.

CATARRH Treat as for Bronchitis.

COAT IN POOR CONDITION Add ¼ teaspoon of the following blend to each feed:

Olive oil	1 tablespoon
Wheatgerm oil	1 tablespoon
Carrot oil	5 drops
Evening primrose oil	5 drops

CUTS AND BITES Bathe the area with a solution of salt water to which 2 drops of thyme have been added, then apply 1 neat drop of lavender.

CYSTS Apply 1 neat drop of lavender or tea tree.

EAR PROBLEMS Drip the following formula into the ear as well as massaging around the ear:

Tea tree	1 drop
Lavender	1 drop
Chamomile	1 drop

Diluted in 1 teaspoon warm olive oil

RHEUMATISM Massage the area with the following:

Ginger	5 drops
Rosemary	2 drops
Chamomile	5 drops

Diluted in 2 tablespoons vegetable oil

SKIN PROBLEMS Apply the following oil over the affected area:

Evening primrose oil	2 teaspoons
Lavender oil	5 drops
Chamomile oil	5 drops

Diluted in 2 tablespoons vegetable oil

♦ CHAPTER 18 ♦
GARDENS FOR THE FUTURE

EACH GENERATION CARETAKES the land for the next. Our generation and the couple preceding us have brought environmental catastrophe.

Wise land management in the future must take its guidance from nature itself and nowhere in the natural world do we find monoculture. Nature likes to mix a few varieties within a given space. Analysis of the symbiotic relationship between the range of varieties in a natural environment shows a harmony and coexistence which should be a lesson to anyone concerned with plant growth. If we accept this principle, and accept our responsibility to maintain the goodness of the earth, with the sensible utilization of the widespread ability of plants and plant products to enhance and protect each other, we might just be able to hand on to our descendants the beautiful planet that was once handed to us.

We are hampered in this ideal by our ignorance about plants and about the symbiotic relationships they set up between themselves. Scientists know very little indeed, for example, about the role of aroma in nature, and yet in the plant world aroma is a matter of life and death. Reproduction, "the birds and the bees," is about pollen being transported from one plant to another—and in this aroma plays a vital role. The most highly scented flowers tend to be fertilized by butterflies and moths, while fruity aromas attract beetles, and those plants with an unpleasant, fishy aroma attract dung- and flesh-flies. And aroma also protects a plant by making it repugnant or even poisonous to certain insects. Our scientific knowledge about this whole subject is so far very limited, and that may be partly due to the fact that aroma is extremely difficult to describe, yet alone catalog.

It is not known to what extent defensive aromatic action occurs in plant life. The seminal work on this subject was done as recently as 1982 when two biologists from Washington University, Drs. Orians and Rhoades, discovered a sophisticated biochemical communication system operating in willow and alder trees. They deliberately infested these with predatory caterpillars and webworms and the trees began to produce terpenes and tannins from their leaves, while also changing their protein content. The insects now found the leaves unpalatable and indigestible and began to die. The trees also managed to communicate a warning to trees of the same species, although unconnected by branch or root systems, so that they too began to make the chemical changes needed to protect themselves from the common enemy. The scientists believe that scented chemicals deliver the warning message by air—in other words aroma molecules.

This phenomenon has since been found to occur in other plants, and as time progresses we will no doubt be able to build up a catalog of information based on scientific observation. It will, however, be much longer before a comprehensive picture can be painted of the effect aromatic molecules have on those organisms that are much tinier than caterpillars and more difficult to observe—bacteria and viruses, both of which can have a deleterious effect on plants. But the work needs to be done, because the proven antibacterial and antiviral properties of certain aromatic essences indicate that they were working on this level in the plants from which they were extracted. Aroma molecules may exert an influence on plants in even less obvious ways such as wavelength and electromagnetism—as, indeed, they do on animals and humans.

When we understand more about the role aroma plays in nature we may be in a better position to explain why one crop does so well when planted next to another. Mutually beneficial relationships are already well established, if not yet well understood, and used commercially. In Bulgaria, roses are inter-cropped with garlic and onion, which not only protect the roses from predators and fungi but enhance their fragrance—while growing strong themselves. Carrots have for centuries been known to do well when grown alongside marigolds, and at Ryton Research Centre, in Coventry, England, they have observed that this growing relationship deters whitefly from going near the carrots.

Why one plant variety should help another is not always easy to determine. It could be that the predator of one is discouraged from the area by the aroma of another; or that the color of one plant attracts the insect needed to pollinate another. It may simply be that one plant has a root system that goes deep and takes nutrients from the lower levels of soil while its thriving bedmate is shallow-rooted and left free to extract the nutrients from the upper layers. Or perhaps one variety excretes just the nutrients that its neighbor requires. In some cases it may be that the antibacterial and antiviral properties contained in the aromatic substances work to protect neighboring plants from micropests. Or the symbiotic benefits may be far simpler, one plant merely providing the shade and protection that its neighbor needs. And as well as discovering the reasons for positive relationships, we need to find out why some plants have a negative impact upon one another.

Clearing Out the Garden Shed ◆◆◆◆◆◆

The average gardener's shed contains enough poison to kill off his family and neighbors several times over. This may be in the form of pesticides, fungicides, or wood preservatives. If you have any products in your shed which contain the following, they should be thrown out immediately because health risks have been shown to be involved in their use: paraquat is contained in fourteen products for garden and agricultural use in the United Kingdom; Lindane, an insecticide, is included in one hundred and thirty products in the United Kingdom with a wide range of uses including wood treatment in the home; 2.4.5.T (phenoxy herbicide) comes in eleven forms in the United Kingdom, including products sold to gardeners; chlordane/Heptachlor is an insecticide found in twelve products, especially those sold to kill ants and earthworms.

The list of dangerous chemicals sold in Britain is much longer than this and many concerned parties ask why, if they are so dangerous, they are on sale at all—especially when all of these and many others have been banned in other countries. This is a question I cannot answer and I would refer the reader who requires further information on this subject to Pesticide Action Network International, whose address may be found in the appendix.

Under no circumstances should you use chemical pesticides in the home, and as chemical sprays travel as fast as bad news, ask your neighbors to let you know when they intend to spray their garden so that you can make sure your windows are closed.

Using Essential Oils in Your Garden ◆◆◆◆◆◆◆

Essential oils play several roles in the garden. They can be natural pest deterrents, and as pests carry disease in the form of bacteria and viruses, the oils are a form of preventative medicine for your garden. More than this, the known antibacterial and antiviral properties of certain essential oils indicate that one of their jobs in the plant from which they were extracted was to provide direct protective measures against bacteria and viruses. Fungi and mold are other problems that essential oils deal with quickly and effectively.

Strong healthy plants resist disease, and the essential oils, working on the same principles that apply to the biochemical and electromagnetic aspects of intercropping, build up the health of plants. This seems not only to affect the yield, which is increased, but the fragrance or flavor of flowers, fruit, and vegetables. For example, as companions in the cooking dish or salad bowl, tomato and basil are well known, but basil grown around the tomato plant or basil oil in the watering can will enhance the taste of the tomato before it even leaves the plant.

In Holland, the Dutch plant protection service uses French marigolds to deter nematode worms in the public parks but they could just as easily chop up this plant and scatter it around the affected area, or use the essential oil of tagetes in the watering can. Roses love to be in the company of garlic, basil, or thyme and you can either plant these around the rose bush or use their essential oil when watering them.

THE NATURAL INSECT REPELLENTS

Insect	Repellent Plant or Plant Tea	Essential Oil
ANTS	Spearmint, tansy, pennyroyal, peppermint Grow the plants near the doors of a house either in the ground or in pots. Also put the essential oil on cotton-wool balls and place by the doors. Spray the oils along shelves where the ants are seen, and on their nests.	**Spearmint, Peppermint, Pennyroyal, Garlic, Citronella**
APHIDS (*see also individual species*)	Nasturtium, spearmint, stinging nettle, southernwood, garlic, potatoes, parsley, basil, horseradish	**Spearmint, Peppermint, Cedarwood, Hyssop**
BEAN BEETLE	Potatoes, thyme	**Thyme, Garlic, Peppermint**
BLACK FLY	Stinging nettle, basil, lavender	**Lavender, Tagetes, Tansy**
CABBAGE ROOT FLY	Thyme, sage	**Thyme, Sage**
CABBAGE WHITE BUTTERFLY	Sage, rosemary, hyssop, thyme, peppermint, celery, mint, wormwood, southernwood	**Peppermint, Sage, Rosemary, Hyssop, Thyme**
CARROT FLY	Rosemary, chives, sage, thyme, leeks	**Tansy, Rosemary, Tagetes**
CATERPILLARS	Celery, celeriac family, tomatoes	**Spearmint, Pennyroyal, Peppermint**
CUTWORM	Oakleaf, bark	**Thyme, Sage**
EEL WORM	Marigold	**Tagetes**
FLEA BEETLE (BLACK)	Wormwood, mint, lettuce	**Peppermint, Lemongrass, Spearmint, Rue, Lavender**
FLEAS	Lavender, mint	**Lemongrass, Citronella, Pennyroyal, Rue, Tansy, Lavender**
FLIES	Rue, tansy, wormwood, tomatoes Rue is very helpful grown around composts, manure piles, and barns.	**Rue, Lavender, Citronella, Peppermint, Tansy**

THE NATURAL INSECT REPELLENTS (continued)

Insect	Repellent Plant or Plant Tea	Essential Oil
GNATS	Pennyroyal	Tagetes, Spearmint, Citronella, Patchouli
GREENFLY	Garlic	Lavender, Tagetes, Tansy
LICE	Spearmint, pennyroyal, peppermint, nettle, basil	Spearmint, Peppermint, Cedarwood, Pennyroyal, Rue
MOSQUITOES	Sassafras, pennyroyal, wormwood, southernwood, rosemary, sage, santolina, lavender, mint Castor oil plants are good for a sunny patio.	Lavender, Pennyroyal, Sassafras, Citronella, Lemongrass, Tansy
MOTHS	Wormwood, southernwood, rosemary, sage, santolina, lavender, mint, tansy	Spearmint, Lavender, Hyssop, Citronella, Peppermint
NEMATODES	Marigolds	Tagetes, Sage, Citronella
PLANT LICE	Stinging nettles	Rue, Spearmint, Peppermint
SLUGS	Garlic, chives, wormwood	Garlic, Cedarwood, Hyssop, Sassafras, Pine
SNAILS	Garlic	Cedarwood, Sassafras, Pine, Garlic, Patchouli
TICKS	Rue	Citronella, Lemongrass, Thyme, Sage, Pennyroyal, Rue
WEEVILS	Garlic	Cedarwood, Rue, Sandalwood, Patchouli
WHITE FLY	Marigolds, tomatoes	Tagetes, Tansy, Lavender, Sage
WOOLLY APHIDS	Nasturtium	Sandalwood, Patchouli, Pine

Thyme and lavender are marvelous at protecting all vegetables in the patch, and again, plant them near the vegetables or use their oil in the watering can. To find out which plants and essential oils to use for deterring particular insects, refer to the list on page 368.

You will see there that ants can be deterred by peppermint and, indeed, they hate it and will go to great lengths to avoid it. To clear a nest, just put 2 neat drops of peppermint oil directly onto the nest and wait for the exodus. If ants are coming into your house, put 1 or 2 drops of peppermint oil on the threshold, or wherever they enter. You can create a mobile barrier with a peppermint plant in a pot that can be placed at the back door and moved as the ants get smart and try to find another entrance point. Alternatively, chop the leaves of a peppermint plant and scatter them to create a barrier. As mice hate peppermint too, these same methods can be used to discourage them. Indeed peppermint is a useful plant or oil to have for deterring all sorts of insects including the cabbage white butterfly. Again, scatter the dried leaves or use the essential oil in the watering can. Sage can be used in both these ways against this butterfly.

Of course, certain insects are essential for pollination, including bees, wasps, and butterflies, and using essential oils in your garden will attract these useful insects. Bees especially like coriander.

Essential oils not only control pests and make your crop stronger and better tasting or more fragrant, they will make your own time in the garden altogether more enjoyable. Mosquitoes have an aversion to the aroma of lemongrass, citronella, or lavender oils, among others, and their use in the garden can take the sting out of hot summer nights. But all flying insects are a nuisance in the garden, especially if you are having a barbecue. The answer again is lemongrass or citronella essential oil which may be used in several different ways. Add 3 drops to a cereal bowl of water and soak some ribbons in this before attaching them to the branches of trees. You need to pay particular attention to clearing the area under trees and over water as flying insects, including gnats and midges, love lurking around there. The pond can be cleared by putting some of the soaked ribbons on a pole and sticking this in the middle, or you may find it easier and prettier to put a couple of neat drops of lemongrass or citronella onto an artificial flower or water lily and float that on the pond. If you have candles or flares outside, simply drop the essential oil onto the wax at the top, just as it begins to melt. If you have an outside light, put 1 drop of essential oil onto the bulb before you turn it on, or even earlier if you wish, and as the bulb heats up the aroma molecules will be released into the immediate area and the flying insects will decide that there must be better places to hang out. If your summer evenings are being spoiled by moths, use the same procedures with lavender oil, which they hate.

You can see from the previous paragraph that there are many ingenious ways to use essential oils in the garden, and you may be able to devise yet more ways than those listed below to make use of these exceedingly helpful gardener's mates.

Sprays

Sprays are used as insect deterrents, to banish fungi and mildew, or to encourage growth. Unless otherwise stated, use 4–8 drops of essential oil in 1 gallon of water for spraying onto flowers, fruit, and vegetables.

Hanging Strips

Place 1 drop of neat essential oil on a strip of material and hang it from a stick or a branch. This method is particularly effective when hung from branches of trees and saves the arduous task of spraying such a large area. Renew as needed.

Cotton Wool

This method can be used to deter insects or burrowing animals such as moles. Place 3 drops of essential oil on a cotton-wool ball and place it in the burrow or on the nest and repeat as needed.

Cartons

This method is good for deterring slugs, snails, mice, cats, and dogs, and all ground-moving insects. Bury an old plastic food carton such as a yogurt or margarine container into the ground so that its top is level with the ground. Use 4 drops of essential oil in the carton and renew as needed. Cats and dogs dislike a powerful aroma because it puts them off the scent. It will discourage them from urinating on the area, but not necessarily from walking over newly sown seeds, for example. Use the strong essential oils of peppermint, spearmint, thyme, or eucalyptus. Remember though that dogs like lavender, and although tradition has it that cats do not like oranges, they do like the essential oil of orange, so don't use that.

String

String soaked in a solution of water and essential oil may be strung between rows of vegetables to deter flying insects such as cabbage white butterflies. Use the appropriate essential oil from the chart.

Garden Teas ◆◆◆◆◆◆◆◆◆◆

There are several ways to make garden teas, which are the gentle way to transport the "active principle" of a herb or flower to another plant. The tea plant or material should be picked in the morning as early as possible, before the sun starts to evaporate the essential oil and before the flower blooms, and while the growth factor is still incorporated in the stem, bud, and leaf. Older plants are not as effective as younger ones.

Herb and Flower Teas

Use 1 cup of dried or fresh herb or flower to 2 cups of water. Boil the water, pour onto the plant material and leave to stand for at least four hours. Strain off the liquid and store. Use 2 tablespoons of this tea diluted in 1 gallon of water in a watering can or garden spray.

For a more concentrated tea, fill a jar with the herb or flower material, cover with boiling water, leave to stand overnight, strain off, and use as above.

Essential Oil Teas for the Garden

Add 8 drops of essential oil to 2½ cups water, boil and leave to cool. Use 2 tablespoons to 1 gallon of water in the usual watering methods.

Other Methods of Pest Control ◆◆◆◆◆◆◆

Gardeners have devised all manner of ingenious ways to foil unwelcome insects, and given the determination to avoid chemical solutions, I have no doubt we could think up even more. One of the simplest ways to protect seedlings is to cut the bottom off plastic bottles and push them a couple of inches into the ground, around the plant. These can then be watered through the open hole at the top.

Cabbages can be protected from the larvae of the cabbage white butterfly by having tin foil wrapped around their stalks. Another barrier method involves carpet underlay—cut into squares of about 6 inches and make a cut on one side and a hole in the middle and place these around the vegetable at the time of planting. This simple method will save you hours of wondering whether the cabbage root fly is ruining your crop. Carrot flies hate mothballs and these can be crumbled up and scattered around on the soil. They also appear to have an aversion to creosote, which can be put on string which is hung between the rows of carrots. It also helps if you plant before May and after June, thus avoiding the main activity period of the carrot fly.

We have so far been discussing tactics in the Battle of the Insects from the point of view of deterrents, and the essential oils certainly provide a method that would be acceptable to Buddhists. But there are those among you who are made of harder stuff and won't mind seeing your insect enemies die a horrible death. Once you have decided to take this option, a whole range of possibilities is open to you. Wasps, for example, can be made to do the damage to themselves if you simply fill jam jars with water, while they are still unwashed, and hang them up, especially around fruit trees. The wasps suddenly turn into kamikaze pilots and dive-bomb into the jars where, of course, they drown! The same principles apply when dealing with slugs with the beer trick. Bury old margarine or yogurt containers so that the top of the container is level with the ground, fill them with beer or cider and stand back and watch as the smell of the beer attracts the slugs which fall into the beer, get drunk, and drown.

Slugs have an acute sense of smell and hate garlic in any shape or form. The essential oil of garlic is so aromatically powerful as to be rather unpleasant to handle and an easier option may be to break a garlic bulb into its cloves and place these in the ground, especially along the edges of the garden where slugs often lay their eggs. French gardeners use crushed garlic: add 1 tablespoon to a watering can, mix well, and water the areas where the slugs are causing their damage. You can also protect the plants that attract the slugs—usually the thickest and most succulent plants you have—by laying a protective barrier of pine needles or holly around them. Save the needles from your Christmas tree, ready for your battle next summer. This method works for the simple reason that slugs aren't too fond of dragging their soft little tummies over the sharp prickly carpet presented by pine needles and holly leaves. Oak mulch is another surface the slugs are not too keen on, but any prickly substance will do the job of persuading them to take their slimy selves somewhere else.

Slugs have obviously made a lot of enemies over the years because so many methods of dealing with them have been devised, but most insects can be thwarted in their endeavors to devour your crop and lay their eggs so that their offspring can do the same. Whether you plan to frustrate or annihilate, the secret of success in the battle is to know your enemies—their likes and dislikes, their natural enemies and how to attract them, their life cycle, the parameters of their movements, and so forth. With that information it should be possible to construct a battle plan that ensures you win.

Birds ♦♦♦♦♦♦♦♦♦♦♦♦♦♦♦♦♦♦♦

Birds have a poor sense of smell and taste, so although planting violets or lavender among soft fruits has been reported to discourage them from going near, it's a mystery as to why this should work (although one can't help noticing that these two plants are of similar color, if not intensity of color). Nets or criss-crossed string or cotton across flower or vegetable beds and between fruit trees will deter birds, but the Royal Society for the Protection of Birds asks that these be colored so that the birds can see them, and strung tightly so that their legs do not get entangled in them.

Molds and Fungi ♦♦♦♦♦

Treated with the antifungal essential oils, molds and fungi growing on trees, plants, and flowers do not survive for long and appear simply to disappear. Use 10 drops to every gallon of water in your usual gardening spray equipment:

ANTIMOLD AND ANTIFUNGI OILS

Patchouli	**Cinnamon**
Tea tree	**Niaouli**

You can also use garden teas in spraying equipment (see page 371). Elderflower tea discourages molds on everything, while chive tea is particularly good with the gray, dusty mold that blights the delicate rose. Nettle tea treats mildew on cucumbers and horsetail tea helps to protect the plant against many types of fungus due to its high silica content.

The Friendly Bunch ♦♦♦

Certain aromatic plants have a beneficial effect on most flowers and vegetables when grown among them. However, you do not actually have to cultivate this friendly bunch to take advantage of their capacity to enhance your garden because their essential oil can be used in the watering can instead. You will only need 6 drops of essential oil to 2 gallons of water. This is not a great deal but remember that each drop of essential oil has been distilled from a large number of the original plants. Add the 6 drops of essential oil to a gallon bucket of warm water and swish it around well. Leave it to cool, then take half this amount and put it in a gallon watering can. Fill the can up with cold water and, again, mix around well. If you use a spray, simply take half the volume you need from the bucket and half from the tap.

The African marigold, Tagetes minuta and patula, was considered sacred by the Aztecs and associated with their god of agriculture—no doubt because grown next to so many plants, the marigolds increased their crop. Sage is beneficial to many vegetables, as is lavender, but lavender bushes should be grown around the borders of vegetable patches, rather than between them, simply because they are so permanent. Tarragon can be grown everywhere because it doesn't leech the soil of nutrients, as many other plants do. Yarrow increases the aromatic quality of all herbs and therefore makes a good companion for medicinal plants and herbs. Valerian is good for most plants because it contains phosphorus and attracts earthworms. The root can be dried and grated and steeped to make a seductive tea which aids in sleep. The root, however, if bruised, attracts cats which will relieve themselves by the plant and necessitates digging up the soil. Foxglove has a good effect on all plants when grown in a border at the back of the beds. There is no essential oil of foxglove so make a tea and use that in the watering.

THE GOOD COMPANIONS

Vegetable	Herb	Flower	Other Vegetable	Essential Oils	Fruit
ASPARAGUS	Parsley		Tomatoes	Basil Parsley	
BEANS, GREEN, DWARF	Savory	Beetroot Celery		Lavender Basil Savory Strawberries	Strawberries
BEANS, BROAD	Savory		Potatoes Sweet corn	Lavender Basil Savory	
BEANS, RUNNER	Savory		Potatoes Sweet corn	Lavender Basil Savory	
BEETROOT	Marjoram		Onions Dwarf beans	Celery Marjoram	
BROCCOLI	Valerian	Nasturtium	Cabbage Peas Tomatoes	Basil Thyme	
CABBAGE	Peppermint Sage Rosemary Feverfew		Cucumber Celery Tomatoes	Peppermint Sage Thyme Clary-sage Chamomile	Rhubarb
CARROTS	Chives		Peas Leeks Lettuce	Sage	
CAULIFLOWER	Thyme		Runner beans Celery Carrots	Celery Thyme	
CELERY	Yarrow		Cabbage Leeks Dwarf beans Celeriac Tomatoes Cauliflower	Geranium Yarrow	

THE GOOD COMPANIONS (continued)

Vegetable	Herb	Flower	Other Vegetable	Essential Oils	Fruit
CUCUMBER	Chives	Sunflower	Peas Cabbage	Sage Yarrow	
LEEKS	Valerian		Celery Carrots	Celery Hyssop	Strawberries
LETTUCE		Tagetes	Carrots	Carrot Tagetes	
ONIONS	Chamomile Summer savory	Roses	Beetroot Tomatoes	Chamomile Savory	Strawberries
PEAS	Caraway	Nasturtium	Sweet corn Carrots Broccoli Radishes Cucumber	Geranium Carrot	
POTATOES	Horseradish	Foxgloves	Beans (all) Sweet corn Cabbage Peas	Basil Sage	
RADISHES	Chervil Parsley		Carrots Peas Lettuce	Parsley Savory	
SWEDE	Sage	Marigolds	Turnip	Sage Tagetes	
SWEETCORN	Savory Chamomile	Marigolds	Broad beans Runner beans Peas Potatoes	Savory Tagetes	
TOMATOES	Basil Chives Parsley	Marigolds Tagetes Foxgloves	Asparagus Celery Broccoli Cabbage	Tagetes Basil	Goose-berries

THE GOOD COMPANIONS (continued)

Fruit	Herb	Flower	Vegetable	Essential Oils	Other Fruit
APPLES	Southern-wood Chives	Nasturtiums Wallflowers Foxgloves Lavender	Legumes	**Lavender** **Artemisia**	Elm
GRAPES	Hyssop	Clematis		**Hyssop** **Lavender**	
STRAWBERRIES	Borage Nettles Mint Thyme	Leeks Spinach Lettuce	Sage Rosemary Mint		
FLOWERS:					
ROSES	Garlic Parsley Chives	Mignonette Lupins Marigolds	Onions	**Basil** **Hyssop**	
CEREALS:					
RYE	Chamomile	Pansies		**Chamomile**	
WHEAT	Chamomile			**Chamomile**	

Nature's Nursemaids ◆◆

Hyssop helps other plants which are suffering from bacterial invasion, and as such an event is unforeseen when laying out the garden, using hyssop essential oil in a plant-spray is the perfect method of dealing with this problem. Chamomile is another plant which helps sick plants to recover—either move your chamomile plants next to the ailing patient or spray it with chamomile essential oil. Once the plant has recovered, spray on alternate days only.

Nobody likes to find stinging nettles in his garden and yet these are the great unappreciated nurses of the plant world. Whenever you find nettles growing somewhere inconvenient or unwelcome, cut them down and make a tea which can become the standby emergency "medicine" for all your plants.

Just as there are plants that find each other's company mutually beneficial, there are those that do not thrive close to each other. Sometimes we can explain why—because they are competing for resources, for example, or attract insects

THE BAD COMPANIONS

Vegetable	Herb	Flower	Other Vegetable	Fruit/ Cereal
BEANS, GREEN (all)	Garlic Fennel	Gladioli	Beetroot Kohlrabi Onions Shallots	
BEETROOT		Marigolds	Tomatoes Spinach	
CABBAGE			Onions	Strawberries
CABBAGE, RED			Tomatoes	
CARROT	Dill			
CUCUMBER			Potatoes	
LETTUCE	Parsley			
PEAS	Garlic	Gladioli	Onions	
POTATOES		Sunflowers	Onions Pumpkin Cucumber	Raspberries
RADISHES	Hyssop			
TOMATOES			Kohlrabi	
FRUIT:				
CHERRIES			Potatoes	Wheat
STRAWBERRIES			Cabbage	
FRUIT TREES (general)				Oats

and microorganisms that harm each other—but sometimes the reasons are unclear, as yet. Certain planting arrangements just do not work well. Growing any type of bean near onions, garlic, and shallots, for example, is a grouping in which none will do well, whatever the soil and weather conditions. Perhaps you can find in the list above the answer to one of your most mystifying gardening failures. Fennel and rue are generally bad for all plants—they should be grown on their own, so I suppose in gardening terms they are the outcasts.

Trees and Fruits ◆◆◆◆◆◆◆◆◆◆◆◆

In companion gardening terms, trees have their friends too. All the following help trees to flourish if grown nearby: chives, horseradish, garlic, tansy, southernwood, nasturtium, and the stinging nettle. Nasturtiums planted around the base of a tree, or encouraged to grow up its trunk, will protect it from aphids. They also have a discouraging effect on scab and molds on apple trees. Chives too prevent apple scab. Wallflowers, either grown around apple trees or made into a tea and sprayed onto them, have a similarly protective and beneficial action. Legumes in general help all trees and can be encouraged to grow up their trunks, while beans particularly increase the growth of apricot trees.

Southernwood planted around the tree repels fruit tree moths, while tansy keeps away flying insects in general. On the other hand, bees are vital to pollination and they can be encouraged by planting coriander between the trees. An old wives' tale holds that hanging mothballs on a tree is effective in keeping insects at bay, but I prefer to use lavender. Make little bags by soaking cotton-wool balls in lavender oil and putting them in the corners of a plastic bag, cutting the corners off and sealing them. Then pierce the bags with a pin a few times so that the odor can escape but not evaporate completely, and hang them in the branches. You can also use fresh or dried lavender tied in little gauze bags.

It's a great shame to go to all the trouble of protecting your trees and bringing in a terrific crop if the whole effect is ruined by bad storage. The most heartbreaking story I heard along these lines came from a Jersey flower grower who decided to branch out into tomatoes and thought he would send both crops to Covent Garden market in the same container. When it was opened up at the other end, a huge pile of rotting vegetation met the horrified buyers! Flowers and fruit do not store well together, even for a few hours. Apples don't do well if stored near potatoes (and they don't like growing near each other, either). Ripe apples give off a gas called ethylene which brings forward the ripening of flowers and vegetables and has other effects not always easy to see—for example, carrots stored by apples lose their sweetness.

Brown rot is the scourge of fruit farmers but they have four very good friends in horseradish, garlic, onion, and chive. These can either be grown between the fruit or made into a tea and used to water or spray the fruit plants.

Stinging nettles are a very useful plant because they contain nitrogen, silica, iron, proteins, phosphates, folic acid, mineral salt, and trace elements, and when grown between any type of currant, whether black, red, or white, they will bring in a bigger and tastier crop.

Strawberries do very well grown beside dwarf beans, spinach, borage, and lettuce. The borage encourages bees which are needed for pollination. Lettuces and strawberries both entice slugs, but these can be sent scuttling at double speed if you use pine needles for bedding. Indeed pine needles make a better option than straw not only as a slug deterrent but because they make a very warm bedding material and contain more nutrients than straw, which is dead, and will do more for the quality of your earth. As an added bonus, the pine needles give strawberries the flavor of wild strawberries—a trick not entirely unknown to certain catering suppliers.

Flowers and Indoor Plants ◆◆◆◆

As we all know, trying to buy a rose that smells like a rose is today often a fruitless task. Breeders seem more concerned with the look of the flower than its aroma. And yet it is the aroma which gives a flower its natural resistance to pests, which is why old roses do so well without the need for pesticides.

The most sensational rose crop in the world comes from Bulgaria. The Bulgarians have always inter-cropped their roses with garlic, onions, parsley, mignonette, and lupins. The fact is that with companion gardening you simply do not need to use chemicals and, moreover, you increase the fragrance as well as the health of the flower.

Of course, flowers have their little pests, as vegetables do, and with roses the problems are mildew and black spot. These can be treated using the relevant essential oil listed on page 374. As a general rule the oils used against fungi work well with flowers, although I have had some truly remarkable results from using geranium and lemongrass oil on roses. There is only one important point to remember—a particular flower will loathe being sprayed with the essential oil of its relatives, so don't use rose oil to spray your roses unless you want a flower strike on your hands!

Bicarbonate of soda used in the watering can has a miraculous effect on sweet peas and other flowers. It increases the size and number of blooms and enhances their fragrance. You only need to give flowers this treatment once a month: use ¼ teaspoon of bicarbonate of soda to 1 gallon of water, and water the roots. Do not exceed this amount—under-use rather than over-use. This same dilution can also be used as cut flower water.

Once cut, certain flowers seem to have a deleterious effect upon one another when in the vase. Lily of the valley and narcissus, for example, will quickly die if put together. Although daffodils and tulips are very often displayed together as they flower at the same time, they actually make the life of the other shorter. Grow or buy them both by all means, but display them at opposite ends of the room. Mignonette seems to have a bad effect on most cut flowers, and placed in a vase with them will invariably make the other flowers wither long before their time.

The vase life of any flower is easy to prolong with any number of effective methods. One of the simplest is to add white or brown sugar to the water, but do not use more than a quarter of a teaspoon of sugar to a quart of water. A copper penny dropped into the bottom of the vase will prolong the life of some flowers—this works well with roses, for example. Flowers of the daffodil family, such as narcissus and jonquil, last longer if a pinch of salt is added to the water—but no more than a pinch. Tea brewed in a teapot need never go to waste. Any leftover tea can be added to water in china vases—not glass for obvious reasons—while the tea leaves make an excellent mulching material for any plant in the garden. Foxgloves made into a tea which is added to the flower water provide an excellent feed for flowers, but this again must be used in moderation. First, make your infusion of foxglove tea by cramming a jar with fresh foxglove flowers and filling it with hot water. (You will need only half the quantity if the flowers are dried, and you can do this by hanging them upside down in the shed.) Leave the flowers to infuse for forty-eight hours: this then is your tea. It can be filtered and rebottled if there is a danger of the flowers rotting because you are going to leave the jar a long time before using the tea. From this jar take 1 teaspoon of liquid to each quart of vase water.

House plants and plants in window boxes can be watered with dilutions of milk or beer. It is important to realize that only tiny quantities of these are of benefit, so when you have finished with a carton or bottle of milk or a can of beer, fill it with water and swish it around so that the dregs become mixed in with the water and use this to water the plants. It is thought that the plants benefit from the proteins in milk and the hormones in the hops.

Essential oils that are too old to use for medicinal purposes, that is after about two years, can be used to wash out plant pots. This will kill off the plant bacteria and viruses that destroyed the plant you are now having to replace! There is no point in letting the disease carry on to your nice, new plant. Indoor plant growth will be encouraged by using a few drops of geranium, frankincense, or lemongrass in a water-spray. Basil and lemongrass used in the spray are very effective against aphids.

Herbs ◆◆◆◆◆◆◆◆◆◆◆◆◆◆◆◆◆

Herbs are so useful as an inter-crop between vegetables and flowers that the specialist herb garden should really become a thing of the past. But that is not because they don't grow well together—they do, with a few exceptions. It is not a good idea, for example, to grow sweet basil and rue together, or coriander and fennel.

Good companions of the herb variety are rosemary and sage, and anise and coriander; while all herbs benefit from having yarrow or stinging nettles nearby. Generally speaking, herbs like sunny, well-drained conditions although this can be difficult to arrange when inter-cropping. Try the following among your vegetables and flowers: lavender, sage, basil, thyme, marjoram, chamomile, hyssop, chervil, and tarragon. Cabbage, broccoli, brussels sprouts, and kale are just some of the vegetables that produce large, good quality produce when scattered among the herbs and flowers. Sweet corn does particularly well near dill.

The Soil ◆◆◆◆◆◆◆◆◆◆◆◆◆◆

CHALKY SOIL is most probably alkaline, and may need a lot of compost. Several herbs and plants do particularly well in this type of soil.

Hyssop
Marjoram
Chicory
Rosemary
Summer savory
Salad burnet
Lavender

SANDY SOIL is most likely to have a problem with retaining moisture and the nutrients will be draining away. A good compost to enrich the soil would be very useful. The herbs that do well in sandy soil are many and they will help to replenish lost nutrients. The following herbs can be distilled to produce essential oils that are in demand—making cultivation an even better idea, especially in Third World countries.

Anise
Fennel
Marjoram
Chamomile
Lavender
Borage
Coriander
Tarragon
Evening primrose
Cumin
Thyme

CLAY sticks to your garden fork and Wellington boots in winter and crusts like pottery clay in the summer sun. Compost helps to drain the soil. Herbs need good long roots in these conditions, and these in turn help to break up the soil.

Peppermint	**Spearmint**
Comfrey	**Melissa**
Angelica	

WET, MARSHY SOIL could be called "boggy" because it holds the moisture. Although certain herbs definitely do not like their feet to be continually wet, there are those which do especially well in these bog-type conditions.

Valerian	**Sweet flag**
Marshmallow	(from which orris root is extracted)

MOIST LOAM is a rich soil which retains water even in hot weather. This is a good soil for the gardener and herbs do well in it.

Angelica	**Peppermint**
Valerian	**Spearmint**
Parsley	**Melissa**
Soapwort	**Sorrel**

LOAM is also a rich soil, and is full of nutrients. It may need to be drained. A good range of useful herbs can be grown in it.

Basil	**Parsley**
Caraway	**Dill**
Thyme	**Rosemary**
Chives	**Sage**
Coriander	**Lovage**
Chervil	**Rue**
Fennel	

Getting the Best from Your Soil

Fertile soil is the key to good gardening and if you feed it, rather than the plants, your plants will take care of themselves. This is a very big subject and not within the scope of this book, but here are a few tips you might find helpful.

Nitrogen helps to promote growth and strength and it can be put into the ground by natural means. Lupins produce a lot of nitrogen and are often the first plants to grow on barren waste, for example after a volcanic eruption, leading the way for other plants to follow and take up the nitrogen they left behind. Legumes have bacterial nodules on their roots which bring nitrogenous compounds into the soil. Beans, peas, clover, alfalfa, and soya fall into this group. Mustard is a fast growing "green manure" which adds nitrogen to the soil. Sow it between May and August wherever you have spare land and within four to six weeks it will be ready to dig in.

Sapogin-rich plants help nearby crops. Sapogin is a lather-producing substance used as a substitute for soap by vegans and others. Soapwort is the best known example, but other sapogin-rich plants are spinach, runner beans, tomatoes, potatoes, primroses, carnations, and camellias. The brassica family of cabbage loves sapogin, so plant your spinach and cabbage crops on the same piece of land on alternate years.

Crop rotation is very important to gardens and even the most modern farmers are coming around to the view that the old-fashioned method of putting a different crop on a piece of land each year is just what the doctor orders for their nutrient-deficient soils, recovering from the leeching effects of monoculture. Heavy feeders need to be alternated with light feeders. The heavy feeders, as their name implies, suck up nutrients in the soil. Among this group are the cabbage family, cauliflowers, most green leafed vegetables, sweet corn, cucumber, and celery. Light feeders include beans, peas, and tomatoes, and although tomatoes generally like to stay in the same place, you can move them as much as you like if you plant basil around them.

The whole idea of crop rotation is to allow each plant to extract what it needs and to return to the soil its own particular nutrients, alternating these with other crops which have other needs and thus enabling them to make their own unique contribution to the makeup of the soil. Some plants are not a crop as such but are very good for the soil. Nettles are a prime example, and if you leave a patch of land bare over one season, don't worry if the weed seems to take over—it will be doing your soil a power of good. Dandelions are also good for the soil and will benefit the next plant grown there. These other so-called weeds, including couch grass, help to prepare the soil for fruit trees in particular.

"Green manure" need not be green at all. Banana skins contain calcium, magnesium, sulphur, phosphates, sodium, and silica, all of which make them excellent fertilizers for roses and peonies, among other plants—just dig them in around the base. Roses can be given a stronger perfume by digging in garlic and onion leftovers—collect the discarded skins and what not when you top and tail them and save them for future good use. Melon leaves are full of calcium and make a good mulching material.

Mulch put directly around plants protects them and retains moisture; it also, when laid on ground between the plants, hinders the growth of weeds. Wet straw, grass, and leaves are all traditional mulching materials, but why not use forest bark or wood chippings between the beds, especially where slugs are to be found. Lay your mulching material when the soil is moist and warm, in the spring before the weeds start growing. Black plastic, dug in at the edges or held down with stones, makes an excellent mulch for vegetable patches. Old newspaper, cardboard, or carpeting make good mulching material; just make sure the pieces overlap properly and that it's all held down with bricks, stones, hay, grass clippings, or whatever. Instead of mulching, you could grow a crop of marigolds and lupins which impede the growth of weeds—and look far more attractive than black plastic!

Everyone who makes compost has his own theory as to the best method of doing so, but basically all you need is vegetable and animal waste, moisture, air, warmth, activators, and earthworms. Good materials for the compost heap are dandelions, chamomile, valerian, seaweed, elderberry, all leaves, and especially comfrey and nettles which are good activators and help the fermentation process. Bad materials are pine needles, conifer cuttings, twigs and other woody materials, diseased plants, and grass cuttings if used in excess.

For flower bulbs or shrubs that need a lot of water but have deep roots and tend to get over-thirsty in dry weather, sink into the ground an old pipe or length of hose, alongside the plant. This provides a way of watering that ensures the water reaching the roots.

Finding the most propitious time to plant seeds is another area of gardening that attracts many theories. One of the more eccentric methods employed in centuries past by farmers in the English Midlands involved sitting bare-bottomed on the ground to test the temperature of it. An even older method is to plant by the moon, and although this might sound like an old wives' tale, a great number of high-tech farmers throughout the world take the principle seriously enough to apply it to large-scale farming methods. When you think about it, the idea is not so strange.

The waxing and waning of the moon not only pulls the tides of huge oceans and creates a pull in such small volumes of water as a cup of tea (which has been observed scientifically), but affects those other aspects of creation which are largely composed of water—you, me, and all the plants in our gardens. The planets are silent influences upon us all, and although the agreed beneficial effect of planting according to the moon has been put down to the simple fact that one tends to get heavy rain after the new and full moons and the first and third quarters, thus seeds germinate more quickly, there is undoubtedly more to it than this. There is only one way to decide whether moon planting works or not, and that is to do it yourself. Plant one row of cabbages, for example, by the moon and the next not, and see if there is any difference. *Old Moore's Almanack* gives the full list of dates, and these are very specific. For example, in October 1989 there are four planting days and on the 13th and 14th you are supposed to plant between 8:10 and 10:35 am, or 12:40 to 4:25 pm or 5:35 to 6:35 pm. There are also those who maintain that growing north-south gives different results than planting east-west. This again is thought to be due to electromagnetic forces and their pull on living organisms, so why not try both and see if you can see a difference.

All life begins with the seed, but these days seed companies are more than likely to be owned by chemical companies which have great fun interfering with the genes of plants and devising a symbiotic relationship between them and the chemicals they would like us to use on them! What all this interference will do in the long run is frightening to imagine, and gardeners who wish to rely on the evolved wisdom of nature herself, rather than on the financial considerations of chemical companies and the "plant designers" who work for them, should get their seeds or cuttings from a known source. It may be time to form seed banks and seed and cutting cooperatives to provide us with the raw materials for our natural gardens. The catalogs for these should include a description of the aroma and taste of the product. It is a shame that no provision for this exists in commercial catalogs and that plants are described only in terms of color, size, and shape.

The Perfect Crop ◆◆◆◆◆

For the farmer, growing plants which can be distilled into essential oils makes tremendous economic and ecological sense. In growing any plant one contributes to the oxygen circulating in the atmosphere. Once distilled, the first-grade oils can be sold to promote physical and mental health, while second-grade oils can be used in the fragrance industry. The spent material and the unused portion of the plant can be dried and used to fire the distilling apparatus the next time around. The ashes can be put back into the earth, providing a whole wealth of nutrients such as potassium and trace elements, so that you end up with excellent soil and strong, disease-resistant plants. Other spent material could be used as compost or animal feed. It costs nothing after the initial capital outlay for the still, which could be shared on a cooperative basis between several farms. Essential oils can be put to so many uses that the market for them is wide—and growing.

Because making essential oils makes such good sense to the Third World farmer who cannot afford fertilizers and fuel, some Western governments are beginning to get involved in exporting the knowledge and equipment necessary for them to do so. This provides a cash crop which is of interest to the medical, cosmetic, and food industries, as well as to consumers such as you or me. These same governments, and others, could also consider the high percentage of imports of essential oils in their own countries and aim to cut this figure by encouraging farmers to grow these useful crops.

Knowledge about the symbiotic relationship between plants can also help to increase the yield of essential oil in those plants grown for the purpose. Have a look at the Good Companions list, but meanwhile don't forget the humble stinging nettle. It has been shown to have a significant effect on the production of the following plants when grown nearby:

PLANT	INCREASE IN YIELD (pecentage)
Angelica	80
Valerian	20
Marjoram	10–20
Sage	10
Peppermint	10

As can be seen from the scope of this book, essential oils are in demand for medicinal purposes—for both humans and animals—for cosmetic, hair and beauty products, fragrances in perfumes and colognes, flavorings for food, preservatives, for cleansing and air freshening materials, pest deterrents, fungicides, and plant feeds. Their diversity, and the fact that they enhance the whole environment, must make them the perfect crop.

♦ APPENDIX 1 ♦

THE ESSENTIAL OIL CHARTS

THE BACTERIA BUSTERS

COMMON NAME	ANTIBIOTIC	ANTISEPTIC	ANTIVIRAL	ANTIFUNGAL
BALSAM DE PERU	◆			◆
BAY		◆		
BERGAMOT	◆	◆		
BOIS DE ROSE		◆		
CAJEPUT		◆		
CAMPHOR		◆		
CARDAMON		◆		
CEDARWOOD		◆		
CELERY (WILD)		◆		
CELERY		◆		
CHAMOMILE GERMAN	◆	◆		
CHAMOMILE ROMAN	◆	◆		
CINNAMON	◆	◆	◆	
CITRONELLA		◆		
CLARY-SAGE		◆		
CLOVE	◆	◆	◆	
CUMIN		◆		
CYPRESS		◆		
ELEMI		◆		
EUCALYPTUS	◆	◆		
EUCALYPTUS LEMON	◆	◆	◆	◆
EUCALYPTUS RADIATA	◆	◆	◆	◆
GARLIC	◆	◆	◆	
GERANIUM		◆		
GINGER		◆		
HYSSOP	◆	◆		
JUNIPER		◆		◆
LAVENDER	◆	◆	◆	◆
LEMON	◆	◆		◆
LEMONGRASS		◆		
LIME	◆	◆		

THE BACTERIA BUSTERS

COMMON NAME	ANTIBIOTIC	ANTISEPTIC	ANTIVIRAL	ANTIFUNGAL
MANDARIN		♦		
MARJORAM		♦		
MYRTLE	♦	♦		♦
NIAOULI	♦	♦		
NUTMEG	♦	♦		
ONION	♦	♦	♦	♦
ORANGE		♦		
OREGANO	♦	♦	♦	
PARSLEY		♦		
PATCHOULI	♦	♦		♦
PEPPERMINT		♦		
PETTIGRAINE, LEMON		♦		
PETTIGRAINE, ORANGE		♦		
PIMENTO		♦		♦
PINE	♦	♦		
RAVENSARA	♦	♦	♦	
ROSE		♦		
ROSEMARY		♦		
SAGE		♦		♦
SANDALWOOD		♦	♦	♦
SARRIETTE	♦	♦		♦
SAVORY		♦		♦
SPEARMINT		♦		
TEA TREE	♦	♦	♦	♦
TEREBINTH	♦	♦		
THYME	♦	♦	♦	♦
VERBENA		♦		
VETIVER		♦		
WINTERGREEN		♦		
YLANG-YLANG		♦		

BEAUTY OILS

	EYES	HANDS	FEET	NAILS	NECK	LIPS
Lemon	◆	◆	◆	◆	◆	◆
Lavender	◆	◆	◆	◆		◆
Grapefruit				◆		
Carrot	◆	◆	◆	◆	◆	
Cypress				◆		
Rosemary		◆		◆		
Eucalyptus peppermint				◆		
Pettigraine					◆	
Tea tree				◆ *(Nail-bed Infections)*		◆
Tagetes			◆	◆		
Oregano				◆		
Thyme			◆ (linalol)	◆ (all)		
Ravensara				◆		
Myrrh				◆		
Patchouli		◆		◆		
Calendula			◆	◆		◆

BEAUTY OILS

	EYES	HANDS	FEET	NAILS	NECK	LIPS
Fennel	◆		◆			
Chamomile	◆ (German)		◆ (all)			◆ (all)
Geranium		◆			◆	◆
Rose		◆			◆	◆
Sandalwood		◆				
Neroli		◆				
Lime		◆				
Eucalyptus lemon		◆				
Orange					◆	
Basil					◆	
Palma rosa	◆	◆	◆		◆	◆
Clary-sage					◆	
Vetiver					◆	
Lemongrass					◆	
Bois de rose	◆					
Eucalyptus radiata				◆		

BEAUTY BODY OILS

	DRY SKIN	GREASY SKIN	GENERAL OILS	DISTURBED SKIN	SENSITIVE SKIN
Bezoin	♦				
Palma rosa	♦		♦		
Patchouli	♦		♦		
Carrot	♦		♦		
Geranium	♦		♦	♦	♦
Pettigraine	♦				
Bois de rose	♦				
Lavender	♦	♦	♦	♦	♦
Chamomile German	♦			♦	♦
Rose	♦				
Chamomile Roman	♦		♦	♦	
Orange		♦			
Lemon		♦			
Clary-sage		♦		♦	
Jasmine		♦	♦		
Neroli		♦	♦		
Nutmeg		♦			
Cypress		♦			
Ylang-ylang		♦	♦		
Frankincense			♦		
Sandalwood	♦		♦		
Niaouli				♦	
Eucalyptus lemon				♦	
Eucalyptus peppermint				♦	
Thyme linalol				♦	
Myrrh				♦	
Bergamot		♦			

TONING/SLIMMING OILS

	GENERAL	DIURETICS	FOR CELLULITE	FOR BREASTS	FOR FLABBY ARMS
Orange	◆				
Basil	◆		◆		
Sage	◆		◆	◆	
Thyme	◆				
Pettigraine	◆				
Lime	◆				
Lemongrass	◆			◆	
Grapefruit	◆	◆	◆		
Rosemary	◆		◆		
Lavender	◆				
Juniper		◆	◆		◆
Celery		◆	◆		
Fennel		◆		◆	◆
Cypress		◆	◆	◆	◆
Lemon		◆	◆		
Oregano		◆	◆		
Thyme (all)			◆		
Patchouli			◆		
Cedarwood			◆		
Clary-sage				◆	
Angelica				◆	
Spearmint				◆	
Geranium				◆	
Carrot	◆			◆	◆
Hop				◆	
Parsley				◆	
Lavender					◆

FACIAL SKIN OILS / 1

	OILY	DRY	DEHYDRATED	HYDRATED	SENSITIVE	DISTURBED
Chamomile	◆	◆ (blue)			◆ (blue)	◆
Carrot	◆	◆	◆	◆	◆	◆
Lemon	◆	◆		◆		◆
Geranium	◆	◆	◆	◆	◆	◆
Lavender	◆		◆	◆	◆	◆
Hyssop		◆		◆		◆
Palma rosa	◆	◆		◆		◆
Patchouli	◆	◆		◆		◆
Benzoin	◆	◆				
Marjoram	◆					
Peppermint	◆					
Orange	◆					
Rosemary	◆	◆				
Sandalwood		◆		◆		◆
Fennel				◆		
Rose		◆		◆		
Cypress	◆			◆		
Neroli		◆				
Jasmine	◆					
Bois de rose		◆				
Pettigraine	◆					
Ylang-ylang	◆					
Frankincense	◆					
Juniper	◆					◆
Clary-sage						◆

FACIAL SKIN OILS / 2

	ENERGIZING	FOR DERMATITIS	FOR ACNE	FOR ECZEMA (DRY)	(WET)	FOR WRINKLES
Lemon	♦		♦			♦
Eucalytpus radiata			♦			
Juniper			♦			
Lavender		♦	♦			
Palma rosa	♦		♦			♦
Patchouli			♦			
Sandalwood			♦			♦
Clary-sage			♦			♦
Bergamot	♦			♦		
Chamomile		♦		♦	♦	
Carrot	♦	♦		♦	♦	♦
Geranium				♦		♦
Hyssop		♦		♦	♦	
Rosemary				♦		♦
Juniper					♦	
Myrrh					♦	
Rose						♦
Orange						♦
Neroli						♦
Bois de rose						♦
Galbanum	♦					♦
Pettigraine			♦			
Violet leaf	♦		♦			♦

FACIAL SKIN OILS / 3

	FOR PSORIASIS	NORMAL	FOR BROKEN CAPILLARIES	COMBI- NATION OILY / DRY	COMBI- NATION DRY / OILY	REVITAL- IZING
Calendula	◆			◆		
Violet leaf						◆
Galbanum						◆
Fennel						◆
Parsley			◆	◆		
Chamomile	◆	◆	◆	◆	◆	
Cypress			◆			◆
Geranium		◆	◆	◆		
Hyssop			◆			
Bergamot	◆					
Lemon		◆			◆	◆
Palma rosa		◆		◆		
Sandalwood		◆			◆	
Rose		◆	◆	◆	◆	◆
Neroli		◆			◆	◆
Carrot		◆	◆	◆	◆	◆
Bois de rose		◆		◆		◆
Lavender	◆	◆		◆		
Pettigraine				◆		
Benzoin						◆

THE ESSENTIAL OILS

COMMON NAME *LATIN NAME*	TYPE OF PLANT	PART FROM WHICH THE ESSENTIAL OIL IS OBTAINED	COUNTRIES OF ORIGIN
Angelica *Angelica archangelica*	Herb	Seeds/Roots	China, Spain, USSR, Egypt
Aniseed *Pimpinella anisum*	Herb	Seed Pod	Central and South America, Indonesia, India
Basil *Ocimum basilicum*	Herb	Whole Plant	Europe, United States, Réunion, Madagascar, Seychelles
Bay *Pimenta racemosa*	Tree	Leaves	West Indies, South America
Benzoin *Styrax benzoin*	Tree	Trunk	Java, Sumatra, Borneo, Thailand
Bergamot *Citrus bergamia*	Tree	Peel of Fruit	Italy, Morocco, Guinea
Birch *Betula lenta*	Tree	Bark	USSR, Holland, Germany
Black Pepper *Piper nigrum*	Vine	Berries	India, Indonesia, Brazil, Southeast Asia
Bois de Rose *Aniba rosaeodora*	Tree	Wood	Brazil, Mexico
Camphor *Cinnamomum camphora*	Tree	Wood	Borneo, Sumatra, China, Japan
Cardamom *Elettaria cardamomum*	Plant	Seeds	Guatemala, India
Carrot *Daucus carota*	Vegetable	Root, Seeds	England, France, Europe
Cedarwood *Cedrus Atlantica*	Tree	Wood	North America
Chamomile German *Matricaria chamomila*	Herb	Flowers, Leaves	England, Hungary, South America, France
Chamomile Roman *Athemis nobilis*	Herb	Flowers, Leaves	England, France, Hungary, Bulgaria, Yugoslavia

AROMATHERAPEUTIC HOME USE	SOME OTHER USES
Coughs, Colds, Fevers, Flatulence, Indigestion	Confectionery, Pharmaceutics
Indigestion, Coughs, Bronchitis, Catarrh	Pharmaceutics, Dentistry
Bronchitis, Fatigue, Colds, Loss of Concentration, Migraine, Gout, Aches and Pains	Food Industry, Pharmaceutics
Sprains, Colds, Flu, Insomnia, Rheumatism	Perfumery
Coughs, Itching, Arthritis, Colds; as a Sedative	Pharmaceutics, Cosmetics
Fevers, Acne, Tension, Wounds, Coughs, Stress; as an Antidepressant	Pharmaceutics, Perfumery, Cosmetics
Gout, Rheumatism, Eczema, Ulcers	Perfumery, Pharmaceutics
Colds, Aches and Pains, Influenza, Flatulence, Rheumatism	Pharmaceutics
Tonic, Coughs, Headaches; as an Antidepressant	Perfumery
Coughs, Colds, Fevers, Rheumatism, Arthritis	Pharmaceutics
Nausea, Coughs, Headaches, Aches; as a Digestive and Tonic	Perfumery, Pharmaceutics, Food Industry
Gout, Ulcers, Flatulence, Eczema, Psoriasis; as a Diuretic	Food Industry, Pharmaceutics
Bronchitis, Catarrh, Acne, Arthritis; as a Diuretic	Pharmaceutics, Cosmetics
Nerves, Migraine, Acne, Inflammation, Insomnia, Menstrual Problems, Dermatitis, Eczema, Psoriasis, Inflammatory Diseases, Burns	Pharmaceutics, Cosmetics
Nerves, Migraine, Acne, Inflammation, Insomnia, Menstrual Problems, Dermatitis	Pharmaceutics, Cosmetics

THE ESSENTIAL OILS

COMMON NAME *LATIN NAME*	TYPE OF PLANT	PART FROM WHICH THE ESSENTIAL OIL IS OBTAINED	COUNTRIES OF ORIGIN
Cinnamon *Cinnamomum zeylanicum*	Tree	Twigs, Leaves	Sri Lanka, India, Madagascar
Citronella *Cymbopogon nardus*	Grass	All parts	Madagascar, South America
Clary-sage *Salvia sclarea*	Herb	Flowering Tops	Spain, USSR, France
Clove *Eugenia caryophyllata*	Tree	Flower Buds	Philippines, Molucca Islands, East and West Indies
Coriander *Coriandrum sativum*	Herb	Seeds of Ripe Fruit, Leaves	USSR, India, Italy, Morocco, Tunisia, United States
Cumin *Cuminum cyminum*	Herb	Seeds, Fruit	Mediterranean, India, Sicily, Morocco
Cypress *Cupressus sempervirens*	Tree	Leaves, Twigs	Mediterranean
Dill *Anethum graveolens*	Herb	Seeds, Fruit	Mediterranean
Eucalyptus *Eucalyptus globulus*	Tree	Leaves, Twigs	Australia, Tasmania, China, Spain, California, Brazil
Eucalyptus Lemon *Eucalyptus citriodora*	Tree	Leaves, Twigs	Australia, Tasmania
Eucalyptus Peppermint *Eucalyptus dives*	Tree	Leaves, Twigs	Australia, Tasmania
Eucalyptus Radiata	Tree	Leaves, Twigs	Australia, Tasmania
Fennel *Foeniculum vulgare*	Herb	Seeds	Japan, India, Mediterranean, Russia, Romania, Northern Europe

AROMATHERAPEUTIC HOME USE	SOME OTHER USES
Flu, Rheumatism, Warts, Coughs, Colds, Viral Infections	Pharmaceutics, Dentistry, Food Industry, Perfumery
As an Insecticide, Deodorant, Tonic, Stimulant	Perfumery, Household Products
Depression, Nerves, Sore Throat, Aches and Pains, Debility; as a Sedative	Pharmaceutics, Cosmetics, Perfumery
Nausea, Flatulence, Bronchitis, Arthritis, Rheumatism, Toothache, Diarrhea, Infections; as an Analgesic and Antiseptic	Pharmaceutics, Perfumery, Food Industry
Indigestion, Influenza, Fatigue, Rheumatism, Flatulence, Nervousness; as an Analgesic	Pharmaceutics, Veterinary, Perfumery
Indigestion, Headache, Liver Problems; as a Stimulant	Food Industry, Perfumery, Veterinary
Menopausal Problems, Circulatory Conditions, Rheumatism, Colds, Whooping Cough, Nervous Tension, Hemorrhoids, Wounds; as an Astringent	Pharmaceutics, Perfumery
Flatulence, Indigestion, Constipation, Nervousness, Gastric Upsets, Headaches	Pharmaceutics, Perfumery, Cosmetics, Food Industry
Sore Throats, Coughs, Bronchitis, Sinusitis, Skin Infections, Ulcers, Sores, Rheumatism, Aches and Pains; as an Antiseptic and Antiinflammatory	Pharmaceutics, Veterinary
Dandruff, Scabs, Sores, Candida, Asthma, Fever, Fungal Infections, Skin Infections, Sore Throats; as an Antiseptic	Pharmaceutics, Perfumery
Ulcers, Sores, Coughts, Colds, Fever, Respiratory Problems, Viral Infections, Headaches, Flu, Rheumatism, Arthritis	Pharmaceutics, Veterinary
Viral Infections, Colds, Coughts, Bronchitis, Whooping Cough, Rheumatism, Muccular Strains; as an Antiseptic	Pharmaceutics, Veterinary
Digestive Problems, Menopausal Problems, Obesity, Constipation, Kidney Stones, Nausea; as a Diuretic	Pharmaceutics, Food Industry, Veterinary

THE ESSENTIAL OILS

COMMON NAME *LATIN NAME*	TYPE OF PLANT	PART FROM WHICH THE ESSENTIAL OIL IS OBTAINED	COUNTRIES OF ORIGIN
Frankincense *Buswellia thurifera*	Tree	Bark	Somalia, China, Ethiopia, Southern Arabia
Galbanum *Ferula galbaniflua*	Plant	Bark	Iran, Lebanon, Cape of Good Hope
Geranium *Pelargonium graveolens*	Plant	Leaves, Stalks, Flowers	Réunion, Madagascar, Egypt, China, France, Algeria, Morocco, USSR
Ginger *Zingiber officinale*	Plant	Roots	China, Japan, India, West Africa
Grapefruit *Citrus paradisi*	Tree	Rind of Fruit	Israel, United States
Hops *Humulus lupulus*	Plant	Buds and Flowers	Northern Europe, Russia, Spain, United States, New Zealand
Hyssop *Hyssopus officinalis*	Herb	Leaves, Flowering Tops	Southern Europe, Brazil, Palestine
Immortelle (Italian Everlasting) *Helichrysum angustifolium*	Flower	Flowering Tops	Europe
Jasmine *Jasminum Officinale*	Bush	Flowers	France, Egypt, China, Algeria, Morocco
Juniper *Juniperus Communis*	Bush	Berries	Europe, North America, North Asia, North Africa
Lavender *Lavendula* *Angustifolium, officinalis*	Plant	Flowering Tops	England, France, Tasmania, Yugoslavia
Lemon *Citrus Limonum*	Tree	Rind of Fruit	Brazil, Israel, United States, Argentina

AROMATHERAPEUTIC HOME USE	SOME OTHER USES
Sores, Wounds, Fevers, Coughs, Colds, Stress, Bronchitis, Laryngitis, Nervous Conditions, Tension	Pharmaceutics, Religion
Bronchitis, Respiratory Problems, Swelling, Inflammations, Tension, Nervous Conditions	Perfumery
Depression, Menstrual Problems, Diarrhea, Diabetes, Sores, Neuralgia, Bleeding, Circulatory Conditions, Eczema, Sore Throats, Nervous Tension, Kidney Stones	Pharmaceutics, Perfumery, Cosmetics
Rheumatism, Muscular Aches and Pains, Sprains, Broken Bones, Colds, Nausea, Diarrhea, Alcoholism, Digestive Disorders	Perfumery, Food Industry
Tonic, Obesity, Kidney and Liver Problems, Migraine, Depression; as a Tonic and Aid in Drug Withdrawal	Food Industry, Cosmetics, Perfumery
Neuralgia, Bruising, Menstrual and Menopausal Problems, Rheumatism; as a Nerve Tonic, Diuretic, Sedative, and Analgesic	Food Industry, Pharmaceutics
Bruises, Rheumatism, Arthritis, Coughs, Colds, Sore Throat, Viral Infections, Blood Pressure, Circulatory Problems, Nervous Tension, Asthma; as a Tonic	Perfumery, Food Industry
Bacterial Infections, Rheumatism, Muscular Aches and Pains, Weakness, Lethargy, Depression, Respiratory Problems, Colds, Flu, Fever; as a Fungicide	Pharmaceutics, Perfumery
Nervous Tension, Depression, Menstrual Problems, Laryngitis, Anxiety, Lethargy; as a Relaxant	Perfumery, Cosmetics
Liver Problems, Obesity, Rheumatism, Acne, Coughs, Ulcers, Urinary Infections; as a Diuretic	Pharmaceutics, Perfumery, Food Industry
Burns, Inflammation, Cuts, Wounds, Eczema, Dermatitis, Fainting, Headaches, Influenza, Insomnia, Hysteria, Migraine, Nausea, Nervous Tension, Infections, Bacterial Conditions, Sores, Ulcers, Acne, Boils, Asthma, Rheumatism, Arthritis	Pharmaceutics, Perfumery, Cosmetics
Sore Throat, Nervous Conditions, Blood Pressure, Digestive Problems, Gallstones, Debility, Fever, Anxiety; as a Tonic, Astringent, and Antiseptic	Food Industry, Pharmaceutics, Cosmetics, Perfumery

THE ESSENTIAL OILS

COMMON NAME *LATIN NAME*	TYPE OF PLANT	PART FROM WHICH THE ESSENTIAL OIL IS OBTAINED	COUNTRIES OF ORIGIN
Lemongrass *Cymbopogon citratus*	Grass	Whole Plant	Brazil, Sri Lanka, Central Africa
Lime *Citrus aurantifolia*	Tree	Rind	Brazil, Mexico, Italy, West Indies
Mace *Myristica fragrans*	Tree	Peel of Fruit	Sri Lanka, West Indies, Java, Sumatra
Mandarin *Citrus Nobilis*	Tree	Rind of Fruit	Italy, Brazil, Spain, Argentina, China
Marjoram *Origanum marjorana*	Herb	Flowering Tops, Leaves	Hungary, Egypt, Spain, France, Germany, Portugal
Melissa *Melissa officinalis*	Herb	Leaves	Mediterranean, Europe
Myrrh *Commiphora myrrha*	Tree	Bark/Resin	Somalia, Ethiopia, North Africa
Neroli (Orange Blossom) *Citrus bigaradia, aurantium*	Tree	Flowers	France, Egypt, Italy, Morocco, Tunisia
Niaouli *Melaleuca viridiflora*	Bush	Leaves, Twigs	Australia, Tasmania, East Indies
Nutmeg *Myristica fragrans*	Tree	Seed	Java, Sumatra, Indonesia, West Indies
Orange *Citrus aurantium*	Tree	Rind of Fruit	United States, Brazil, France, Spain
Oregano *Origanum vulgare*	Herb	Leaves, Flowering Tops	North Africa, Europe, Egypt, Asia

AROMATHERAPEUTIC HOME USE	SOME OTHER USES
Infections, Headaches, Sore Throats, Respiratory Problems, Fevers; as a Tonic, Antiseptic, and Insect Repellent	Pharmaceutics, Perfumery
Fevers, Rheumatism, Sore Throats, Headaches, Anorexia, Alcoholism, Depression, Anxiety; as an Astringent and Tonic	Confectionery, Food Industry, Perfumery
Indigestion, General Weakness, Bacterial Infections, Gout, Rheumatism, Arthritis; as an Aid to Circulation	Dentistry, Perfumery, Food Industry
Insomnia, Nervousness, Liver Problems, Digestive Weakness, Anxiety; as a Tonic and Tranquilizer	Food Industry, Perfumery
Sprains, Bruises, Colds, Rheumatism, Intestinal Cramps, Menstrual Problems, Anxiety, Asthma, Bronchitis, Insomnia, Circulatory Disorders, Muscular Problems	Pharmaceutics, Food Industry
Nervousness, Bacterial Infections, Fungal Infections, Diarrhea, Eczema; as a Sedative and Cardiac Tonic	Pharmaceutics, Perfumery
Wounds, Mouth Ulcers, Dermatitis, Bacterial Infections, Bronchitis, Diarrhea, Fungal Infections, Candida	Pharmaceutics, Dentistry
Depression, Anxiety, Hysteria, Diarrhea, Nervous Tension, Menopausal Problems, Dermatitis; as a Cardiac Tonic	Perfumery, Cosmetics, Food Industry
Cuts and Wounds, Infections, Bacterial Disease, Sore Throats, Burns, Respiratory Problems, Acne; as an Antiseptic	Pharmaceutics, Cosmetics
Nausea, Vomiting, Muscular Aches and Pains, Rheumatism, Arthritis, Nervousness, Insomnia; as a Heart Stimulant	Pharmaceutics, Food Industry
Depression, Anxiety, Constipation, Nervous Conditions, Muscular Spasm; as a Tonic, Sedative, and Antiseptic	Food Industry, Perfumery
Bronchitis, Viral Infections, Rheumatism, Respiratory Problems, Muscular Pain, Digestive Problems	Food Industry

THE ESSENTIAL OILS

COMMON NAME *LATIN NAME*	TYPE OF PLANT	PART FROM WHICH THE ESSENTIAL OIL IS OBTAINED	COUNTRIES OF ORIGIN
Palma rosa *Cymbopogon martini*	Grass	Whole Plant	Brazil, Central America
Parsley *Petroselinum sativum*	Herb	Seeds	Europe
Patchouli *Pogostemon patchouli*	Plant	Leaves	China, Indonesia, Madagascar, Japan
Peppermint *Mentha piperata*	Herb	Whole Plant	America, Europe, China
Pettigraine *Citrus aurantium*	Tree	Leaves, Twigs	France, Italy, Paraguay, Brazil
Pimento *Pimenta officinalis*	Tree	Berries, Twigs	West Indies, Réunion, India
Pine *Pinus sylvestris*	Tree	Needles, Twigs	Europe, USSR, North America
Ravensara *Ravensara aromatica*	Bush	Leaves	Australia, Madagascar
Rose Bulgar *Rosa Damascena*	Bush	Flowers, Petals	Bulgaria
Rose Maroc *Rosa Damascena*	Bush	Flowers, Petals	Morocco
Rosemary *Rosmarinus officinalis*	Herb	Flowers, Leaves	Spain, France, Yugoslavia, Japan
Sage *Salvia officinalis*	Herb	Flowers, Leaves	Mediterranean, China

AROMATHERAPEUTIC HOME USE	SOME OTHER USES
Skin Infections, Anorexia; as a Tonic	Perfumery, Cosmetics
Nervous Conditions, Kidney Problems, Menstrual Problems, Menopausal Problems; as a Sedative and Diuretic	Pharmaceutics, Perfumery
Skin Inflammations, Fungal Infections, Acne, Eczema, Dandruff; as an Antiseptic, Diuretic, and Insecticide	Perfumery, Cosmetics
Inflammation, Nausea, Indigestion, Fevers, Flatulence, Headaches, Migraine, Liver Problems, Arthritis; as a Stimulant	Pharmaceutics, Food Industry
Anxiety, Insomnia, Depression; as an Antiseptic, Tonic, and Aid to Convalescence	Perfumery, Cosmetics
Flatulence, Indigestion, Cramps, Intestinal Problems, Colds, Rheumatism, Muscular Strains, Depression; as a Tonic and Tranquilizer	Pharmaceutics, Perfumery
Bladder and Kidney Problems, Rheumatism, Respiratory Problems, Chest Infections, Colds, Catarrh, Sore Throats, Circulation Problems, Muscular Aches and Pains; as a Diuretic	Pharmaceutics
Viral Infections, Liver Infections, Lung Infections, Respiratory Problems; as an Antiseptic	Pharmaceutics
Anxiety, Depression, Circulatory Problems, Menopausal Problems; as an Antiseptic and Tonic	Perfumery, Cosmetics
Menstrual Disorders, Depression, Stress, Tension, Circulatory Conditions; as a Tonic and Sedative	Perfumery, Cosmetics
Gout, Headaches, Fatigue, Rheumatism, Skin Infections, Muscular Aches and Pains, Sprains, Dandruff, Alopecia, Obesity, Spinal Injuries; as a Nerve Stimulant, Heart Tonic and Liver Decongestant, Analgesic	Pharmaceutics, Veterinary
Sores, Bacterial Infections, Bronchitis, Catarrh, Rheumatism, Arthritis, Sprains, Fibrositis; as an Astringent	Pharmaceutics, Veterinary

THE ESSENTIAL OILS

COMMON NAME *LATIN NAME*	TYPE OF PLANT	PART FROM WHICH THE ESSENTIAL OIL IS OBTAINED	COUNTRIES OF ORIGIN
Sandalwood *Santalum album*	Tree	Wood	India, Indonesia
Spearmint *Mentha spicata*	Herb	Leaves, Flowering Tops	Europe, Mediterranean, Russia, United States
Tagetes *Tagetes patula*	Plant	Flowers	Northern Africa
Tea Tree *Melaleuca alternifolia*	Tree	Leaves, Twigs	Australia, Tasmania
Thyme, Red *Thymus vulgaris*	Herb	Leaves, Flowering Tops	Mediterranean, Egypt
Thyme Linalol	Herb	Leaves, Flowering Tops	Mediterranean
Valerian *Valeriana officinalis*	Plant	Roots	Europe, Northern Asia, Japan, Mexico
Vetiver *Vetiveria zizanoides*	Grass	Roots	Indonesia, Philippines, Comoro Islands
Violet Leaves *Viola odorata*	Plant	Leaves	Italy, France, England, Greece
Yarrow *Achillea millefolium*	Herb	Leaves, Flowering Tops	Europe, Africa, North America
Ylang-ylang *Cananga odorata*	Tree	Flowers	Indonesia, Philippines, Comoro Islands

AROMATHERAPEUTIC HOME USE	SOME OTHER USES
Acne, Catarrh, Cystitis, Menstrual Problems, Depression, Skin Infections, Fungal and Bacterial Infections; as a Sedative	Perfumery, Pharmaceutics
Flatulence, Indigestion, Intestinal Cramps, Fevers, Nausea, Colic, Hemorrhoids	Food Industry, Cosmetics, Pharmaceutics
Fungal Infections, Skin Infections, Cuts, Sprains, Strains, Wounds, Circulatory Problems; as an Antiseptic	Pharmaceutics
Fungal Infections, Viral and Bacterial Infections, Colds, Influenza, Cold Sores, Warts, Verrucas, Inflammation, Acne, Burns, Candida, Shock, Hysteria	Pharmaceutics, Veterinary
Bacterial Infections, Urinary Infections, Rheumatism, Viral Infections, Lethargy, Sores, Wounds; as a Stimulant and Tonic, and to Raise Immunity	Pharmaceutics, Veterinary
As above	Pharmaceutics
Sedative, Calming, Nervous Conditions, Trembling, Neuralgia, Insomnia, Palpitations; as a Sedative and Tranquilizer	Veterinary, Pharmaceutics
Nervousness, Insomnia, Rheumatism; as a Muscular Relaxant, Antiseptic, and Tonic	Perfumery
Inflammations, Kidney Problems, Obesity, Skin Infections, Fibrositis, Rheumatism; as an Analgesic and Liver Decongestant	Perfumery
Inflammations, Cramps, Constipation, Circulation, Rheumatoid Arthritis, Menstrual Problems; as an Astringent	Pharmaceutics
Palpitations, Anxiety, Depression, High Blood Pressure; as a Sedative and General Tonic	Perfumery

Formulations

R1 Used for arthritis, rheyumatism, muscular sprains, strains, neuralgia, and overexercised muscles.

AV1 (Dermatect) An antiviral, used in all viral conditions.

B1 Used for all bronchial tract disorders, cartarrh, and mucus conditions.

RE1 Used for rejuvenation of mature skins, skin care, and general facial tone.

For all these formulations, see list of suppliers on page 413.

♦ APPENDIX 2 ♦
AROMASSAGE

Aromassage can be part of a healing process, or a way to apply essential oils to the right places. It is neither complicated nor difficult. Anyone can do it, to their friends, their families, and even to themselves.

Effleurage

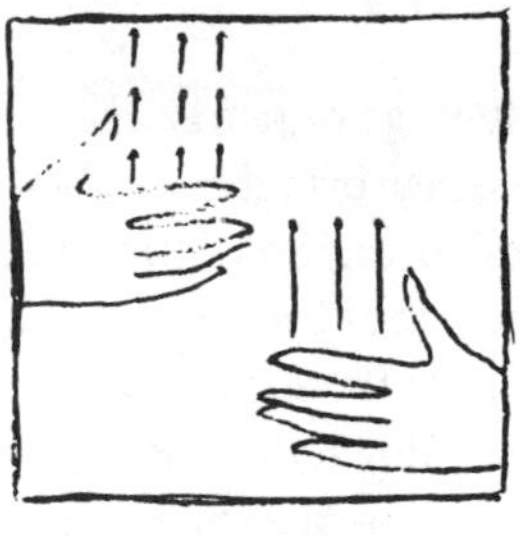

Effleurage is possibly the most useful movement in Aromassage. It is a series of gentle, soothing strokes, which enable the essential oils to penetrate the body, causing relaxation and calm throughout. Use your whole hands, not just your fingers, in strokes that can be either long or short, firm or gentle. Muscles will be relaxed and nerve endings soothed, circulation increased, stress and tension relieved.

Keep your hands relaxed but firm in this movement.

Petrissage

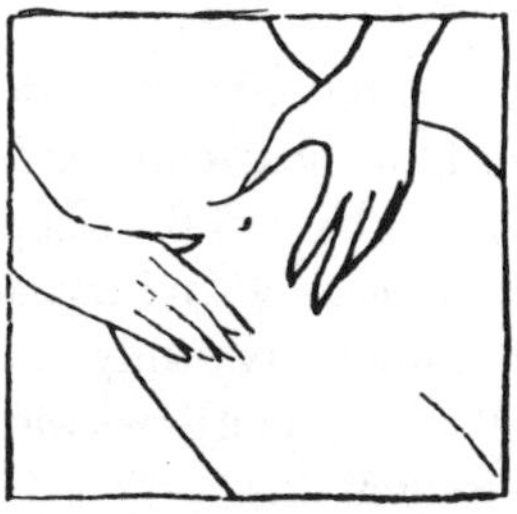

Petrissage is like gently kneading dough. Each movement should be slow and careful, never causing pain. These movements are often helpful on fatty areas, and on backs. They can relax the muscles, increase circulation, help lymphatic flow, and aid the release of trapped toxins.

Use slight pressure on your thumbs in this movement.

Head Massage

When using Aromassage on the scalp, put the oil on the fingertips and use the fingers, working all over the scalp.

For Migraine and Headaches

Massage around the base of the neck and work upwards to the base of the scalp. Continue massaging this area for a few moments. Use your fingers in firm effleurage strokes to apply the appropriate essential oils.

For the Neck

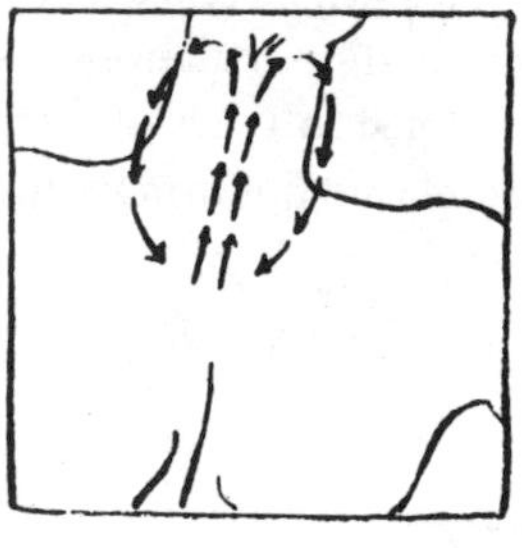

Use small, firm circular movements, working from the base of the neck, either side of the vertebrae, to the base of the scalp. Work to the sides of the neck and repeat the movements, this time very gently, and work down again. Repeat several times with the appropriate essential oils.

For the Shoulders

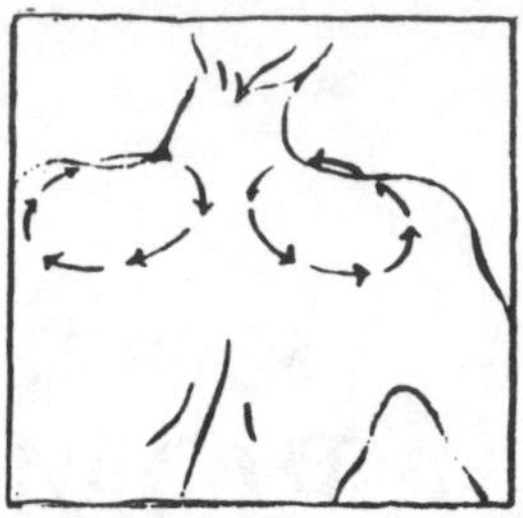

Aromassage into the muscles with effleurage and petrissage movements. Using your thumbs and palms, make firm strokes from the shoulder to the neck and back again.

For the Arms

Aromassage up towards the armpit, using effleurage or petrissage, on the fatty or muscular areas only.

For the Back

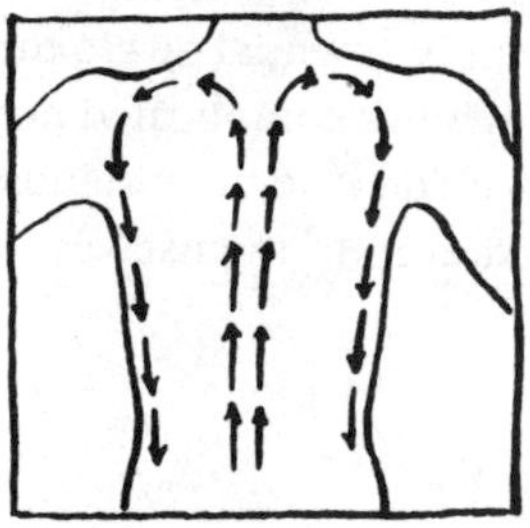

Firm or gentle effleurage or petrissage can be used. Do not massage over the vertebrae. Start from the lumbar region of the back, and with two hands stroke all the way up to the shoulders. Slide the hands over the shoulders and return down the sides of the back. Repeat this movement as many times as you like. The longer the aromassage, the more relaxing it is.

For the Abdomen

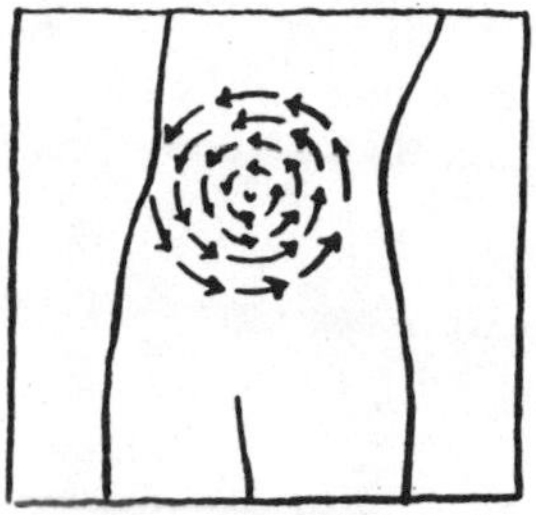

Use circular movements only, in a clockwise direction. Effleurage is the best stroke to use for this.

For the Legs

Always aromassage legs upwards. Use effleurage alone or with petrissage on the fatty or muscular areas only (never over varicosed areas).

For Women's Reproductive Problems

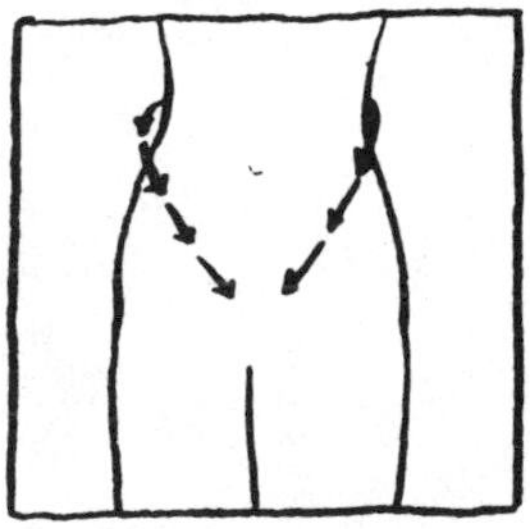

Aromassage using effleurage movements. Begin at the lower back and slide over the hips. Now slide each hand separately over the abdomen, and repeat the whole process.

For the Feet

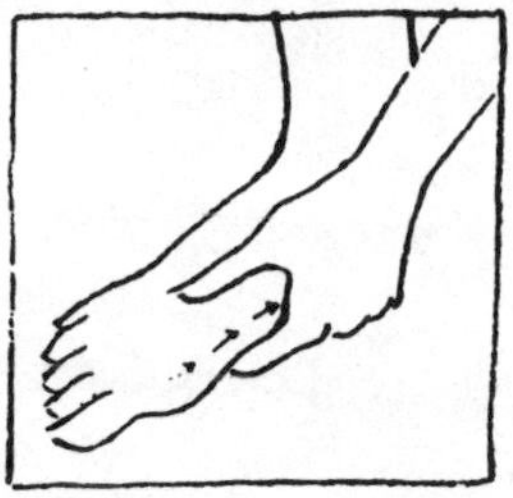

Aromassage from the toes to the heel, thumbs under the foot and fingers on top. You will find this very soothing.

All massage should be carried out with the flow of the body, that is, towards the heart.

When massaging children and invalids use gentle, comforting effleurage movements.

After an aerobic workout, petrissage movements are useful to release toxins and keep muscles supple.

♦ APPENDIX 3 ♦

ADDRESSES AND BIBLIOGRAPHY

Useful Addresses ♦♦♦♦♦

Valerie Ann Worwood would be pleased to hear readers' comments and how they have used the information contained within this book, but is unable to reply to letters. Please write to: PO Box 210, Romford Essex RM7 7DW UK

Aromatherapy Service and Reputable Suppliers

Essentially Yours International
Mail order service with fully comprehensive aromatherapy product list including all essential oils and products mentioned in this book and other related items — for both the public and professionals.

For a catalog, please send a stamped, self-addressed envelope to:

Essentially Yours, Ltd. England
366-368 London Road
Westcliff on Sea,
Essex SS0 7H2 UK
Tel. 0702 390625

Essentially Yours North America
PO Box 81866
Bakersfield, CA 93380

Essentially Yours Canada
254 Hart Street
Coquitlam, B.C. CANADA V3K4A6

Aroma Vera Inc.
PO Box 3609
Culver City, CA 90231

Original Swiss Aromatics
PO Box 606
San Rafael, CA 94915

Aromatherapy Courses

For details of Valerie Ann Worwood's lectures and seminars in the USA please contact the address below:

Correspondence and professional aromatherapy training, workshops, seminars, and short courses for the non-professional.

The International Academy of Holistic Studies UK/USA
PO Box 210
Romford, Essex RM7 7DW UK

Aromatherapy Seminar
3384 Robertson Place
Los Angeles, CA 90034

Pacific Institute of Aromatherapy
PO Box 606
San Rafael, CA 94915

For a list of Registered Aromatherapists write to:

Europe
The International Federation of Aromatherapists
Department of Continuing Education
Room 8, Royal Masonic Hospital
RavensCourt Park
London W6 OTN UK
Tel. 081-864-8066

USA
American Aromatherapy Association
PO Box 1222
Fair Oaks, CA 95628

Bibliography ♦♦♦♦♦♦♦♦♦

Baerheim, Svendson, Scheffer, *Essential Oils and Aromatic Plants.* Dr. W. Junk, 1985.

Bardeau, Fabrice, *La Médecine Aromatique.* Robert Laffont, Paris, 1976.

Belaiche, P., *Traits de Phytothérapie et d'Aromathérapie,* 3 vols. Librairie Maloine, Paris, 1979.

Bernadet, Marcel, *La Phyto-Aromathérapie Pratique.* Editions Dangles, St. Jean de Braye, 1983.

Culpeper, *Complete Herbal.* W. Foulsham & Co., London, 1952.

Duraffourd, Paul, *The Best of Health (Thanks to Essential Oils).* Cevic, 1984.

Franck, Gertrude, *Companion Planting.* Thorsens, 1983.

Gattefosse, R. M., *Antiseptiques Essentials.* Desforges, Girardot, 1931.

Grieves, Maud, *A Modern Herbal.* Jonathan Cape, London, 1979.

Hutchens, Alma, *Indian Herbology of North America.* Merco, 1973.

Huws, Ursula, *VDU Hazards Handbook.* London Hazards Centre Trust Ltd., 1987.

Leyel, C. F., *Cinquifoil — Herbs to Quicken the Five Senses.* Faber, London, 1957.

Maury, M., *The Secret of Life and Youth.* MacDonald, 1964.

Moncrieff, R. W., *Odour Preferences.* Grampian Press, 1966.

Rouvière, A., Meyer, M.C., *La Santé par les Huiles Essentials.*

Valnet, Jean, *The Practice of Aromatherapy.* C.W. Daniel Co., Saffron Walden, 1982.

Valnet, J., Duraffourd, P., Lapraz, *Phytothérapie et Aromathérapie.* Presses de la Renaissance, Paris, 1978.

Van Toller, Dodd, *Perfumery.* Chapman and Hall, 1988.

Waal, M., *Medicinal Plants of the Bible.* Samuel Weiser Inc., New York, 1980.

Wells, Billot, *Perfumery Technology.* Ellis Horwood Publications, 1975.

Worwood, V. A., *Aromantics.* Pan Books, London, 1987.

• INDEX •

C

About the Author

VALERIE ANN WORWOOD is an aromatherapist, a reflexologist, a member of the London and counties society of Physiologists, and as Chairman of Research is an active member of the International Federation of Aromatherapists. She runs her own clinic in Romford, England, conducts research on aromatherapy and its effects on endometriosis and infertility, and is a consultant to several natural beauty and health clinics. In addition, she lectures all over the world on the benefits of aromatherapy and essential oils.

Dr. Worwood has long been interested in natural medicines. Her study of essential oils was stimulated by her discovery of just how effective their medicinal qualities are, and this interest has led her to making a full exploration of all their life-enhancing qualities.

New World Library is dedicated to publishing books and cassettes that help improve the quality of our lives.

For a catalog of our fine books and cassettes, contact:

New World Library
58 Paul Drive
San Rafael, CA 94903
Phone: (415) 472-2100
FAX: (415) 472-6131

Or call toll free:
(800) 227-3900
In Calif.: (800) 632-2122